EVALUATION AND TREATMENT
OF THE INFERTILE MALE

EVALUATION AND TREATMENT OF THE INFERTILE MALE

Edited by

GRACE M. CENTOLA

*Department of Obstetrics and Gynecology,
University of Rochester Medical Center,
Rochester, New York, USA*

and

KENNETH A. GINSBURG

*Department of Obstetrics and Gynecology,
Wayne State University, Hutzel Hospital,
Detroit, Michigan, USA*

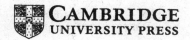

CAMBRIDGE
UNIVERSITY PRESS

PUBLISHED BY THE PRESS SYNDICATE OF THE UNIVERSITY OF CAMBRIDGE
The Pitt Building, Trumpington Street, Cambridge, United Kingdom

CAMBRIDGE UNIVERSITY PRESS
The Edinburgh Building, Cambridge CB2 2RU, UK
40 West 20th Street, New York NY 10011–4211, USA
477 Williamstown Road, Port Melbourne, VIC 3207, Australia
Ruiz de Alarcón 13, 28014 Madrid, Spain
Dock House, The Waterfront, Cape Town 8001, South Africa

http://www.cambridge.org

First published 1996
First paperback edition 2004

A catalogue record for this book is available from the British Library

Library of Congress cataloguing in publication data

Evaluation and treatment of the infertile male / edited by Grace M.
Centola and Kenneth Ginsburg.
p. cm.
Includes index.
ISBN 0 521 45059 4 (hardback)
1. Infertility, Male. I. Centola, Grace M. II. Ginsburg,
Kenneth
[DNLM: 1. Infertility, Male – diagnosis. 2. Infertility, Male –
therapy. WJ 709 E92 1996]
RC889.E94 1996
616.6'92–dc20
DNLM/DLC
for Library of Congress 95-43213 CIP

ISBN 0 521 45059 4 hardback
ISBN 0 521 60273 4 paperback

To Nick and Michael for their support, patience and unending humor,
and to Mom and Dad for their constant love and support
G.M.C.

For Mom and Dad, who made it possible
For Bonnie, who helped it happen
And for Kate and Kevin, who make it all worthwhile
K.A.G.

Contents

Preface

Infertility is defined as one year of unprotected intercourse without a conception. Infertility is a couple phenomenon, affecting both partners due either to medical or surgical problems, psychological issues, or both. It occurs in 1 in every 5, or 20% of couples. Of this 20%, 40% of cases are thought to be due primarily to female factors, 40% primarily to male factors, and 20% to both male and female factors.

During the last decade there has also been increased research into the causes and treatments of infertility. Many anatomical, physiological, biochemical, psychological and genetic abnormalities have been identified as associated with human reproduction, and infertility in the female. Yet, factors related to male fertility, such as sperm maturation, sperm capacitation and fertilization, remain a mystery. The study of male fertility – andrology – is currently at the same place that gynecologic infertility was twenty years ago. Many physicians' offices and clinics are not equipped to evaluate and treat the large range of infertility problems. Residents often spend very little time with the fertility specialist, in the fertility clinic or andrology laboratory. The ability to thoroughly evaluate, diagnose and treat male factor infertility are essential parts of the physician's education.

The focus of this book is the evaluation and treatment of the infertile male. It is aimed at the office-based physician who needs a reference on the basic aspects of the investigation, evaluation and diagnosis of the male partner. Current treatment options are provided. Although it is not expected that all physicians will have such treatment options readily available in their offices or affiliated hospitals, we hope that this text will provide the information needed to initiate treatment, and at the very least locate appropriate referral centers. This text should be useful to the general gynecologist and urologist, as well as the primary care physician who is often involved in the initial evaluation of the infertile couple.

Management of the infertile couple is a team effort – andrologists, gynecologists, urologists, as well as family practitioners and psychologists, often join forces for the evaluation, diagnosis, and treatment of the couple. This team approach is reflected in the diverse array of contributors to this book. We have assembled national leaders in the field of infertility, including urologists, andrologists, and reproductive endocrinologists. We hope to provide both physicians and residents with a general basic knowledge of male dysfunction, what tests are available and when they should be employed, how to interpret the results, and ultimately how to treat the dysfunction.

G.M.C.
K.A.G.

Contributors

Deborah J. Anderson, PhD
Department of Obstetrics and Gynecology and Reproductive Biology, Brigham and Women's Hospital, Harvard Medical School, Boston, Massachusetts, USA

Caleb A. Awoniyi, PhD
Department of Obstetrics and Gynecology, University of Colorado Health Sciences Center, Denver, Colorado, USA

The late Barbara J. Berg
Formerly at Department of Psychology, Washington State University, Pullman, Washington, USA

Richard A. Bronson, MD
Department of Obstetrics and Gynecology, Director of Andrology, Health Sciences Center, State University of New York, Stony Brook, New York, USA

Lani J. Burkman, PhD
Department of Gynecology and Obstetrics, State University of New York, Buffalo, New York, USA

William Byrd, PhD
Department of Obstetrics and Gynecology, University of Texas Southwestern Medical Center, Dallas, Texas, USA

Grace M. Centola, PhD
Department of Obstetrics and Gynecology, Director, Andrology Laboratory, University of Rochester Medical Center, Rochester, New York, USA

Charles C. Coddington, MD
The Jones Institute for Reproductive Medicine, Eastern Virginia Medical School, Norfolk, Virginia, USA

Russell O. Davis, PhD
Department of Reproductive Medicine, Rockford Health Systems, Rockford, Illinois, USA

Jean L. Fourcroy, MD, PhD
Division of Metabolism and Endocrine Drug Products, Food and Drug Administration, Department of Health and Human Services, Rockville, Maryland, USA

Kenneth A. Ginsburg, MD
Department of Obstetrics and Gynecology, Wayne State University, Hutzel Hospital, Detroit, Michigan, USA

David F. Katz, PhD
Duke University, Raleigh, North Carolina, USA

Kristine E. Klinger, RNC
Department of Obstetrics and Gynecology, Wayne State University, Hutzel Hospital, Detroit, Michigan, USA

Susan G. Mikesell, PhD
Private Practice, Washington, DC, USA

Valerie Montgomery Rice, MD
Department of Obstetrics and Gynecology, Wayne State University, Hutzel Hospital, Detroit, Michigan, USA

Harris M. Nagler, MD
Director, Department of Urology, Beth Israel Medical Center, Mount Sinai School of Medicine, New York, New York, USA

Sergio Oehninger, MD
The Jones Institute for Reproductive Medicine, Eastern Virginia Medical School, Norfolk, Virginia, USA

William R. Phipps, MD
Department of Obstetrics and Gynecology, University of Rochester Medical Center, Rochester, New York, USA

Joseph A. Politch, PhD
Department of Obstetrics and Gynecology and Reproductive Biology, Brigham and Women's Hospital, Harvard Medical School, Boston, Massachusetts, USA

B. Jane Rogers, PhD
Director, Infertility Diagnostics, 19592 Clubhouse Road, Gaithersburg, Maryland, USA

William D. Schlaff, MD
Department of Obstetrics and Gynecology, Chief, Reproductive Endocrinology, University of Colorado Health Sciences Center, Denver, Colorado, USA

Rebecca Z. Sokol, MD
Division of Endocrinology, Harbor-UCLA Medical Center, Torrance, California, USA

Don P. Wolf, PhD
Oregon Regional Primate Center, Beaverton, and Departments of Obstetrics and Gynecology and of Physiology, Oregon Health Sciences University, Portland, Oregon, USA

1

Andrology

GRACE M. CENTOLA

History of andrology

According to *Taber's Cyclopedic Medical Dictionary*, 'andrology' is defined as the study of diseases of men, especially of the male genital organs (Thomas, 1989). Introduction of the term 'andrology' is credited to a gynecologist, Harald Siebke, a Professor of Gynecology in Bonn, Germany (Schirren, 1984). Professor Siebke used this term first in 1951 with the intention of demonstrating that the male and female are equally important in reproduction. Truer words have never been spoken! Although andrology refers to a study of male infertility, in the broadest sense, andrologists not only study the clinical aspects of male fertility, but also study the biological mission of the sperm, from production in the testes, to interaction with, and penetration of the oocyte at the time of fertilization.

Andrology as a science has made tremendous developments in the past 40 to 50 years. There are now national and international membership organizations (The American Society of Andrology), as well as national and international peer-reviewed journals (*Journal of Andrology, Andrologia*) devoted specifically to the field of andrology.

Leeuwenhoek and the discovery of spermatozoa

For centures, the theories of generation presented by Aristotle (reviewed by Schierbeek, 1959) were universally accepted. Aristotle believed that the male principle contained the efficient *cause* of generation and the female the material of it. Aristotle, in discussing whether semen comes from all parts of the body, wrote that the nature of semen is to be distributed to the whole of the body. Furthermore, Aristotle pointed out that the potential parts of the whole organism were found in the semen, not in the female. For centuries, the theories of Aristotle were dominant, although many other scholars, such as Paracelsus,

1

theorized that half the semen came from the female and half from the male. In 1651, William Harvey published a book *Exercitationes de Generatione Animalium*, on reproduction in animals. In this text, Harvey shared Aristotle's belief that the influence of the sperm on the development of the embryo was due to the vital force contained in the semen, and this compares to the secret force of the heavenly bodies upon all life on earth (Schierbeek, 1959). The Dutch biologist, Reinier de Graaf, wrote in 1671–2 that the impregnation was caused by an *aura seminalis*, or a volatile part of the semen.

These ancient theories were considered the truth at the time that Anton van Leeuwenhoek discovered 'little animals' or 'animalcules' in water. In November 1677 he wrote of his discovery of living animals in semen (Schierbeek, 1959). He judged these animalcules to have tails, and to be in such great numbers, that 'a thousand were moving in an amount of material the size of a grain of sand', moving forward by the action of their tails. The discovery of spermatozoa by Leeuwenhoek was one of his most important discoveries, and for 46 years he continued to examine these animalcules. Leeuwenhoek finally concluded that the female supplies the nutrients for preservation of the sperm, while the male sperm forms the fetus. He surmised that the woman provides a receptacle for the semen, and the feeding of the sperm. He went on to state that the shape of the human body is included in the animal of the male seed, and that there were male and female animalcules. He speculated that in the future it would be possible to see the entire shape of a full-grown body in the animalcule. It was a long time before the theories of Leeuwenhoek were accepted, particularly since other scholars wrote of other theories.

In 1749, Buffon declared that the spermatozoa were generated by putrefaction; in 1814, Johannes Muller wrote that they might be parasites! With the development of the cell-theory, the spermatozoa became thought of as body cells, and it was then evident that Leeuwenhoek had made a very important discovery of animalcules in semen.

Leeuwenhoek was probably the first to discuss infertility, without really knowing it. In 1673 he wrote that there must be 'so many thousands of animalcules for every single egg . . . in order that one animalcule out of many may hit the little dot or spot in the yolk' (Dobell, 1932; Schierbeek, 1959). He compared this to what we might call the 'struggle for existence' or 'survival of the fittest'. In 1685, Leeuwenhoek wrote that 'frigidity in some men, is either a want [in them] of the *animalia seminalis*, or a weakness in the animals which renders them unable to live long in the womb' (Dobell, 1932; Schierbeek, 1959).

We have come a long way since the time of Leeuwenhoek but, alas, we have a long way yet to go.

Table 1.1 *Summary of diagnostic sequence evaluation of the infertile male and treatment options*

Couple consultation	Good history, including coital habits, prior fertility, exposure history
Gynecologist *Female*	Physical examination, menstrual history, obstetric history, general health history, endocrine evaluation, post-coital testing, evaluation of tubal and peritoneal factors
Andrologist/urologist *Male*	History and physical examination, semen analysis

General aspects of the evaluation of the male

Infertility is defined as 1 year of unprotected intercourse without a conception. Often, the gynecologist is the first health professional to have contact with the infertile couple. Evaluation of the infertile couple should be in an orderly, logical manner, that is both cost effective and medically efficient (Table 1.1). Concurrent with the initial evaluations of the female (see Chapter 18), the physician will request examination of the male, first using the semen analysis (see Chapters 3 and 4). Referral to a urologist may result depending on the results of this initial laboratory evaluation (see Chapter 14).

The patient's history is the cornerstone of the evaluation of the infertile couple, and should include not only reproductive history, sexual history and family history, but also past medical and surgical history, and exposure to toxic chemicals. A comprehensive physical examination is a useful adjunct (Gangi & Nagler, 1992), and should include a search for evidence of endocrine dysfunction (demasculinized body habitus, thyroid enlargement, gynecomastia, etc.) and reproductive tract abnormality (varicocele, cryptorchidism, hypospadias, etc.). Once a comprehensive history is available for both partners, a plan of diagnostic tests and treatments can be individualized to the particular couple's treatment option as indicated below (see Tables 1.2–1.6). Although the general physical examination is done on all men, key factors in the history and physical examination are indicated for each semen abnormality.

Conclusion

The evaluation of the infertile male necessitates a comprehensive examination of those factors known to be associated with infertility. A careful and complete history is essential. A minimum of three semen analyses can then direct the pathway for further evaluations and treatment. Sperm washing and intrauterine insemination is a widely used and successful treatment with even

Table 1.2 *Evaluation and treatment options: abnormal sperm count*
(oligozoospermia)

1. Concentrate on environmental exposure and injuries
2. Physical examination: anatomy of genital tract; presence of varicocele
3. Endocrine evaluation: potential therapy with gonadotrophins (Chapter 13)
4. Intrauterine insemination of washed sperm (Chapters 7, 8)
5. Varicocelectomy, i.e., internal spermatic vein ligation
6. Assisted reproductive techniques (ART): IVF, GIFT, micromanipulation (SUZI, ICSI) (Chapters 10, 11)

Notes:
IVF, *in vitro* fertilization; GIFT, gamete intra-fallopian tube transfer; SUZI, subzonal insertion; ICSI, intracytoplasmic sperm injection.

Table 1.3 *Evaluation and treatment options: abnormal motility*

1. Concentrate on environmental exposure and injuries; heat factor (waterbed, hot tubs?)
2. Presence of increased numbers of leukocytes in semen (Chapter 16): treatment with antibiotics, then re-evaluation
3. Immunologic assessment: antisperm antibodies (Chapter 5)
4. Physical examination: presence of varicocele – varicocelectomy (Chapter 14)
5. Intrauterine insemination with washed sperm (Chapter 7)
6. Assisted reproductive techniques (ART) (Chapters 10, 11)

Table 1.4 *Evaluation and treatment options: abnormal volume*

1. Consider infection: treat with antibiotics, then re-evaluation
2. If no sperm in urine, assess semen fructose to evaluate congenital absence of seminal vesicles, vas deferens. Referral to urologist; vasogram to determine presence of or patency of vas deferens
3. Post-ejaculation urinalysis for possible retrograde ejaculation. If there is retrograde ejaculation, evaluation for neurologic or anatomic cause. Correct if possible. Can use postejaculation urine processing and recovery of motile sperm for insemination
4. If volume is high, can consider split semen insemination; sperm washing and intrauterine insemination
5. Drugs to increase the amount of semen/seminal fluid and influence antegrade ejaculation

Table 1.5   *Evaluation and treatment options: azoospermia*

1. Semen fructose to determine congenital absence of vas deferens, seminal vesicles. Referral to urologist
2. If fructose present, evaluate plasma FSH (high – testicular failure), consider referral to endocrinologist; consider donor insemination or adoption
   If FSH low: referral to endocrinologist for evaluation of pituitary function, and possible endocrine treatment (Chapter 13)
   If FSH normal: evaluate for obstruction; testicular biopsy for spermatogenic function
3. Depending on results, and ability to correct endocrine dysfunction or obstruction, consider sperm washing and intrauterine insemination (if sperm appears in ejaculate), donor insemination or adoption, or ART

Table 1.6   *Evaluation and treatment options: unexplained infertility*

1. Consider functional evaluation of sperm: sperm penetration assay, hemizona assay, acrosome status, acrosin assay (Chapter 9)
2. Consider sperm washing and intrauterine insemination with ovulation induction (Chapter 7)

severely oligozoospermic men. Assisted reproductive techniques, although costly, may be the only options for certain couples. In others, no treatment is effective and discussion of therapeutic donor insemination is warranted.

It is essential that the physician take an individual approach to each couple, considering the options appropriate to that couple. The result is a logical approach to the evaluation of the infertile male based on this series of diagnostics tests and treatment options (Gangi & Nagler, 1992).

References

Dobell, C. (1932). *Antony van Leeuwenhoek and His 'Little Animals'*. New York: Harcourt, Brace.
Gangi, G.R. & Nagler, H.M. (1992). Clinical evaluation of the subfertile male. In *Infertility and Reproductive Medicine Clinics of North America*, ed. M. Diamond & A. DeCherney, vol. 3(2), pp. 299–318. Philadelphia: W.B. Saunders.
Schierbeek, A. (1959). *Measuring The Invisible World: The Life and Works of Antoni van Leeuwenhoek*, pp. 81–107. New York: Abelard-Schuman.
Schirren, C. (1984). Andrology: origin and development of a special discipline in medicine. Reflection and view in the future. *Andrologia*, 17(2), 117–25.
Thomas, C.L. (ed.) (1989). *Taber's Cyclopedic Medical Dictionary*, p. 90. Philadelphia: F.A. Davis.

2

Sperm–egg interaction

DON P. WOLF

Introduction

This chapter presents an overview of the cell–cell interactions at fertilization, designed to provide a context for the chapters that follow which address the diagnostic and therapeutic procedures employed in the treatment of male infertility. The many original literature citations augmented with recent references, especially to human studies, should be helpful to the reader interested in a more detailed or specific understanding of the underlying physiology and biochemistry (see Dunbar & O'Rand, 1991; and reviews by Yanagamachi, 1988; Saling, 1991; and Green, 1993).

The players and their transport

A discussion of sperm–egg interaction *per se* would not be appropriate without a few comments to set the stage. Successful fertilization is dependent upon the timely presence of mature gametes in the ampullary oviduct, the normal site of fertilization.

In general terms, the production of fertile sperm requires the concerted activity of the male genital tract with contributions from the testis, epididymis and accessory glands. At the testicular level, spermatogenesis, modulated by endocrine/autocrine/paracrine processes that require approximately 74 days in man, results in the production of and release to the epididymis of large numbers of differentiated sperm cells on a relatively consistent basis. Gamete production in the adult male is continuous, rather than cyclical as in the female. Spermatogenesis and its regulation are complex and poorly understood, and may be influenced by such unrelated parameters as age, scrotal temperature, diet, exercise, stress, smoking, the use of cytotoxic or recreational drugs, toxicant exposure and viral infection.

Sperm recovered from the testis are not functionally mature but acquire motility, zona binding ability and fertilizing capacity during passage through the epididymis. During epididymal transit, fertility potential increases in sperm recovered from the caput to the cauda of the epididymis, a consequence of successive androgen-induced protein interaction with the sperm plasma membrane. Sperm transit time through the epididymis is relatively short, being estimated at 3.8–4.3 days (Johnson & Varner, 1988), and the storage capacity of this organ is probably limited to approximately 200 million cells.

Mature sperm leave the epididymis and vas deferens at emission, when they are mixed with accessory gland secretions, forming the ejaculate. The secretions provide a vehicle for transport, and include energy sources, decapacitation factors, and buffering agents that support sperm survival during early stages of transport in the female genital tract when protection from the acidic environment of the vagina is needed. Sperm access to the relative protection of the cervix and its mucus then occurs and cervical sperm provide a reservoir for transport to the upper genital tract. Although both rapid and slow transport have been described, the former is not considered physiologically significant (Overstreet, 1983). The fertile lifetime of human sperm in the female genital tract is at least 2 days, which justifies the recommended intercourse frequency of every 2 days during the periovulatory period for couples attempting to achieve pregnancy.

The fertile human oocyte, when ovulated, is arrested at metaphase II of meiosis. Nuclear maturation can be readily assessed in the laboratory of an assisted reproductive technology program. However, cytoplasmic competence, which may be equally important, cannot readily be assessed. The oocyte, although biochemically competent, is relatively inactive but poised to respond to the activation stimulus provided by the fertilizing sperm. A discussion of cell cycle arrest in mammalian oocytes and the interplay between nuclear and cytoplasmic maturation can be found in Eppig (1993).

Sperm capacitation

Freshly ejaculated non-capacitated sperm are incapable of fertilizing the mature oocyte but must undergo a series of poorly defined events which culminate in the acquisition of ability to fertilize. The unique characteristics of capacitated sperm include hyperactive motility, and the capability to acrosome react and bind to the zona pellucida (ZP). The individual steps in sperm–egg interaction from capacitation through egg activation are illustrated in Fig. 2.1.

One early, measurable hallmark of capacitation is the motility transition from progressive, typified by sperm trajectories observed in semen, to non-progressive, most commonly seen in washed sperm (see Chapter 4). The

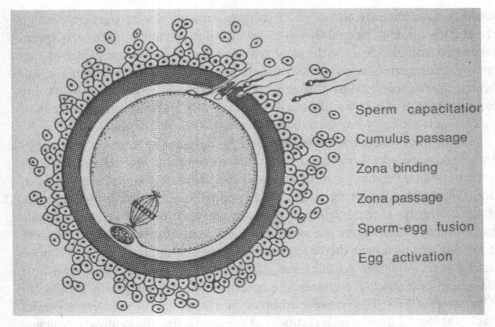

Fig. 2.1. A schematic illustration of the individual steps in mammalian sperm–egg
interaction (see the text for details).

association between hyperactivation and capacitation is species-specific,
varying from minimal in the mouse to absolute in the rhesus monkey where
induction of these phenomena by washed sperm exposure to dibutyryl cyclic
adenosine monophosphate and caffeine is critical to fertility (Boatman &
Bavister, 1984). The functional significance of hyperactivation may be related
to the increased mechanical forces generated by the high-amplitude flagellar
beat at the penetration site on or in the ZP (Katz *et al.*, 1993). In the human,
sperm hyperactivated motility is initiated as they leave the seminal plasma
(Robertson *et al.*, 1988). Fertility success may be maximized by asynchronous
capacitation/hyperactivation. The regulation of sperm motility is beyond the
scope of this discussion but the interested reader is referred to the review by
Cummins & Yovich (1993).

Sperm capacitation is accomplished *in vitro* in many species, including man,
by simply removing seminal plasma and resuspending washed cells in a suitable
medium containing serum or albumin. Although the molecular basis for this
process is unknown, one current line of thinking focuses on membrane fluidity
and organizational changes secondary to alterations in membrane lipid
composition (see below, and Ravnik *et al.*, 1993).

Cumulus passage

The existence of precontact sperm–egg communication (sperm chemotaxis) in mammals, a phenomenon known to occur in animals with external fertilization, is a subject of continuing controversy (Eisenbach & Ralt, 1992).

The first step in actual sperm–egg interaction involves cumulus passage, a process that may require only a few minutes for capacitated sperm. The hyaluronic-acid-rich matrix responsible for the structural integrity of the cumulus persists for some time after fertilization but is readily dispersed by hyaluronidase, an enzyme present both in sperm and in the oviductal epithelium. The requirement for acrosomal hyaluronidase in sperm passage through the cumulus is variable and incompletely understood. For example, in capacitated hamster sperm the hyaluronidase inhibitor, Myocrisin, prevents *in vivo* or *in vitro* penetration into the cumulus (Cummins & Yanagamachi, 1986), while motile sperm from sea urchins, frogs or a mutant variety of the alga *Chlamydomonas*, all of which lack hyaluronidase, are capable of penetrating hamster cumuli (Talbot *et al.*, 1985). While cumulus presence is critical to oocyte/embryo transport in the oviduct its premature dispersal *in vitro* is without effect on fertilization. Indeed, mechanical or chemical disruption of the cumulus is used in male factor treatment during *in vitro* fertilization (IVF) to facilitate sperm access to the oocyte or in assessing oocyte maturity.

Sperm–zona interaction

A major barrier to sperm seeking access to an oocyte is the ZP, a glycoprotein-rich layer produced by and surrounding the oocyte. This sperm–zona interaction represents a very important step in fertilization, forming the molecular basis for species recognition and specificity. Mammalian zonae are typically comprised of three glycoproteins designated ZP 1, 2 and 3, with molecular weight ranges in the mouse of 180–200, 120–140 and 70–96, respectively (Wassarman, 1991). Most ZP glycoproteins contain both *N*- and *O*-linked sugars, with microheterogeneity in oligosaccharide side chains, their composition, length and position on the polypeptide backbone. Zonae in many species are readily solubilized by reducing agents, acidic culture media, protease or heat exposure. The susceptibility to denaturation can change following oocyte aging or fertilization.

Attachment

Sperm–zona attachment, or the relatively loose, reversible association between the plasma membrane overlying the acrosome and the ZP, has been studied extensively in the hamster (Hartmann, 1983). This step is not highly species specific, requires approximately 30 minutes and is without clearly defined physiologic importance.

Binding

The tight binding between acrosome-intact, capacitated sperm and the ZP is mediated by a primary sperm receptor present throughout the ZP in the ZP3 glycoprotein molecule. This acquired binding capacity is another hallmark of the capacitated cell. It can be demonstrated shortly after removal from the epididymis or from the seminal fluid, and is a calcium-dependent event (Storey & Kopf, 1991). Evidence for a sperm receptor was originally based on the results of a competitive sperm binding assay where sperm binding to intact ZP could be inhibited by solubilized whole ZP or purified ZP3 from unfertilized oocytes but not from embryos (Bleil *et al.*, 1981). Sperm receptor activity is retained in low molecular weight, pronase digests of ZP3, and is characterized by a specific class of *O*-linked oligosaccharides containing an α-linked galactose residue at the nonreducing terminus (Wassarman, 1991).

While the ZP's sperm receptor is well defined (and the ZP3 gene cloned), the nature of complementary components on the mammalian sperm head remains elusive despite the availability of several candidate molecules or sites. On the basis of the biochemical characteristics of the primary sperm receptor (ZP3 oligosaccharide), carbohydrate-binding capacity is implied. Candidates for such sperm surface binding proteins include galactosyl transferase (Shur & Hall, 1982) and mannosidase (Benoff *et al.*, 1993). Other possibilities that may not proceed through a carbohydrate-binding mechanism include a protease inhibitor sensitive site and a 95 kDa tyrosine kinase signalling receptor (Saling, 1991; Moore *et al.*, 1993).

Sperm–zona binding can be evaluated clinically using the hemizona binding assay. The test employs oocytes that have failed to fertilize *in vitro*, providing matched hemizonae for study. That this specific sperm–zona binding can be demonstrated after such manipulation attests to the remarkable resiliency of the zona sperm receptor.

Induction of acrosomal exocytosis

Following the establishment of tight binding between acrosome-intact sperm and the zona receptor, sperm undergo an acrosome reaction in preparation for zona passage. The time requirement for this event may be considerable, and even rate limiting, and its timely occurrence is critical since a premature or a delayed reaction results in no penetration. While both acrosome-reacted and acrosome-intact human sperm have been observed on the human zona surface, it is presumably the intact cell which is uniquely capable of interacting with the receptor (Cross *et al.*, 1988).

The ZP3 glycoprotein molecule is also implicated in acrosomal exocytosis. However, the activity, in this case, depends on the molecule's *O*-linked oligosaccharides and polypeptide chain; pronase digestion destroys this activity (Wasserman, 1991). Purified ZP3, following solubilization, has been used to induce acrosomal loss in many species, including human. Moreover, recombinant ZP3 with this activity has been isolated from transformed rodent and primate cells (Beebe *et al.*, 1992).

The ability of human sperm to respond to inducers of acrosomal exocytosis (ZP3, progesterone, follicular fluid, high salt or ionophore) may eventually be used to improve fertility potential in the context of the assisted reproductive technologies. At present, however, induction of the reaction is of academic interest or, at best, used for diagnostic purposes to evaluate sperm fertility potential.

The signal transduction mechanisms involved in the sperm's acrosomal response to ZP3 are not well understood. A GTP-binding regulatory protein (G-protein) may be involved (Storey & Kopf, 1991). In any event, the consequence of binding or signal reception is an increase in intracellular calcium ion concentration. Extracellular calcium is a prerequisite for exocytosis, and calcium uptake may result from the activation of voltage-dependent calcium channels (Florman *et al.*, 1992).

Zona penetration

Following zona binding and the initiation of acrosomal exocytosis, zona penetration by these acrosome-reacted sperm involves the action of mechanical forces generated by hyperactivated motility and of acrosomal-associated enzyme(s), presumably localized to the inner acrosomal membrane. Most evidence supports limited proteolysis of the zona glycoprotein matrix by acrosin, a trypsin-like protease (Dunbar *et al.*, 1991). Thus, neutralizing acrosin activity with trypsin inhibitor can block human sperm penetration of the zona in oocytes that failed to fertilize in IVF without adverse effects on motility or sperm binding to the zona (Liu & Baker, 1993). Maintenance of sperm binding during zona passage is achieved by interaction between the sperm's inner acrosomal membrane and secondary sperm receptors localized in ZP2 (Wassarman, 1991).

Sperm–egg fusion

Membrane fusion is a key event in sperm incorporation and fertilization, for it not only allows a paternal genomic contribution to the zygote but triggers a sequence of intracellular events that are essential for subsequent embryonic development (see below). While this process has not been studied as extensively as sperm–zona interaction, the specificity of membrane fusion, in general, would suggest the involvement of unique recognition molecules for both fusion partners with events proceeding through several sequential steps: binding and adhesion, capping and cytoskeletal redistribution, and fusion followed by egg activation (Green, 1993). Evidence suggests that such a specific cell surface ligand/receptor mechanism exists in the sea urchin, where a sperm ligand (bindin) mediates sperm recognition of and binding to the egg. A specific transmembrane protein, only recently described, may serve as the egg's receptor for sperm (Foltz *et al.*, 1993).

For the acrosome-reacted mammalian sperm, the existence of a sperm ligand is suggested by antibody experiments where sperm–egg fusion in zona-free oocyte assay systems is inhibited by monoclonal or polyclonal antibodies that bind to the equatorial segment (Saling & Lakoski, 1985; Rochwerger *et al.*, 1992) or to a specific postequatorial protein, PH30. PH30 has been characterized as a disintegrin-like protein thought to contain fusigenic peptide sequences (Blobel *et al.*, 1990). One of the interesting characteristics of these putative binding proteins is their tendency to migrate to the equatorial segment or postacrosomal region following the acrosome reaction. Thus, the acrosome reaction not only results in the release of proteolytic enzymes, but also involves the repositioning of the binding site protein close to the sperm head region involved in initiating fusion with the egg plasma membrane.

Evidence also exists for specific sperm binding sites mediating fusion in the mammalian egg's plasma membrane. The evidence for oocyte-associated binding sites includes the following: (1) simple and complex saccharides impair penetration of zona-free eggs; (2) protease treatment of zona-free eggs inhibits sperm–egg interaction and causes modification of a 94 kDa egg plasma membrane protein, recovery of which is associated with fertility restoration (Kellom *et al.*, 1992); (3) pretreatment of zona-free eggs with a sperm binding protein of epididymal origin reduces sperm–egg fusion in a protein-concentration-dependent manner (Rochwerger *et al.*, 1992); and (4) fibronectin or components of the complement system inhibit human sperm binding to zona-free hamster eggs (Fusi *et al.*, 1991).

Mechanism of egg activation

In marine invertebrates, the first measurable response to sperm addition, within a second or two, is a dramatic, transient shift in egg membrane potential (the fertilization potential) which creates an electrical block to polyspermy. No equivalent fertilization potential has been measured in mammalian eggs, although transient hyperpolarizations occur over much longer time frames (Jaffe & Cross, 1984).

In all cases, however, a transient but dramatic increase in intracellular calcium concentration occurs after sperm–egg fusion, in the form of a calcium wave which is the primary intracellular signal responsible for the initiation of development. Experimental observations that support this conclusion include: (1) measurable increases in intracellular calcium ion concentrations at fertilization; (2) egg activation following manipulations or exposures that artificially increase intracellular calcium; and (3) the inhibition of egg activation by exposures that suppress the natural rise in calcium.

The exact mechanism by which sperm–egg fusion triggers increased cytosolic calcium is unknown. Possibilities include the sperm bringing in calcium or a factor that directly initiates calcium release or interacts with a classical signal transduction mechanism such as a G-protein (Williams *et al.*, 1992), as well as the involvement of specific signaling intermediates or second messengers. For example, inositol 1,4,5-trisphosphate (InsP3) can act as a second messenger in animal eggs, as has been shown by direct InsP3 injection experiments. Moreover, antibody to the InsP3 receptor can block the calcium release induced in eggs by InsP3 injection or by sperm (Miyazaki *et al.*, 1992). In this scenario, sperm–egg fusion would be receptor-coupled to phospholipase C activation. Subsequent hydrolysis of membrane phosphoinositides results in the production of water-soluble InsP3 which diffuses to intracellular sites of calcium sequestration and stimulates calcium release, acting as a calcium ionophore. The diacylglycerol produced by phospholipase C action also stimulates protein kinase C, whose activity may, in turn, mediate the pH change that occurs moments after fertilization in the oocytes of some species. Another possible second messenger in animal eggs is cyclic ADP-ribose. This molecule, first found in sea urchin eggs, is not only more potent than InsP3 in releasing calcium but is active in a number of mammalian cell types which contain the biochemical machinery required for its synthesis and degradation (Galione, 1993).

Responses to egg activation

Within a few minutes after fusion in mammals, cortical granule (CG) exocytosis secondary to increased cortical calcium concentrations occurs in a wave around the egg cortex, originating at the site of sperm entry. These early events have been associated with the establishment of a block to polyspermy, a response which is critical since the polyspermic embryo does not develop normally.

The block to polyspermy response can occur at two levels: the egg plasma membrane (primary) and the ZP (secondary; also called the zona reaction). Reliance on one versus the other or both of these responses is species specific. Thus, while a primary block is apparent in zona-free mouse and intact rabbit oocytes, no such response can be demonstrated in the hamster. By marine invertebrate standards, the primary response in mammalian oocytes is relatively slow, and may involve an alteration in the ability of the oocyte plasma membrane to allow sperm adhesion (Horvath *et al.*, 1993).

The CG-mediated secondary response has been extensively studied and is expressed by unique but related mechanisms in different species. For instance, in sea urchins the conversion of the vitelline to fertilization layer involves protein crosslinking mediated by CG ovoperoxidase, whereas in the amphibian *Xenopus laevis* the analogous conversion is mediated by a CG lectin (Schmell *et al.*, 1983). In most mammals major reliance on maintaining the monospermic condition resides with a secondary block response, delayed in time (30 or more minutes post-fusion) but, nonetheless, effective under *in vivo* conditions where sperm presence at the site of fertilization may be limited to a few cells. A CG role in this response is implied not only from temporal considerations but also directly from the demonstration that fertility can be reduced in eggs treated with isolated CG contents (Wolf & Hamada, 1977). Two changes have been implicated in the mouse oocyte's secondary block to polyspermy: inactivation of the ZP3 sperm receptor by a CG glycosidase(s) and conversion of the ZP2 secondary receptor by a CG protease (Wassarman, 1991). In the human, a fertilization-associated modification in ZP1 has been described (Shabanowitz & O'Rand, 1988).

Following sperm–egg fusion, sperm incorporation and processing represents a major activity for the oocyte. In mammals, the entire sperm, including the flagellum, is normally incorporated. Decapitation occurs, closely followed by breakdown of the nuclear envelope, dispersion of the condensed chromatin (requiring disulfide bond reduction) and, subsequently, development of a pronuclear envelope in preparation for male pronucleus formation. Studies on these events are largely descriptive in nature and the reader is referred to Longo (1985) for a review and additional detail.

Another response of the activated oocyte is the resumption of meiosis and subsequent events that culminate in the formation of the female pronucleus, pronuclear migration and eventual breakdown and, finally, syngamy. This response may involve calcium-mediated, cell cycle control mechanisms. Also implicated are the activity of protein kinases and phosphatases (the degree of phosphorylation) as well as the activity of substrates such as maturation-promoting factor, cytostatic factor and cyclins (Parrish *et al.*, 1992).

The activation of development is also dependent upon the recruitment of maternal mRNAs stored in the oocyte, their translation, and the production of fertilization-associated proteins. While these events can be documented, their regulation and implications for development are, at present, only poorly understood (Williams *et al.*, 1992).

Acknowledgments

The secretarial contribution of Carol Gibbins is recognized along with the editorial assistance of Drs Baha Alak and Andrew Weston. Supported in part by NIH RR00163 grant. Publication No. 1967 of the Oregon Regional Primate Research Center.

References

Beebe, S.J., Leyton, L., Burks, D., Ishikawa, M., Fuerst, T., Dean, J. & Saling, P. (1992). Recombinant mouse ZP3 inhibits sperm binding and induces the acrosome reaction. *Dev. Biol.*, **151**, 48–54.

Benoff, S., Cooper, G.S., Hurley, I., Napolitano, B., Rosenfeld, D.L., School, G.M. & Hershlag, A. (1993). Human sperm fertilizing potential *in vitro* is correlated with differential expression of a head-specific mannose-ligand receptor. *Fertil. Steril.*, **59**, 854–62.

Bleil, J.D., Beall, C.F. & Wassarman, P.M. (1981). Mammalian sperm–egg interaction: fertilization of mouse eggs triggers modification of the major zona pellucida glycoprotein, ZP2. *Dev. Biol.*, **86**, 189–97.

Blobel, C.P., Myles, D.G., Primakoff, P. & White, J.M. (1990). Proteolytic processing of a protein involved in sperm–egg fusion correlates with acquisition of fertilization competence. *J. Cell Biol.*, **111**, 69–78.

Boatman, D.E. & Bavister, B.D. (1984). Stimulation of rhesus monkey sperm capacitation by cyclic nucleotide mediators. *J. Reprod. Fertil.*, **71**, 357–66.

Cross, N.L., Morales, P., Overstreet, J.W. & Hanson, F.W. (1988). Induction of acrosome reactions by the human zona pellucida. *Biol. Reprod.*, **38**, 235–44.

Cummins, J.M. & Yanagimachi, R. (1986). Development of ability to penetrate the cumulus oophorus by hamster spermatozoa capacitated *in vitro*, in relation to the timing of the acrosome reaction. *Gamete Res.*, **15**, 187–212.

Cummins, J.M. & Yovich, J.M. (1993). Sperm motility enhancement *in vitro*. *Semin. Reprod. Endocrinol.*, **11**, 56–71.

Dunbar, B.S. & O'Rand, M.G. (1991). *A Comparative Overview of Mammalian Fertilization*. New York: Plenum Press.

Dunbar, B.S., Prasad, S.V. & Timmons, T.M. (1991). Comparative structure and function of mammalian zonae pellucidae. In *A Comparative Overview of Mammalian Fertilization*, ed. B.S. Dunbar & M.G. O'Rand, pp. 97–114. New York: Plenum Press.

Eisenbach, M. & Ralt, D. (1992). Precontact mammalian sperm–egg communication and role in fertilization. *Am. J. Physiol.*, **262**, C1095–101.

Eppig, J.J. (1993). Regulation of mammalian oocyte maturation. In *The Ovary*, ed. E.Y. Adashi & P.C.K. Leung. New York: Raven Press, pp. 185–208.

Florman, H.M., Corron, M.E., Kim, T.D.-H. & Babcock, D.F. (1992). Activation of voltage-dependent calcium channels of mammalian sperm is required for zona pellucida-induced acrosomal exocytosis. *Dev. Biol.*, **152**, 304–14.

Foltz, K.R., Partin, J.S. & Lennarz, W.J. (1993). Sea urchin egg receptor for sperm: sequence similarity of binding domain and hsp70. *Science*, **259**, 1421–5.

Fusi, F., Bronson, R.A., Hong, Y. & Ghebrehiwet, B. (1991). Complement component C1q and its receptor are involved in the interaction of human sperm with zona-free hamster eggs. *Mol. Reprod. Dev.*, **29**, 180–8.

Galione, A. (1993). Cyclic ADP-ribose: a new way to control calcium. *Science*, **259**, 325–6.

Green, D.P.L. (1993). Review. Mammalian fertilization as a biological machine: a working model for adhesion and fusion of sperm and oocyte. *Hum. Reprod.*, **8**, 91–6.

Hartmann, H.F. (1983). Mammalian fertilization: gamete surface interactions *in vitro*. In *Mechanism and Control of Animal Fertilization*, ed. J.F. Hartmann, pp. 325–64. New York: Academic Press.

Horvath, P.M., Kellom, T., Caulfield, J. & Boldt, J. (1993). Mechanistic studies of the plasma membrane block to polyspermy in mouse eggs. *Mol. Reprod. Dev.*, **34**, 65–72.

Jaffe, L.A. & Cross, N.L. (1984). Electrical properties of vertebrate oocyte membranes. *Biol. Reprod.*, **30**, 50–4.

Johnson, L. & Varner, D.D. (1988). Effect of daily spermatozoan production but not age on transit time of spermatozoa through the human epididymis. *Biol. Reprod.*, **39**, 812–17.

Katz, D.F., Davis, R.O., Drobnis, E.Z. & Overstreet, J.W. (1993). Sperm motility measurement and hyperactivation. *Semin. Reprod. Endocrinol.*, **11**, 27–39.

Kellom, T., Vick, A. & Boldt, J. (1992). Recovery of penetration ability in protease-treated zona-free mouse eggs occurs coincident with recovery of a cell surface 94 kD protein. *Mol. Reprod. Dev.*, **33**, 46–52.

Liu, D.Y. & Baker, H.W.G. (1993). Inhibition of acrosin activity with a trypsin inhibitor blocks human sperm penetration of the zona pellucida. *Biol. Reprod.*, **48**, 340–8.

Longo, F.J. (1985). Pronuclear events during fertilization. In *Biology of Fertilization*, vol. 3, *The Fertilization Response of the Egg*, ed. C.B. Metz & A. Monroy, pp. 251–98. Orlando, FL: Academic Press.

Miyazaki, S., Yuzaki, M., Nakada, K., Shirakawa, H., Nakanishi, S., Nakade, S. & Mikoshiba, K. (1992). Block of Ca^{2+} wave and Ca^{2+} oscillation by antibody to the inositol 1,4,5-trisphosphate receptor in fertilized hamster eggs. *Science*, **257**, 251–5.

Moore, A., Penfold, L.M., Johnson, J.L., Latchman, D.S. & Moore, H.D.M. (1993). Human sperm–egg binding is inhibited by peptides corresponding to the core region of an acrosomal serine protease inhibitor. *Mol. Reprod. Dev.*, **34**, 280–91.

Overstreet, J.W. (1983). Transport of gametes in the reproductive tract of the female mammal. In *Mechanism and Control of Animal Fertilization*, ed. J.F. Hartmann, pp. 499–543. New York: Academic Press.

Parrish, J.J., Kim, C.I. & Bae, I.H. (1992). Current concepts of cell-cycle regulation and its relationship to oocyte maturation, fertilization and embryo development. *Theriogenology*, **38**, 277–96.

Ravnik, S.E., Albers, J.J. & Muller, C.H. (1993). A novel view of albumin-supported sperm capacitation: role of lipid transfer protein-1. *Fertil. Steril.*, **59**, 629–38.

Robertson, L., Wolf, D.P. & Tash, J.S. (1988). Temporal changes in motility parameters related to acrosomal status: identification and characterization of populations of hyperactivated human sperm. *Biol. Reprod.*, **39**, 797–805.

Rochwerger, L., Cohen, D.J. & Cuasnicu, P.S. (1992). Mammalian sperm–egg fusion: the rat egg has complementary sites for a sperm protein that mediates gamete fusion. *Dev. Biol.*, **153**, 83–90.

Saling, P.M. (1991). How the egg regulates sperm function during gamete interaction: facts and fantasies. *Biol. Reprod.*, **44**, 246–51.

Saling, P.M. & Lakoski, K.A. (1985). Mouse sperm antigens that participate in fertilization. II. Inhibition of sperm penetration through the zona pellucida using monoclonal antibodies. *Biol. Reprod.*, **33**, 527–36.

Schmell, E.D., Gulyas, B.L. & Hedrick, J.L. (1983). Egg surface changes during fertilization and the molecular mechanism of the block to polyspermy. In *Mechanism and Control of Animal Fertilization*, ed. J.F. Hartmann, pp. 365–413. New York: Academic Press.

Shabanowitz, R.G. & O'Rand, M.G. (1988). Characterization of the human zona pellucida from fertilized and unfertilized eggs. *J. Reprod. Fertil.*, **82**, 151–61.

Shur, B.D. & Hall, N.G. (1982). A role for mouse sperm surface galactosyltransferase in sperm binding to the egg zona pellucida. *J. Cell Biol.*, **95**, 574–9.

Storey, B.T. & Kopf, G.S. (1991). Fertilization in the mouse. II. Spermatozoa. In *A Comparative Overview of Mammalian Fertilization*, ed. B.S. Dunbar & M.G. O'Rand, pp. 167–216. New York: Plenum Press.

Talbot, P., DiCarlantonio, G., Zao, P., Penkala, J. & Haimo, L.T. (1985). Motile cells lacking hyaluronidase can penetrate the hamster oocyte cumulus complex. *Dev. Biol.*, **108**, 387–98.

Wassarman, P.M. (1991). Fertilization in the mouse. I. The egg. In *A Comparative Overview of Mammalian Fertilization*, ed. B.S. Dunbar & M.G. O'Rand, pp. 151–65. New York: Plenum Press.

Williams, C.J., Schultz, R.M. & Kopf, G.S. (1992). Role of G proteins in mouse egg activation: stimulatory effects of acetylcholine on the ZP2 and $ZP2_f$ conversion and pronuclear formation in eggs expressing a functional m1 muscarinic receptor. *Dev. Biol.*, **151**, 188–96.

Wolf, D.P. & Hamada, M. (1977). Induction of zonal and egg plasma membrane blocks to sperm penetration in mouse eggs with cortical granule exudate. *Biol. Reprod.*, **17**, 350–64.

Yanagamachi, R. (1988). Mammalian fertilization. In *The Physiology of Reproduction*, vol. 1, ed. E. Knobil & J.D. Neill, pp. 135–85. New York: Raven Press.

3

Routine semen analysis

GRACE M. CENTOLA

Introduction

The routine semen analysis is the most important source of information on the fertility status of the male partner. Although gradually being replaced by more sophisticated computer-aided semen analysis methods (CASA; see Chapter 4), most hospital and private laboratories rely on the traditional, manual light microscopic method of assessing semen. Although an important part of the couple-based fertility evaluation, the semen analysis is more an assessment of the *potential* for fertility, rather than a test of actual fertility. Although only a *rough* estimate of the functional capability of the spermatozoa, routine semen analysis is an *accurate* measure of sperm production and epididymal maturation. A definitive diagnosis of male fertility cannot be made as a result of the semen analysis, and thus more sophisticated tests have become useful to the fertility specialist (see Chapters 6 and 9).

Historically, there has been a lack of standardization of methodologies for the semen analysis, as well as difficulty with interpretation of results. This makes comparison of semen analysis results and patient diagnosis nearly impossible between centers. Recently, the World Health Organization has published a manual (now in its third edition) for the laboratory evaluation of semen which encourages the use of standardized procedures for semen analysis (WHO, 1992). This should result in greater comparability among laboratories, as well as improving the precision, reproducibility and interpretation of the results.

This chapter will describe the standard manual methods for performing a semen analysis. Most importantly, however, information useful for the clinical evaluation of infertile couples will be presented, such as when to request a semen analysis, instructions in preparation for the analysis, and the interpretation of results.

General considerations

It takes approximately 70–90 days for sperm to be formed and to mature in the human testicle and epididymis. Approximately 1 week or more of that time is spent in the epididymis, where sperm gain the capacity for fertilization through both physicochemical and morphological changes. During this time, the maturing spermatozoa are sensitive to a variety of factors. Examples of such exogenous and endogenous factors include fever and illness, stress, ejaculatory frequency and even sitting in a hot tub. When taking a detailed fertility history, the physician should include questions about recent illnesses, social activities, drug and alcohol use, prescription medications, and coital frequency. Recent studies suggest that stress causes a decrease in sperm count, and an increase in fertilization failure in an *in vitro* fertilization program (Harrison *et al.*, 1987).

The routine semen analysis provides the clinician with information which may direct further evaluation and treatment of the couple. The results of the semen analysis, for example, can be compared with results of a well timed post-coital test to determine the need for further evaluations or even for the use of intrauterine insemination (IUI). It is important that a minimum of two or three semen analyses be performed at a 3–4 week interval to eliminate any unexplainable variations. A repeat semen analysis 1 week after the first analysis is only useful in that it may show collection error. Combined data from the multiple semen analyses can then be critically evaluated prior to instituting a logical diagnostic and treatment plan.

Specimen collection

The laboratory performing the analysis should provide clear and concise instructions to the patient regarding the abstinence period, method of collection and delivery to the facility. Ideally, the analysis should be scheduled for no less than 48 hours, and no more than 72 hours, after the last ejaculation. Two or three days is preferred since too short or too long an abstinence period may affect the sperm count and motility, as well as increasing the contaminating cells and debris (Centola, 1993). It is important for each laboratory to establish standards in this regard, since variability in this time period may increase the variability in the results and make comparisons between multiple specimens from individual patients virtually impossible (World Health Organization, 1992; Centola, 1993).

The specimen should be collected by masturbation, without the use of lubricants which might affect the motility and viability of the sperm. The specimen can be collected at home into a sterile container provided by the laboratory and delivered within one-half hour of ejaculation, keeping it warm at body temperature. Special seminal collection condoms, unlike commercially available condoms, can be used for those men who are unwilling or unable to collect the specimen by masturbation (Zavos, 1985). Zavos (1985) reported that the use of these condoms optimizes semen collection, particularly for those with low sperm counts. Incomplete specimens should not be assessed, or, at the very least, the referring physician should be alerted that the results may be in doubt because of faulty collection.

The analysis should begin within 30–40 minutes after ejaculation. Although sperm motility may be maintained even at 1 hour post-ejaculation, it is not recommended that specimens be held longer than 45 minutes prior to motility analysis (Centola, 1993). If held any longer, diminished motility may be reported erroneously.

Evaluation of physical characteristics

At the time of ejaculation the semen is a thick coagulum which, within 5–30 minutes, liquefies becoming very fluid-like or watery. Non-liquefaction is characterized by areas of immobilized sperm within a visible matrix (Overstreet *et al.*, 1992), whereas increased viscosity or thickness of the semen is different from failure to liquefy. The matrix dissolves with liquefaction, and the spermatozoa swim freely in the seminal fluid. Failure of liquefaction within 1 hour of ejaculation is abnormal, although rare, and may require referral for treatment (Overstreet, 1988) by processing and IUI or other laboratory manipulations. Hyperviscosity may inhibit motility, and prevent contact between the ejaculate and the cervix after intercourse. The significance of increased viscosity can be ascertained following the post-coital test. If the post-coital test reveals good concentration of motile sperm in midcycle mucus (8–10 freely progressive sperm per high-power field in a minimum of four fields) then increased viscosity is probably of no significance. The increased viscosity is often of unknown etiology, although a subclinical infection might be suspected. Clinical examination of the prostate and seminal vesicles may provide information to the clinician, and patients are often treated empirically with antibiotics. Also, use of expectorant medication (i.e., guanefescin) can also help to reduce the hyperviscosity (Centola, unpublished data). Alpha-amylase suppositories used after intercourse have been recommended, but with limited success (A.T.K. Cockett, personal communication). Lastly, sperm processing and IUI (Chapter 8) may be an option in cases of semen hyperviscosity or failed liquefaction.

The semen should be white to whitish-grey in color. When the sperm count is excessively high, the color of the semen is densely white; when the sperm count is severely low or azoospermic (lack of sperm), the semen is clear. Pink to red color may signal the presence of red blood cells in the ejaculate, which is confirmed microscopically. A greenish or yellow color and or a strong odor may signal an infection, which should also be confirmed microscopically. The laboratory performing the analysis should notify the referring physician who should then request a semen or urethral microbiological culture.

The semen volume should be 1.0–5.0 ml (Centola, 1993); the World Health Organization normal volume is >2.0 ml (WHO, 1992). Abnormal volume may be a significant cause of subfertility. Mattox and colleagues (1990) demonstrated that the fertilization rate and subsequent pregnancy rate after *in vitro* fertilization (IVF) were reduced for hypovolemic specimens. High volume may suggest dysfunction of the prostate or seminal vesicles. Homologous artificial insemination, split ejaculate insemination or withdrawal coitus has been suggested by some to enhance contact of the sperm with the cervical mucus in these patients (Howards, 1986). IUI of processed semen may also be an option. Low volume may result from obstruction (see Chapter 15), or congenital absence of the vas deferens. Chronic low volume with concomitant low sperm count may suggest retrograde ejaculation (ejaculation into the bladder) which is common in diabetic men. A post-ejaculatory urine analysis can confirm the presence or absence of sperm in the urine. Significant concentration of sperm in the urine indicates a dysfunction of the bladder neck sphincter, and is cause for referral of the patient to a urologist. Sperm can be recovered from neutralized urine, washed, resuspended in nutrient medium, and used for an IUI. Pregnancy rates following retrograde recovery and IUI are not significantly different from the normal monthly fecundity (Centola, unpublished observations).

Many laboratory semen analyses measure ejaculate pH. The pH should be assessed when a specimen presents with immobilized sperm, which could be a result of the semen being too acidic or too basic. The semen pH should be in the range of 7.0–7.5 (Centola, 1993). Increased or decreased pH may signal accessory gland dysfunction or infection, and warrants urologic referral prior to proceeding with other evaluation or therapy.

Evaluation of quantitative characteristics

Sperm count

Table 3.1 shows the normal semen parameters. The sperm count is an accurate measure of spermatogenesis, and the sperm motility is a rough measure of epididymal maturation and sperm functional capabilities. There is a wide fluctua-

Table 3.1   *Normal values of semen parameters*

Parameter	Normal range
Semen volume	2.0 ml or more
pH	7.2–8.0
Sperm concentration	20 million/ml or more
Total sperm count	40 million or more
Motility	50% or more with forward progression or 25% or more rapid progression, at 1 hour
Morphology	30% or more normal forms
Vitality	75% or more live; excluding vital dye
White blood cells	Fewer than 1 million/ml

Notes:
From WHO (1992).

tion in biweekly sperm concentration, ranging from oligozoospermic (<20 million/ml) to well within normal limits (>40 million/ml) (WHO, 1987). Variations in production of seminal plasma, environmental influences such as injury, illness, toxic exposure, stress and ejaculatory frequency can affect sperm concentration – hence the need for several specimens for analysis (see above).

The normal sperm concentration is greater than 20 million sperm per milliliter, with a total number of sperm (count × volume) of greater than 50 million (WHO, 1987, 1992). Recently, assisted reproductive technologies such as IVF, subzonal insertion, intracytoplasmic injection and IUI have suggested that the normal fertile sperm concentration might be much lower than 20 million/ml. Considering these techniques, 1 spermatozoon is needed for intracytoplasmic injection, 10 for subzonal insertion, 50 000 for *in vitro* fertilization, and 1 million or fewer motile sperm for IUI (Byrd *et al.*, 1987).

If the sperm count is 10 million/ml or greater, it is reasonable to suggest several cycles of IUI prior to further therapy, or referral for ovulation induction or IVF (see Chapters 7, 10 and 11). In severely oligozoospermic specimens (5 million/ml and less) referral to a urologist or reproductive endocrinologist is the logical initial step, where endocrinological evaluation (LH, FSH, testosterone, prolactin), Doppler examination, etc., will be considered (see Chapters 13 and 14). A urologist can also determine whether a testicular biopsy is warranted to determine histological mapping of the testicles and determination of the degree of sperm production by the testicle. Often no cause can be found for the low sperm count. Regardless of etiology, there may be no medical or surgical treatment to enhance the sperm count. Following several cycles of IUI the couple may decide to proceed with other assisted reproductive technologies or donor insemination.

High sperm concentrations (greater than 150 million/ml) may also result in subfertility (Centola, 1993). The high sperm concentration may result in many collisions between motile sperm, or between motile and non-motile sperm, thus affecting the percentage progressive motility. The sperm count should fall within or close to the normal range following repeated analyses. Fluctuations in sperm count over three or more analyses are difficult to explain. A sperm count within 5–7 million of the normal value may result in anxiety on the part of the couple, but is probably of no concern. Many clinicians, however, will conclude after one analysis showing less than 20 million/ml, that there is a male factor, and cease any further evaluation of the female partner. Since what was once termed a 'low' sperm count is no longer considered as such, the clinician should complete the basic evaluation of the female partner (see Chapter 18) and then consider IUI as an alternative option prior to donor insemination or IVF.

Consistency of sperm count is critical. A man with five normal sperm counts and one abnormal count should not be concerned. Furthermore, a man with five abnormal analyses and one normal sperm count should not be considered cured. Consistent low sperm count should be evaluated. Clomiphene, tamoxifen and halotestin treatments have been attempted for treatment of oligozoospermia with limited, if any, success (Centola, 1993; see Chapter 13). In most cases, referral to a urologist or endocrinologist specializing in reproductive disorders is helpful and may provide information useful to the managing clinician.

Sperm motility

The percentage of motile sperm is probably as important, or more important, than the sperm concentration. Sperm motility is important for movement through the female reproductive tract, and for successful sperm–oocyte interaction. However, motile sperm are not essential for fertilization – subzonal insertion or intracytoplasmic sperm injection can be accomplished without sperm motility. Although not all couples are candidates for such assisted techniques, this example demonstrates how normal values for semen variables vary as a function of available technology.

The normal percent motility is 50% with a grade of 2 or better on a scale of 1 (low) to 4 (high) for progressiveness (WHO, 1992). Motility of 40% might not be of concern when the sperm count or the results of the post-coital test are considered. Consistent motilities of less than 40% may be cause for further investigation. Manual assessment of sperm motility is highly subjective. The lack of precision in manual visual assessments has led many to question their clinical utility (Overstreet, 1992). As a result, computer-assisted motion analysis has been suggested as a more objective and precise tool for motility measurement. Computerized motion analysis can provide valuable information relative to the quality of the sperm motion, which only now is becoming important in assessment of fertility (Overstreet *et al.*, 1992; see also Chapter 4).

Many extrinsic factors might affect sperm motility. Increased testicular temperature, such as with the use of hot tubs, hot baths, or even waterbeds, will compromise sperm motility and potentially the sperm count following long-term exposure to the increased temperature. Certain prescription medications, recreational drug use, excessive alcohol and cigarette smoking may compromise sperm motility as well as the sperm count. Exposure to solvents, pesticides, and metals such as lead, mercury or gold may also affect sperm parameters. A change in these lifestyle or recreational habits may improve sperm parameters. Reduced motility might also accompany genital infection. Increased viscosity may affect sperm motility. The presence of antisperm antibodies might also be reflected in a consistent low sperm motility that does not increase with empiric treatment. When all other factors are considered and eliminated, antisperm antibody analysis should be considered (see Chapter 5).

In addition to the above causes of low motility, a varicocele should be considered and excluded (see Chapters 14 and 15). A varicocele, present in approximately 41% of infertile men, is a dilatation of the pampiniform plexus of veins. Its pathophysiology and pathogenesis remain controversial. A clinically significant varicocele is often accompanied by decreased sperm motility and sperm count, and increased numbers of tapered sperm and immature sperm forms. The decision to undergo surgical repair of the varicocele is difficult. Prior to consideration of repair, several cycles of IUI of washed sperm, with or without ovulation induction, can be recommended. If there is no success, further evaluation of the female may continue, as well as consideration of the varicocele repair. That testicular endocrine function is disturbed in men with varicocele is suggested by Hudson and Perez-Marrero (1993), who reported an excessive response to intravenous infusion of GnRH (by increase in LH and FSH) which was related to lower than normal free testosterone levels in certain men with varicoceles. Furthermore, men with clinically insignificant (or incidental) varicoceles had normal GnRH responses, and no improvement following surgical repair of the varicocele. The majority of those with excessive GnRH response showed marked improvement in hormonal and seminal parameters following varicocele repair. Tinga and colleagues (1984) have also shown dramatic improvement in sperm count and motility following varicocele repair.

Morphology

The morphological assessment of seminal cytology is performed on a stained slide by a trained, experienced technologist. An ejaculate contains both normal and abnormal appearing spermatozoa. Morphologically abnormal sperm are probably not functional cells (Morales *et al.*, 1988). Currently, two methods are available for the assessment of morphology: the World Health Organization method (WHO, 1992) and the strict criteria developed by Kruger *et al.* (1987). This strict method is based on exact measurements of the length and width of the sperm head. The percentage of normal sperm using the strict criteria is considerably lower than the cutoff using previous standard methods (14% vs 50%, respectively). The most recent version of the WHO manual (WHO, 1992) suggested a more sophisticated staining and assessment, with a resulting percentage normal morphology of 30% or greater. The objectivity and precision in assessment of morphology is clearly a major concern, since morphology assessment is subject to significant human bias and errors. This lack of objectivity, coupled with problems of standardization, limits the utility of this potentially valuable semen parameter (Overstreet *et al.*, 1992). Computer-aided morphology analysis is currently being investigated by many centers using the computerized semen analyzer (see Chapter 4). However, there are inherent problems of standardization in this methodology also, thus limiting its clinical utility. When assessing sperm morphology, the clinician is urged to employ an experienced technician or laboratory that routinely performs multiple semen analyses on a daily basis. Such experience is invaluable, and may provide some standardization.

The percentage of normal forms does not vary widely. This can be demonstrated by repeated analyses of the same individual's sperm morphology. Experienced laboratories report similar morphologies in repeated 'blind' analyses within the same individual (Centola, unpublished observations).

It is also very important to distinguish between immature forms and contaminating white blood cells in the semen (see Chapter 16). Special staining methods for the detection of white blood cells, particularly granulocytes, are essential. These methods are generally available in specialized andrology laboratories, thus supporting the use of such laboratories for fertility analyses.

Morphological analysis can provide the physician with valuable information on the functional status of the seminiferous epithelium as well as the epididymis. If there is a large percentage of small or pin-head sperm forms, or absence of acrosomal caps (round heads), for example, impairment of spermiogenesis may be suspected. Hormonal analysis, and testicular biopsy, with referral to a reproductive specialist would then be needed (Centola, 1993).

Summary: interpretation of the semen analysis and treatment options

A semen analysis cannot provide all the answers to questions regarding a man's fertility potential. Many examples of successful pregnancies have been reported where one or more of the male partner's sperm parameters was significantly out of the normal range. Furthermore, the interaction between the sperm and the female reproductive tract is essential in determining male fertility potential. Tests of functional capabilities, such as the sperm penetration assay, computerized motion analysis of sperm, and hyperactivation analysis, for example (see Chapters 4 and 9), may provide more specific information to the clinician managing the infertile couple.

Semen analysis initiates the investigation of the infertile male. One semen analysis is insufficient for the clinician to formulate a diagnosis and treatment regimen. We recommend a minimum of two or three analyses at 3–4 week intervals. Analyses should be done by the same laboratory, so that results can be compared in the same individual over time. All laboratory procedures demand precision, sensitivity and reproducibility. In order for reports to be easily intelligible within a laboratory and between laboratories, standardization of testing is essential (Mortimer, 1994).

When reviewing the semen analysis reports, the clinician should be aware of both the intrinsic variability in semen parameters and the effects of extrinsic factors. A significant influence of abstinence on semen characteristics is well established (Mortimer, 1994). Illnesses, particularly febrile illnesses, drug use, exposure to toxic chemicals (solvents, pesticides, heavy metals), and smoking have been known to affect semen quality, and should be taken into consideration when interpreting the results of the semen analyses. Additionally, use of a waterbed, hot tub or sauna, excessive exercise and tight clothing may affect scrotal temperature, and thus affect sperm count and motility. If any of these are documented, the clinician may want to request repeat analyses, allowing an adequate time interval to eliminate the effects of these factors. Thorough and careful history is thus essential when considering the results of the semen analysis.

Surgical treatment of a male's infertility is helpful when there is a documented anatomic or surgically correctable condition. These may include blockage of the vas, previous vasectomy, or clinical varicocele (see Chapters 13, 14 and 15). Medical treatment is very difficult in the male, particularly in the absence of documented endocrine abnormalities. Artificial insemination, such as by the intrauterine route, has been utilized with success in many infertile couples. In cases of low motility or sperm count, low volume, repeated poor post-coital tests, as well as ejaculatory dysfunction and unexplained infertility

Table 3.2   *Summary of treatment for various problems with semen parameters*

Problem	Treatment/consideration
Increased debris/white blood cells	Possible prolonged abstinence or subclinical infection. Consider empiric antibiotics
Hyperviscosity	Possible subclinical infection. Consider antibiotics, cough syrups, IUI; correlate with PCT
Hypovolemia	Possible retrograde ejaculation, accessory gland dysfunction, blockage. Consider urologic referral, AIH, IUI
Hypervolemia	Possible prolonged abstinence. Consider AIH, IUI, withdrawal coitus
Decreased concentration	Possible injury, illness, toxic exposure; decreased abstinence, consider volume and viscosity. Consider testicular biopsy, hormone treatment, IUI, IVF
Decreased motility	Check time of analysis; consider specimen cold shock, waterbed, hot tub/baths, prolonged abstinence, infection, hyperviscosity, sperm antibodies, varicocele. Correlate with PCT. Consider AIH, IUI, IVF. Empiric antibiotics

Notes:
From Centola (1993). Interpretation is based on a general summary of a minimum of two or three analyses performed at 3–4 week intervals.
IUI, intrauterine insemination; PCT, post-coital test; AIH, artificial insemination by husband; IVF, *in vitro* fertilization.

(both male and female), IUI provides a relatively inexpensive, easily accomplished and successful option. Sperm processing (washing) to remove seminal contaminants and prostaglandin should be done by an experienced laboratory. Many techniques are available for sperm washing, and individualized attention to each ejaculate is very important. Ovulation timing is critical. For a review of sperm washing procedures and the use of IUI for infertile couples see Chapters 7 and 8. IVF, with or without micromanipulation, may be useful in cases of low sperm count or motility, or in cases where no other treatment has been successful (see Chapters 10, 11). Use of donor semen may be an option in cases of azoospermia, but should also be considered where other treatment options have failed.

In conclusion, it is important for the clinician who initiates the investigation of the infertile couple to study the results of multiple semen analyses very carefully before formulating a treatment regimen (Table 3.2). The results of the semen analyses should be considered in the light of a complete medical and social history, as well as post-coital testing. Only then can the clinicians make educated and informed decisions with regard to the course of further evaluation and therapy.

References

Byrd, W., Ackerman, G.E., Carr, B.R., Edman, C.D., Yuyick, D.S. & McConnell, J.D. (1987). Treatment of refractory infertility by transcervical intrauterine insemination of washed spermatozoa. *Fertil. Steril.*, **48**, 921–7.

Centola, G.M. (1993). Conventional semen analysis. In *Decision Making in Reproductive Endocrinology*, ed. W.D. Schlaff & J.D. Rock, pp. 433–7. Boston: Blackwell Scientific.

Harrison, K.L., Callan, V.J. & Hennessey, J.F. (1987). Stress and semen quality in an *in vitro* fertilization program. *Fertil. Steril.*, **48**, 633–6.

Howards, S.S. (1986). Semen analysis: routine techniques. In *The Male Factor in Infertility: Pathophysiology, Evaluation and Treatment*. Postgraduate Course, 42nd Annual Clinical Meeting, The American Fertility Society. Birmingham: The American Fertility Society.

Hudson, R.W. & Perez-Marrero, R.A. (1993). Free testosterone (T) and sex hormone binding globulin (SHBG) levels in men with varicoceles. Proceedings of the American Fertility Society and the Canadian Fertility Society, 11–14 October, p. 528. Birmingham: The American Fertility Society.

Kruger, T.F., Acosta, A.A. & Simmons, K.F. (1987). New method of evaluating sperm morphology with predictive value for human *in vitro* fertilization. *Urology*, **30**, 248.

Mattox, J.H., Graham, M.C., Partridge, A.B. & Marazzo, D.P. (1990). Impact of hypospermia on outcome in an IVF program. *J. Androl.*, **11**, 56.

Morales, P., Katz, D.F. & Overstreet, J.W. (1988). The relationship between the motility and morphology of spermatozoa in semen. *J. Androl.*, **9**, 241.

Mortimer, D. (1994). *Practical Laboratory Andrology*. New York: Oxford University Press.

Overstreet, J.W. (1988). Semen liquefaction and viscosity problems. In *Contemporary Management of Impotence and Infertility*, ed. E.A. Tanaagho, T.F. Lue & R.D. McClure, p. 311. Baltimore: Williams and Wilkins.

Overstreet, J.W., Davis, R.O. & Katz, D.F. (1992). Semen evaluation. In *Infertility and Reproductive Medicine Clinics of North America: Male Infertility*, vol. 3, ed. M.P. Diamond & A.H. DeCherney, pp. 239–40. Philadelphia: W.B. Saunders.

Tinga, D.J., Jager, S., Bruijnen, C.L.A.H., Kremer, J. & Mensink, H.J. (1984). Factors related to semen improvement and fertility after varicocele repair. *Fertil. Steril.*, **41**, 404.

World Health Organization (1987). *WHO Laboratory Manual for the Examination of Human Semen and Semen–Cervical Mucus Interaction*, 2nd edn. Cambridge: Cambridge University Press.

World Health Organization (1992). *WHO Laboratory Manual for the Examination of Human Semen and Sperm–Cervical Mucus Interaction*, 3rd edn. Cambridge: Cambridge University Press.

Zavos, P.M. (1985). Seminal parameters of ejaculates collected from oligospermic and normospermic patients via masturbation and at intercourse with the use of silastic seminal fluid collection device. *Fertil. Steril.*, **44**, 517–20.

4

Computer-aided sperm analysis: a critical review

RUSSELL O. DAVIS and DAVID F. KATZ

Introduction

Commercially available computer-aided sperm analysis (CASA) was introduced to research laboratories and laboratory medicine nearly 10 years ago. The first instruments were CellSoft (Cryo Resources, Montgomery, NY) and ExpertVision (later called CellTrak, Motion Analysis Corp., Santa Rosa, CA). There soon followed the HTM-2000 (Hamilton Thorn Research, Beverly, MA), the SM-CMA instrument from Europe (Stromberg-Mika, Bad Feilnbach, Germany), and others. There are now over 120 papers which verify CASA technology for semen analysis or apply it in basic and clinical studies. However, despite this enormous body of work, and the considerable time since its introduction, CASA's potential has not been realized for two basic reasons. First, manufacturers have been unwilling or unable to address a fundamental limitation of the technology, namely the inability of CASA instruments to obtain accurate counts and percent motilities when the concentration of a specimen is greater than about 50×10^6 sperm/ml or less than about 20×10^6 sperm/ml, or when a specimen is laden with debris. These common conditions require laboratories to either dilute, concentrate, or wash specimens, significantly limiting routine clinical application of the technology. Second, professional societies and organizations have been slow to develop and recommend performance and operating standards for CASA instruments. Appeals have been made by industry spokesmen and individual scientists (Schrader *et al.*, 1992; Chapin *et al.*, 1992) to achieve this end, but no stance has been taken by any professional group on the performance, use, calibration, or standardization of CASA technology.

The application of CASA in clinical laboratory medicine is hindered by these continuing technical limitations and the lack of involvement by professional organizations. Significant results have been obtained in basic research that would not have been possible without CASA technology, but their generalization and applications are limited because no standard approach has been used. As a consequence, it remains extremely difficult to verify or repeat experimental findings between instruments or sites, or to interpret them. Such practical and technical limitations have been clearly recognized by the World Health Organization (WHO), which represents CASA as a research tool in its new *Laboratory Manual for the Analysis of Human Semen and Semen–Cervical Mucus Interaction* (WHO, 1992), and not as a device that can automate, objectify, and standardize clinical laboratory semen analysis.

In this review, we assess current knowledge about CASA technology and analyze its technical strengths and weaknesses. We do not review the biological results obtained with CASA, because many problems persist with experimental design, standardization of procedures, and instrument performance. Making use of fundamental engineering principles, and of known factors that affect CASA results, we develop a list of standard operational procedures for the major instruments.

Is CASA necessary?

Since its introduction, the biomedical value of CASA has been questioned and challenged. It continues to be argued that CASA is suitable only for basic research. This view may have arisen because of the high cost of the technology and anxiety over dependence upon computers and automation. However, cost and technical limitations aside, the question remains valid. Is CASA technology necessary to address fundamental biological questions and laboratory quality-control issues in modern fertility research and in the clinical diagnostic laboratory? Two answers suggest that it is.

First, researchers have recognized for many years that there is more biomedical information available in the ejaculate than is revealed by simple properties such as sperm count, the percentage of motile sperm, and a population average estimate of sperm progression. Techniques were developed in the 1970s and the early 1980s to measure the detailed pattern and vigor of individual spermatozoa motion to investigate this source of information. These methods included time-exposure photomicrography (Janick & MacLeod, 1970; Overstreet *et al.*, 1979), manual frame-by-frame analysis of high-speed cine film (Zorgniotti *et al.*, 1958; Philips, 1972), and early applications of digitizing pads and computers to multiple-exposure photomicrographs (Makler, 1980), frame-by-frame analysis of cine film (Katz *et al.*, 1978), and videotape (Katz & Overstreet, 1981). These studies indicated that direct measurement of individual spermatozoa produced more accurate measures of population average values than traditional methods. They also provided a wealth of new information that was especially useful in detecting and studying important cell physiological events involved in sperm transport, capacitation, and oocyte binding. However, a lingering problem was that manual or even semi-automated analyses of individual spermatozoa were prohibitively time-consuming and expensive. Such techniques could never be used for routine clinical analysis and diagnosis. Only by their complete automation could such objective methods be made widely available.

Second, numerous studies have shown that subjective, visual measures of sperm count, percent motility, and morphology are inaccurate and imprecise (Jequier & Ukome, 1983; Dunphy *et al.*, 1989; Neuwinger *et al.*, 1990*a*). Sperm count has been the most widely assessed variable because, together with seminal volume, it is perhaps the most amenable parameter to objective, visual measurement. Nevertheless, large coefficients of variation (CVs) have been reported for between-technician (44%) and within-technician (33%) variability for sperm count (Jequier & Ukome, 1983; Dunphy *et al.*, 1989). In one study, several specimens were evaluated by nine laboratories as part of an external quality control experiment (Neuwinger *et al.*, 1990*a*). Ejaculates were processed by swim-up, then resuspended in phosphate-buffered saline (PBS) with formalin. Aliquots of the fixed specimens were distributed to participating laboratories, which determined count according to the then current WHO guidelines (WHO 1987). High between-laboratory CVs were reported (mean 37.5%), the highest occurring in samples with a low concentration (73%) and the lowest occurring in samples with a high concentration (23%). A low CV (2%) was reported for repeated counts of the same drop by two technicians, and a higher one (10%) for counts of repeated drops from the same specimen. Recent work in our own laboratory, which evaluated the effect of counting method and chamber, gave similar results (Davis, 1992).

Studies of sperm motility have produced similar variability. In one such report, 26 technicians independently analyzed a single specimen visually, and reported percent motilities between 30% and 80% (Jequier & Ukome, 1983). Other studies have reported between-technician CVs of 10–20%. Although important biological information is reflected in sperm motility and movement patterns, this assessment is subjective and imprecise.

From these reports it is evident that obtaining precise and accurate results using traditional, subjective, visual semen analysis methods is difficult at best. However, it is not impossible. Given sufficient effort in developing objective methods, defining standards for technician training, and performing proficiency testing at regular intervals, significant improvements in visual analysis can be made (Mortimer *et al.*, 1986). Whether it is more cost-effective to develop a program to train, test, and certify laboratory technicians for visual

Table 4.1 *Factors that can affect CASA results*

Instrument precision
Instrument accuracy
Microscope
Counting chamber
Diluent or extender
Video framing (or digitization) rate
Physiological state of sperm
Temperature effect on VCL and MOT
Specimen concentration
Presence of debris in the sample
Instrument parameter settings
Digitization threshold (gray scale)
Number of points per track
Number of frames tracked
Number of fields (or sperm) analyzed
Computational algorithms for average path and ALH
Statistical methods
Laboratory supplies
Videotaping (inter-tech variation)
Between-aliquot variation

Notes:
VCL, curvilinear velocity; MOT, percent motility; ALH, amplitude of lateral head displacement.

analysis or to automate many of the assays now being performed remains the question facing experts today.

Applications of CASA

Numerous studies have been performed in which CASA measures of sperm motion have been compared with visual analogs (so-called verification studies). Other work has been undertaken in which characteristic parameters of a specific population have been reported (e.g., CASA values for 'normal' men). Finally, several studies have been performed in which biological results have been reported for treated and untreated groups (e.g., capacitated versus non-capacitated sperm, or normal versus patient populations). Because of the problems summarized in Table 4.1, conclusions from these reports must be viewed with caution.

Many CASA verification studies have concluded that two methods of measurement, e.g., CASA and visual, or two CASA instruments, are in accord. Such conclusions have usually been based on agreement of population means for a given parameter for the two methods. However, no precision estimates have usually been given for the compared techniques, and when the data are examined on a pair-wise basis, large differences are usually found. It should be remembered that the unit of study in semen analysis is not the population average performance of two methods across many specimens, but rather the comparison of individual samples. Only a few studies have employed appropriate statistical techniques when comparing two methods of semen analysis (Mortimer, 1988; Ginsburg *et al.*, 1988; Mortimer *et al.*, 1988; Davis & Katz, 1992; Davis *et al.*, 1992). The same criticism can be applied to studies that report significant differences between groups of patients, or between treated and untreated specimens.

Finally, several studies have attempted to characterize semen parameters of normal men or infertility patients. In many such studies, raw specimens were analyzed that were well above (or below) the concentration range needed for accurate CASA. Consequently, values reported for CASA measures of normal men or patients from such studies should be interpreted with caution.

Problems with CASA

Modern CASA instruments analyze spermatozoan motion by identifying and analyzing magnified video images of live or videotaped cells (Boyers *et al.*, 1989). Numerous factors can significantly affect CASA results (Table 4.1). Some pertain to specimen preparation and observation techniques, while others pertain to the inherent accuracy or precision of CASA instruments. Also of importance are instrument parameter settings and the computational algorithms used. Finally, the statistical procedures employed to analyze CASA data can also significantly affect the quantitative results.

Many of these factors can be controlled and therefore do not present problems for CASA. For example, laboratory supplies (gloves, specimen collection cups, etc.) can be routinely screened for cytotoxicity. The effect of temperature on spermatozoan motility has been known for many years, and can be controlled easily by using a heated microscope stage. Issues such as aliquot variation can be addressed by using standardized protocols for specimen preparation, with appropriate quality control procedures. Variability in counting chambers can be reduced by replacing reusable chambers (e.g., the hemacytometer, Makler chamber) when their recommended life time has been reached, or by utilizing one of the new disposable sperm counting chambers. The accuracy of kinematic parameters, particularly curvilinear velocity (VCL), beat-cross frequency (BCF), linearity (LIN) and the amplitude of lateral head displacement (ALH) (see Table 4.2 for definitions), can be improved by employing a video framing rate that is suitable for the physiological state of the

Table 4.2 *Names, definitions, and standard symbols for kinematic variables measured by CASA*

Symbol	Name	Definition
VSL	Straight-line velocity	Time-average velocity of the sperm head along a straight line from its first position to its last position
VCL	Curvilinear velocity	Time-average velocity of the sperm head along its actual trajectory
VAP	Average path velocity	Time-average velocity of the sperm head along its average trajectory
LIN	Linearity	Linearity of the curvilinear trajectory (VSL/VCL)
ALH	Amplitude of lateral head displacement	Amplitude of variations of the actual sperm-head trajectory about its average trajectory (the average trajectory is computed using a rectangular running average)
BCF	Beat cross frequency	Time-average rate at which the actual sperm trajectory crosses the average path trajectory
CON	Specimen concentration	Concentration of sperm cells in a sample in millions of sperm per milliliter of plasma or medium
MOT	Percent motility	Percentage of sperm cells in a suspension that are motile (in manual analysis, motility is defined by a moving flagellum; in CASA, motility is defined by a minimum VSL for each sperm)

sperm, i.e. their degree of vigor. The stability of kinematic parameters can be improved by tracking all sperm for a sufficient number of video frames. Statistical biases can be eliminated when summary statistics are computed on sperm trajectories of equal length. Finally, the accuracy of estimates of the central tendency and the shape of the population distribution can be increased if a sufficient number of motile sperm are analyzed. Many of these procedures have recently been recommended for human clinical semen evaluation (Davis, 1992), epidemiological studies involving humans (Schrader *et al.*, 1992) and toxicological studies of the rat (Chapin *et al.*, 1992).

Problems with specimen concentration

Inaccuracies of CASA for determining sperm count and percent motility in low and high sperm concentrations have been described in both human and animal studies (Gill *et al.*, 1988; Budworth *et al.*, 1988; Mortimer *et al.*, 1988; Mathur, 1989; Neuwinger *et al.*, 1990*b*; Davis & Katz (1992); Davis *et al.*,

1992). Two factors are responsible for such effects: the confusion of sperm with debris, and the conjoining of sperm trajectories under conditions of high concentration and velocity.

CASA instruments recognize spermatozoa relative to non-sperm objects by their size, shape, luminosity, and movement. Most instruments have little difficulty in accurately detecting cells that are moving above the minimum velocity defined for a motile cell. However, immotile sperm are more difficult to distinguish from seminal debris, because such debris can be similar in size and shape to the sperm themselves. Inaccurate counts at high sperm concentrations are the consequence of the movements of the motile sperm. Swimming cells frequently bump into or cross over each other, and into immotile sperm and debris, creating optical conjunctions. Such conjunctions seriously challenge tracking algorithms. Such difficulties in determining sperm count have been, at least temporarily, mitigated at the laboratory level by diluting or concentrating semen specimens. The effects on CASA results of diluting semen in any medium have been evaluated in only one study (Davis & Boyers, 1992), when it was found that dilution in either homologous seminal plasma or PBS medium had significant effects on motility.

Problems with percent motility

In addition to problems with sperm count, several studies have reported inaccurate CASA results for sperm motility (Gill *et al.*, 1988; Budworth *et al.*, 1988; Mortimer *et al.*, 1988; Mathur, 1989; Davis & Katz, 1992; Neuwinger *et al.*, 1990*b*). Percent motility can be influenced by inaccurate concentration measures, if such measures are biased toward motile or immotile cells (Mortimer & Mortimer, 1988). Moreover, CASA motility measures have usually been compared with motility measures obtained by subjective, visual techniques. In many instances, both methods have not been applied to the same drop of sperm suspension. Hence, variability between drops must be taken into consideration when comparing methods. Given the lack of precision in visual motility measures, as well as the considerable drop-to-drop variation reported in most studies, it is not surprising that visual and CASA measures for percent motility often differ. More importantly, CASA and visual measures of percent motility usually differ because their definitions are not identical. In visual measures, a spermatozoon is usually considered to be motile if its flagellum is twitching, even though it may not exhibit forward progression. In CASA, a spermatozoon must achieve a minimum VSL to be motile (e.g., 10 μm/s). Hence, CASA measures will, by definition, usually be lower than visual estimates of percent motility, no matter how carefully the latter are done.

CASA in laboratory quality control

In addition to the potential clinical utility of CASA technology to male fertility testing, videomicrographic sperm analysis may also be employed advantageously in laboratory quality control protocols. Significant improvements in laboratory quality control have been mandated for US andrology and *in vitro* fertilization laboratories by the Clinical Laboratory Improvement Act of 1988 (CLIA). Quality control consists of a number of procedures which collectively assure that the functions of the laboratory are accomplished within a defined range of consistency and measurement error. These elements of laboratory quality control were recently recommended by the American Fertility Society (1992) in new guidelines for human embryology and andrology laboratories. However, despite these recent efforts to improve laboratory quality control, no such procedures have been defined for CASA, although one manufacturer has distributed a booklet on laboratory quality control and calibration procedures. Some attempts have been made to calibrate CASA instruments on a daily basis, using a standardized solution of fixed cells or synthetic particles to perform counts. However, these procedures are inadequate because they do not simulate the actual working conditions encountered by CASA instruments with live specimens. Another approach has been to analyze live or videotaped specimens. A novel solution to these problems, currently under development in our laboratory, is to create a computer simulation of swimming sperm using the equations of motion where the kinematics of each object are known, *a priori*.

Clinical applications of CASA

The quantitative analysis of sperm movement made possible with CASA analysis is of potential importance on several levels in medicine. On a basic level, study of sperm movement provides an excellent model for evaluating all aspects of normal cellular motility processes. Abnormal sperm motility may be a problem *per se* or it may be an indicator of a defect in spermatogenesis or epididymal maturation. Description of abnormal sperm movement patterns may thus be indicative of disordered energy metabolism or fine structure which in turn are potentially reflective of genetic, toxic, teratogenic or other developmental abnormalities. These alterations in pattern and vigor of sperm movement may translate to clinical disorders in sperm transport and sperm–oocyte interaction leading to subfertility or sterility. If such relationships can be documented, CASA will then provide the clinician with a powerful tool for the diagnosis of male infertility. Computerized methods of sperm motion analysis are more objective than routine semen analysis methods and may have additional advantages in terms of cost per analysis, quality control, etc., accounting for their current popularity as clinical laboratory tools.

Yet at present there are few data to recommend adoption of computerized methods as the standard for routine semen analysis. Using a variety of manual and computer-automated trajectory analysis methods, investigators have attempted to document differences in motion parameters between fertile and infertile semen samples. The strategy has typically been to attempt to correlate one or more averaged characteristics of sperm movement with other abnormalities of sperm function such as capacitation/acrosome reaction, zona pellucida binding or membrane fusion. However, this strategy probably is faulty for two reasons. First, normal ranges for sperm movement parameters have not been established, nor is there consensus on which parameters are most important in describing and analyzing sperm movement under different conditions (e.g., in seminal plasma, in cervical mucus). Further, most studies reported to date have averaged measurements across all sperm examined, hence possibly obscuring alterations in movement between small subpopulations of spermatozoa. Incisive multivariate statistical methods are required to evaluate these (as yet unknown) subpopulations of spermatozoa which will ultimately successfully interact with the cumulus–oocyte complex.

These criticisms aside, differences in the proportion of hyperactivating sperm (as measured by computerized analysis) have been demonstrated between samples from infertile and fertile subjects. In addition, alterations in movement patterns have been correlated with defective *in vitro* sperm penetration into cervical mucus, zona-free hamster oocytes and human oocytes in clinical assisted reproduction programs. It must be emphasized that there are at present limited data regarding the clinical utility of the movement measurements obtained by CASA. These associations, although not proof of cause–effect relationships, point to the potential *future* clinical utility of computerized sperm analysis measurements. Additional studies are necessary to establish which measurements are reflective of normal sperm function, which values are sufficiently outside an established normal range to reasonably conclude that sperm function is disturbed, and prospectively to confirm these relationships in large groups of subjects.

Conclusions

Many areas of medical diagnosis have been revolutionized by recent advances in computer technology and digital image processing. Such technologies, when combined with new surgical and drug delivery systems, have already begun to change the course of medical treatment. It is inevitable that computers, automated laboratory assays, lasers, high-resolution sonography, and other new technologies will be implemented in reproductive biology and medicine (Davis & Boyers, 1992). The role of CASA in these developments is twofold.

First, CASA can significantly improve the accuracy and precision of existing laboratory measures, particularly if standard procedures are followed and if the problems with dilution and thresholding are overcome. Second, and more importantly, CASA has the potential for providing more incisive measures of sperm function and fertility than do traditional sperm population average values. Only a few spermatozoa arrive at the site of fertilization when an oocyte is present, and only one fertilizes the oocyte. It is highly unlikely that population average values of sperm measures in an ejaculate will provide insights into the biologic mechanisms of sperm transport and fertilization. If our goal is to treat infertility, as well as diagnose it, then the mechanisms of fertility must be understood. CASA enables multivariate statistical analyses on individual cell parameters, which can lead to more detailed insights about cell function. Such techniques have already been applied in studies of hyperactivation (Ginsburg *et al.*, 1990) and fertilization rate in IVF (Davis *et al.*, 1991).

Acknowledgment

Supported by NICHD RO1–ES03614.

References

American Fertility Society (1992). Guidelines for human embryology and andrology laboratories. *Fertil. Steril.*, **58**, Suppl 1.

Boyers, S.P., Davis, R.O. & Katz, D.F. (1989). Automated semen analysis. *Curr. Probl. Obstet. Gynecol. Fertil.*, **12**, 165–200.

Budworth, P.R., Amann, R.P. & Chapman, P.L. (1988). Relationships between computerized measurements of motion of frozen-thawed bull spermatozoa and fertility. *J. Androl.*, **9**, 41–54.

Chapin, R.E., Filler, R.S., Gulati, D., Heindel, J.J., Katz, D.F., Mebus, C.A. *et al.* (1992). Methods for assessing rat sperm motility. *Reprod. Toxicol.*, **6**, 267–73.

Clinical Laboratory Improvement Act of 1988 (1992). Final Rule. *Fed. Reg.*, **57**, 7001–290.

Davis, R.O. (1992). The promise and pitfalls of computer-aided sperm analysis. In *Male Infertility*, ed. J.W. Overstreet. Infertility and Reproductive Medicine Clinics of North America. Philadelphia: W.B. Saunders.

Davis, R.O. & Boyers, S.P. (1992). The role of digital image analysis in reproductive biology. *Arch. Pathol. Lab. Med.*, **116**, 351–63.

Davis, R.O. & Katz, D.F. (1992). Standardization and comparability of CASA instruments. *J. Androl.*, **13**, 81–6.

Davis, R.O., Overstreet, J.W., Asch, R.H., Ord, T. & Silber, S.J. (1991). Movement characteristics of human epididymal sperm used for fertilization of human oocytes *in vitro. Fertil. Steril.*, **56**, 1128–35.

Davis, R.O., Rothmann, S.A. & Overstreet, J.W. (1992). Accuracy and precision of computer-aided sperm analysis (CASA) in multicenter studies. *Fertil. Steril.*, **57**, 648–53.

Dunphy, B.C., Kay, R., Barratt, C.L.R. & Cook, I.D. (1989). Quality control during the conventional analysis of semen: an essential exercise. *J. Androl.*, **10**, 378.

Gill, H.S., Van Arsdalen, K., Hypolite, J., Levin, R.M. & Ruzich, J.V. (1988). Comparative study of two computerized semen motility analyzers. *Andrology*, **20**, 433–40.

Ginsburg, K.A., Moghissi, K.S. & Abel, E. (1988). Computer-assisted human semen analysis: sampling errors and reproducibility. *J. Androl.*, **9**, 82–90.

Ginsburg, K.A., Sacco, A.G., Ager, J.W. & Moghissi, S.K. (1990). Variation of movement characteristics with washing and capacitation of spermatozoa. II. Multivariate statistical analysis and prediction of sperm penetrating ability. *Fertil. Steril.*, **53**, 704–8.

Janick, J. & MacLeod, J. (1970). The measurement of human spermatozoan motility. *Fertil. Steril.*, **21**, 140–6.

Jequier, A.M. & Ukome, E.B. (1983). Errors inherent in the performance of a routine semen analysis. *Br. J. Urol.*, **55**, 434.

Katz, D.F. & Overstreet, J.W. (1981). Sperm motility assessment by videomicrography. *Fertil. Steril.*, **35**, 188.

Katz, D.F., Mills, R.N. & Pritchett, T.R. (1978). The movement of human spermatozoa in cervical mucus. *J. Reprod. Fertil.*, **53**, 259–65.

Makler, A. (1980). Use of a microcomputer in combination with the MEP technique for human sperm motility determination. *J. Urol.*, **124**, 372–4.

Mathur, S. (1989). Automated semen analysis. *Fertil. Steril.*, **52**, 343–4.

Mortimer, D. (1988). Computerized semen analysis. *Fertil. Steril.*, **49**, 182–5.

Mortimer, D. & Mortimer, S.T. (1988). Influence of system parameter settings on human sperm motility analysis using CellSoft. *Hum. Reprod.*, **3**, 621–5.

Mortimer, D., Shu, M.A. & Tan, R. (1986). Standardization and quality control of sperm concentration and sperm motility counts in semen analysis. *Hum. Reprod.*, **1**, 299–303.

Mortimer, D., Goel, N. & Shu, M.A. (1988). Evaluation of the CellSoft automated semen analysis system in a routine laboratory setting. *Fertil. Steril.*, **50**, 960–8.

Neuwinger, J., Behre, H.M. & Nieschlag, E. (1990a). External quality control in the andrology laboratory: an experimental multicenter trial. *Fertil. Steril.*, **54**, 308–14.

Neuwinger, J., Knuth, U.A. & Nieschlag, E. (1990b). Evaluation of the Hamilton-Thorn 2030 motility analyser for routine semen analysis in an infertility clinic. *Int. J. Androl.*, **13**, 100–9.

Overstreet, J.W., Katz, D.F., Hanson, F.W. & Fonseca, J.R. (1979). A simple, inexpensive method for objective assessment of human sperm movement characteristics. *Fertil. Steril.*, **31**, 162.

Phillips, D.M. (1972). Comparative analysis of mammalian sperm motility. *J. Cell Biol.*, **53**, 561–73.

Schrader, S., Chapin, R.E. & Clegg, E.D., *et al.* (1992). Laboratory methods for assessing human semen in epidemiologic studies: a consensus report. *Reprod. Toxicol.*, **6**, 275–9.

World Health Organization (1987). *WHO Manual for the Examination of Human Semen and Semen–Cervical Mucus Interaction*, 2nd edn. Cambridge: Cambridge University Press.

World Health Organization (1992). *WHO Laboratory Manual for the Examination of Human Semen and Sperm–Cervical Mucus Interaction*, 3rd edn. Cambridge: Cambridge University Press.

Zorgniotti, A.W., Hotchkiss, R.S. & Wall, L.C. (1958). High-speed cinephotomicrography of human spermatozoa. *Med. Radiog. Photog.*, **34**, 44–9.

5

Antisperm antibodies: diagnosis and treatment

RICHARD A. BRONSON

Immunology of sperm and seminal plasma

During the onset of spermatogenesis at puberty, new developmental antigens make their appearance on the sperm surface (Ishahakia, 1988). Because immune tolerance for self-antigens is expressed neonatally, these newly appearing sperm antigens may be immunogenic. It has been theorized that sequestration of developing sperm by the blood–testis barrier prevents the generation of autoantibodies to sperm (Dym, 1973). Additional evidence has recently been presented that certain testicular auto-antigens exist outside the blood–testis barrier and are accessible to circulating antibodies and immune processing cells. A population of suppressor T lymphocytes has also been identified in the epididymis, suggesting that active immune suppression may play a role in preventing the development of autoimmunity to sperm (El-Demiry & James, 1988).

Immunoinhibitory substances of high and low molecular weight have been detected within seminal plasma (Lord et al., 1977). One factor that is highly immunosuppressive is prostaglandin PGE_2, which is present in high concentrations in semen (Quayle et al., 1989; Szymaniec et al., 1987). The masking of immunodominant antigens on the sperm surface by seminal-plasma-derived coating factors may also play a role. This is suggested by the relative lack of antigenicity of epididymal mouse sperm that have been incubated in seminal fluid as opposed to saline. Semen has also been found to contain populations of suppressor and helper T lymphocytes, which may play roles in modulating the immune response in the vagina, by the secretion of locally active products (Witkin, 1988). Could nature then provide the means, through exposure at coitus to semen-derived factors, that prevent development of immunity to sperm in women? Conversely, would the lack of immunosuppressive activity of seminal fluid lead to the development of antisperm antibodies? These intriguing questions, unfortunately, currently have no answer.

Conditions that result in an alteration in the balance between the exposure of the male immune systems to sperm antigen and immunosuppressive factors might, in theory, lead to antisperm antibody production. Vasectomy is associated with autoimmunity to spermatozoa in 60–70% of men (Alexander & Anderson, 1979), perhaps mediated through the absorption of an increased amount of sperm antigens that cannot be balanced by immunosuppressive factors. Testicular trauma (Haensch, 1973), torsion (Mastrogiacomo *et al.*, 1982), biopsy (Hjort *et al.*, 1974) and tumors (Guazziero *et al.*, 1985) have also been associated with the production of antisperm antibodies. Witkin & Toth (1983) have presented evidence that genital tract infections, which can act as adjuvants for immune activation, are associated with antisperm antibody production. Non-gonococcal urethritis, and in particular that resulting from *Chlamydia*, has been associated with antisperm autoantibodies (Shahmanesh *et al.*, 1986). Even unilateral obstruction of the vas deferens may also be responsible for antisperm antibody production (Hendry *et al.*, 1982). In addition, congenital obstruction of the vas deferens, seen in cystic fibrosis, has been associated with the appearance of antisperm antibodies (D'Cruz *et al.*, 1991).

Animal studies have suggested that a different pathogenesis of autoimmunity to spermatozoa may be related to non-vaginal inoculation with spermatozoa. Under experimental conditions, the rectal insemination of spermatozoa in rabbits elicits a systemic immune response (Richards *et al.*, 1984), and gastric administration to rats of homologous spermatozoa results in antisperm antibody production associated with decreased fertility (Allardyce, 1984). Similar mechanisms may operate in homosexual men and women who engage in oral and anal intercourse. In humans, a higher prevalence of antisperm antibodies has been described in homosexual men than in heterosexual men from infertile couples (Witkin & Sonnabend, 1983; Bronson *et al.*, 1983). In 40–50% of homosexual men, antisperm antibodies can be detected in serum (Wolff & Schill, 1985). Bronson *et al.* (1983) observed a higher prevalence of antisperm antibodies of the IgM class relative to IgG and IgA in sera of homosexual men when compared with men with autoimmunity to sperm from infertile couples. They proposed that these differences might reflect differences in the etiology of autoimmunity to sperm between the two groups. Intrarectal ejaculation may lead to altered processing of antigens, in that a single layer columnar epithelium is much more permeable than the thick epithelium of the vagina. In addition, the population of B lymphocytes and plasma cells in the gastrointestinal tract is different from that present in the reproductive tract (Mestecky & McGhee, 1987), and their reactivity with sperm antigens might be different. Several lines of evidence have been presented that the large intestine is an organ where plasma cells producing the IgA_2 subclass of antibodies prevail (Kett *et al.*, 1986; Crago *et al.*, 1984). As a result, intrarectal deposition of spermatozoa may result in the stimulation of IgM- or IgA_2-producing cells which might then populate the genital tract, leading to the production of anti-sperm antibodies of this isotype and subclass within semen, as opposed to those antibodies typically present in immunologically infertile men (e.g., IgA_1 and IgG).

Local versus systemic immunity to spermatozoa

Evidence exists in humans, as well as other species, that both the male and the female reproductive tracts are able to participate in mucosal immunity, and to secrete antibodies locally, primarily secretory IgA (Mestecky & McGhee, 1987; Ogra & Ogra, 1973; Wira & Stern, 1990; Parr & Parr, 1990). That the male reproductive tract can participate in a local immune response to infections has been suggested by the finding that total IgA concentration is greater than IgG or IgM in the prostatic secretions. Total IgA in the presence of prostatitis has been found to be greater than total IgA in men with urinary tract infection. More than 50% of total prostatic fluid IgA contains secretory component (SC), suggesting either its local production or active transport from serum by prosta-tic epithelium. In prostatitis caused by *E. coli*, 90% of total IgA and IgG is anti-*E. coli* specific. *E. coli* specific IgA concentration is 40 times higher in prostatic fluid than in serum, providing further circumstantial evidence that active IgA transport occurs in the prostate (Fowler & Mariano, 1982).

A mixture of IgA and IgG antisperm antibodies is observed in ejaculates of men with autoimmunity to sperm. Antisperm IgG is derived primarily as a transudate from serum, and its presence in the ejaculate correlates with the titre of circulating antisperm antibodies (Rumke, 1974). The local production of antisperm IgA in the male genital tract has been suggested both by its detection in semen while absent from serum, and by the presence of antisperm antibodies with unique regional binding specificities on the spermatozoan surface differ-ent from those present in serum. As IgA is locally transported across mucosal surfaces through its association with SC, which is produced by epithelial cells, its finding in association with IgA on the sperm surface is presumptive evidence for its local secretion, although not necessarily its local production (Meinertz *et al.*, 1990; Parslow *et al.*, 1985). Meinertz *et al.* (1990, 1991) have detected SC, utilizing a mixed agglutination reaction (MAR) test, on the surface of sperma-tozoa in men with autoimmunity to sperm. Additional evidence for the involvement of local mucosal immunity in the production of antisperm anti-bodies comes from an analysis of IgA subclasses. While monomeric IgA_1 pre-dominates in serum, immunoglobulins of the IgA_2 class, in addition to IgA_1, are present in mucosal secretions such as tears, saliva and colostrum (Delacroix *et al.*, 1983; Crago *et al.*, 1984).

Effects of antisperm antibodies on sperm function

Several landmark observations have documented that experimental animals immunized with spermatozoa exhibit impaired fertility, and that spontaneously occurring antibodies which react with antisperm antibodies (ASA) exist in both men and women (Hjort & Hansen, 1971). It has also become clear that these ASAs are quite common, but in only a small proportion of men and women do they play a role in altering sperm function (Bronson *et al.*, 1984*a*). Many of these naturally occurring antibodies do not bind to the surface of living sperm. These observations suggest them to be cross-reacting antibodies that would not be expected to play a role in human reproduction (Tung *et al.*, 1976). Conversely, antibodies directed against the sperm surface (those ASA that have the potential to cause infertility by binding to fertilization-related antigens) as detected by sperm agglutination testing, MAR and immunobead binding (IBT) are uncommon and occur in only 5–10% of infertile men (Jarow & Sanzone, 1992).

In a long-term study of men with autoimmunity to sperm, followed over a period of 15 years, Rumke & Hellinga (1959) documented that the chance of conception was markedly diminished when the titer of circulating ASA in serum rose above 1:125. No pregnancies occurred at titers of 1:1024 and above. These observations suggest that as the concentration of circulating antibodies rises in serum, the chance of them entering the seminal fluid increases. Indeed, the amount of immunoglobulins bound to the sperm surface at the time of ejaculation depends on several factors. These include: (1) The transudation of ASA into the prostatic and seminal vesicle secretions and their mixing with sperm at ejaculation, (2) local production of antibodies within the genital tract, (3) the pre-ejaculatory binding of ASA to sperm during their passage through the rete testis and epididymis, and (4) the elapsed time since the last ejaculation. In summary, those immunoglobulins bound on the sperm surface reflect the additive effects of several theoretical mechanisms of immunoglobulin secretion within the male reproductive tract.

Evidence supporting the importance of studying the ejaculate in determining the clinical significance of autoimmunity to sperm comes from a comparison of ASA detected in matched sera and semen of infertile men. From our own studies (Landers *et al.*, 1990), as well as those of Hellstrom *et al.* (1988), it is clear that antisperm antibodies may be present in serum, but not on sperm. Conversely, the male as well as the female reproductive tract is capable of local production of ASA, and these antibodies may be detected on sperm while absent in serum. If one were to rely solely on a serologic test to diagnose auto-immunity to sperm the results could be misleading in approximately one-third of cases. These observations reinforce the notion that the presence of humoral antibodies directed against spermatozoa is not relevant to an individual's fertil-ity unless these antibodies are also present within the reproductive tract. As a corollary, tests capable of detecting immunoglobulins on living sperm recov-ered from the ejaculate provide an important means of determining whether autoimmunity to sperm exists, and if it does of determining its clinical signifi-cance.

Also important in assessing the clinical significance of ASA is our current understanding that they are heterogeneous in terms of both their structure and their ability to alter sperm function. They may be of different immunoglobulin classes (IgA, IgG and IgM) which are structurally different molecules inter-acting with complement in different ways (Bronson et al., 1982). At least six different major immunodominant antigens have been detected on human sperm and are recognized by human sera containing ASA (Primakoff et al., 1990). Several studies have shown varying effects of ASA present in sera of infertile men and women on the ability of spermatozoa to bind to and fertilize eggs at the level of both the zona pellucida and the egg itself. Using the penetra-tion of zona-free hamster eggs by human sperm as a model, we and others have shown that certain ASA inhibit their fertilizing ability, while others promote or have no effects on egg penetration. Variable effects on the number of penetrat-ing sperm per oocyte were also seen (Bronson et al., 1989).

The detection of antisperm antibodies

Proof that immunity to sperm plays a role in individual cases of infertility requires documentation that ASA are present in the man's semen or in the woman's serum or reproductive tract fluids. These ASA must be shown to bind to the surface of living spermatozoa in suspension, either through direct analy-sis of the sperm in the ejaculate, or indirectly, by exposing antibody-free sperm to the woman's serum, follicular fluid, utero-tubal secretions or extracts of cer-vical mucus. There must also be evidence of either an alteration in the ability of antibody-coated sperm to enter the female reproductive tract (demonstrated by impaired cervical mucus penetration and diminished sperm survival) or failure to fertilize eggs.

Initial tests to determine the presence of antisperm antibodies involved quali-tative, macroscopic tests. These classic tests included evaluation of sperm-immobilizing antibodies (Isogima et al., 1968) the macroscopic gel test of sperm

Table 5.1 *Relationship between the extent of binding of monoclonal antibody (MAB) to motile spermatozoa and their ability to penetrate bovine cervical mucus* in vitro

MAB reactivity as judged by % sperm binding immunobeads[a]	No. of samples	Location of vanguard spermatozoa (mm)[b] (mean ± SD)
100%	11	17.5 ± 6.2
50% to <100%	7	27.3 ± 11.8
<50%	6	33.0 ± 5.8

Notes:
After Bronson & Cooper (1987).
[a] A population of nearly 100% motile spermatozoa obtained by swim-up were incubated with monoclonal antisperm antibody then washed free of ascitic fluid or culture supernatant and exposed to immunobeads.
[b] Observed following 90 minutes of incubation at 37°C.

agglutination referred to as the Kibrick test (Kibrick *et al.*, 1952), and the microscopic agglutination test of Franklin–Dukes (Franklin & Dukes, 1964) (see reviews by Rose *et al.*, 1976; Korte & Menge, 1990). Several methods are now clinically available to determine whether spermatozoa themselves are coated with antibodies. The MAR (Jager *et al.*, 1978) and IBT (Bronson *et al.*, 1981) are the primary methods utilized in clinical laboratories worldwide. Although these tests allow one to determine, in a semiquantitative way, the extent of immunity to sperm, the precise amount of immunoglobulin associated with an individual spermatozoan surface still cannot be determined. Very recently, however, experimental methods using flow cytometry have been developed that hold promise in this regard by allowing the analysis of large numbers of spermatozoa and quantitation of the amount of antibody bound to their surface.

Clinical assessment of the effects of autoimmunity to sperm

The proportion of spermatozoa in an ejaculate that are coated with immunoglobin varies markedly among men with autoimmunity to sperm. For instance, in 154 consecutive men documented by IBT to have autoimmunity to sperm, half had nearly all their spermatozoa (more than 95%) coated with immunoglobin, while one-fourth had 50–90% of sperm antibody coated. In the remaining one-fourth, less than 50% of the sperm were coated with immunoglobulins. Sperm that are coated with antibody over the majority of their surface exhibit an impaired ability to penetrate cervical mucus, yet remain completely motile in semen (Table 5.1). Only at very high concentrations of ASA in semen will actual sperm agglutination occur. Conversely, sperm coated with antibody over a very limited region, such as the tail-tip, do not appear to exhibit impaired mucus penetrating ability (Wang *et al.*, 1985). Several studies have shown a relationship between ASA binding to spermatozoa and diminished numbers of motile spermatozoa within cervical mucus observed on post-coital testing. Circumstantial evidence has been presented that this impairment is mediated through the Fc portion of the immunoglobulin molecule coating the sperm surface, since proteolytic removal of this portion of the bound immunoglobulins restores sperm mucus penetration and survival.

We have found an inverse correlation between the proportion of sperm that are coated with immunoglobulin and the number present within cervical mucus following sexual intercourse (Bronson *et al.*, 1984*b*). When 100% of sperm are coated with antibody, it is rare to find as many as one or two motile sperm per high-power field in well-timed post-coital tests, despite the presence of hundreds of millions of motile sperm in the ejaculate. This observation suggests that men who have high levels of autoimmunity to sperm should be considered functionally oligozoospermic; that is, their spermatozoa cannot enter the female reproductive tract, although they are present in high numbers in semen. The chance that they will reach the egg and achieve fertilization is therefore diminished. Evidence for this concept has also been obtained through a retrospective analysis of pregnancies in 80 couples, in whom the men were found to have autoimmunity to sperm but were not treated over a 2 year period of observation (Ayvaliotis *et al.*, 1985), all treatment being directed at the female causes of infertility. Only 15.6% of these couples achieved a pregnancy when the majority of sperm were coated with antibody, compared with 63% when less than half the sperm were antibody bound. Prospective analysis of fecundity in such couples is needed to confirm this phenomenon.

The presence of ASA in women may also be associated with altered sperm motion within cervical mucus. In this case, in contrast to the situation in men with autoimmunity to sperm, spermatozoa initially gain entrance into the cervical mucus but then subsequently become immobilized, either shaking in place without forward progression or being completely immobilized (Jager *et al.*, 1984*a,b*). The behavior of sperm within cervical mucus will depend upon the type of antibodies present within mucus and their specificity for the sperm surface. High degrees of binding of non-complement-fixing antibodies to the sperm surface may result in sperm entrapment and shaking in place. Conversely, complement-fixing antibody which promotes sperm plasma membrane damage will lead to their immobilization. Levels of complement within cervical mucus are lower than those present in serum and, in fact, it may take as long as 6–7 hours for sperm immobilization to occur (Price & Boettcher, 1979).

It is for this reason that overnight post-coital testing provides a clearer indication of antibody-mediated sperm damage than does testing a shorter period (2 hours) after coitus.

The immunologic consequences of vasectomy

Approximately 75% of men who have undergone a vasectomy will develop autoimmunity to spermatozoa. Return of fertility is high after vasovasostomy and there is no relationship between the presence of *circulating* antisperm antibodies and pregnancy rates following sterilization reversal. These facts, however, obscure a key question. To what extent do antisperm antibodies that are present in the ejaculate following sterilization reversal influence infertility? Studies of the immunologic consequences of vasectomy indicate that antisperm antibodies of the IgA class, when they appear in the ejaculate following vasovasostomy, are more likely to impair the mucus penetrating ability of the sperm than are IgG, suggesting that this isotype is clinically important. Linnet *et al.* (1981) documented a conception rate in the partners of men who had undergone sterilization reversal, with no evidence of antisperm antibodies in their seminal plasma, of 85% versus 14% for the partners of men whose semen contained antibodies. Parslow *et al.* (1985) confirmed this finding but also documented that fertility is impaired only when high titers of ASA are present in seminal fluid. They showed too that men from infertile couples with spontaneous autoimmunity to sperm, in contrast to vasectomized men, had higher levels of IgA and more SC on their sperm than did men following a vasectomy reversal. They postulated that secretory IgA, in these men, was more likely to compromise sperm function than those antibodies detected in sterilized men following vasectomy.

Recently, Meinhertz *et al.* (1991) studied the ejaculates of 216 men following sterilization reversal using a MAR. The conception rate was 85% in the partners of a subgroup of men with a pure IgG response, while only 43% of men who had IgA on their sperm fathered children. The conception rate was reduced even further when 100% of sperm were coated with IgA (21.7%). The combination of IgA on all sperm and a high serum titer (more than 1:250) detected by agglutination test was associated with a zero conception rate.

Treatment of immunologically mediated infertility

Three approaches have been used to treat infertile couples in whom the man exhibits antisperm antibodies: immunosuppression, intrauterine insemination (IUI) and *in vitro* fertilization (IVF). Although there was initially a high level of enthusiasm for the use of immunosuppressive corticosteroids, current evidence suggests that this approach is effective in only approximately 30% of treated men. The risk-to-benefit ratio of their use is not well established and documentation of their effectiveness is lacking. When carefully timed to follicular maturation in superovulated, hormonally and sonographically monitored cycles, IUI results in an increased chance of pregnancy. However, the likelihood of pregnancy is no greater than 40% within six treatment cycles. If IUI fails, IVF, though technically intense and expensive, offers the greatest likelihood of achieving pregnancy, whether in the presence of autoantibodies on the sperm in men or circulating ASA in women. Early evidence has indicated that gamete intrafallopian transfer (GIFT) may also be effective in treating couples in whom the man has developed antisperm antibodies. These results with assisted reproductive technologies suggest that immunity to sperm has a greater impact on migration through the female reproductive tract than on sperm–egg interaction.

Corticosteroid therapy

The first report in the United States of the successful corticosteroid treatment of a man with autoimmunity to sperm was by Shulman in 1976. Successful treatment was then not judged by an observed quantitative change in the status of autoimmunity, but rather on the rate of pregnancy during treatment (Shulman & Shulman, 1982; Hendry *et al.*, 1986; DeAlmeida & Jouannet, 1981). Given the now well documented spontaneous pregnancy rates among such couples (15% to over 50% during a 2 year period of observation, depending upon the level of immunobead binding), the use of pregnancy as a validation of treatment is misleading unless there are adequate placebo controls (Ayvaliotis *et al.*, 1985).

Some recent reports have documented variable suppression of antisperm antibodies in seminal plasma and reduced antibody binding in some men treated with corticosteroids. In one cross-over study, only one-third of the partners of men with autoimmunity to sperm achieved conception during treatment of the men with corticosteroids versus placebo (Hendry *et al.*, 1990). Hence, it appears that, in the majority, the degree of corticosteroid suppression of autoimmunity to sperm is insufficient to increase the number of antibody-free sperm in semen to a clinically significant level. Given the side-effects of corticosteroids, such as mood changes, leg muscle cramps, hypertension, reactivation of peptic ulcers, alteration of glucose tolerance and rare but disabling aseptic necrosis of the hip, one must remain conservative about their use pending further well-controlled studies.

Intrauterine insemination

The rationale for IUI is the placement of a large population of living spermatozoa within the cornu of the uterine cavity at the entrance of the fallopian tubes. In theory, this should increase the likelihood that sperm enter the fallopian tube and reach the egg. Utilizing sonographic and hormonal monitoring of follicular maturation, insemination can be timed to within a few hours of the expected ovulation (approximately 36 hours following administration of hCG). The accuracy of timing is theoretically important in that antibody-coated spermatozoa have a shortened survival time within the female reproductive tract. Our approach, like that of others, has been to use gonadotropin-stimulated superovulation in conjunction with IUI (Dodson *et al.*, 1987; Kemmen *et al.*, 1987). Since fertilization rates are lower in the presence of antisperm antibodies (whether derived from the male or female), the rationale for superovulation is to increase the absolute numbers of eggs per cycle, increasing the likelihood that at least one will be fertilized. An added benefit in women with ASA is provided by laboratory evidence in subhuman primates that total immunoglobin levels within oviductal secretions, as well as specific antibody titers, decrease when high circulating levels of serum estradiol are achieved. The reported chance of pregnancy has varied widely over the range of 20–40% in different clinical studies, but usually occurs rapidly, within four to six treatment cycles.

In vitro *fertilization*

IVF currently appears to offer the best chance of conception in couples with documented immunity to sperm in whom other treatments have failed. When present in follicular fluid, antisperm antibodies can be removed by washing and any residual ASA that may remain within the cumulus oophorus surrounding the egg usually does not appear to impair sperm penetration. Several older studies have reported pregnancies following IVF, in women with ASA, to be successful at rates comparable to those in absence of ASA (Clarke *et al.*, 1985*a*; Mandelbaum *et al.*, 1987). However, a more critical examination of the results of IVF in women with antisperm antibodies has recently revealed diminished fertilization and pregnancy rates (Vasquez-Levin *et al.*, 1991). In the immune infertile group of women, 44% of eggs (251/569) were fertilized in 50 cycles versus 74.2% for the control women whose eggs were incubated in maternal serum. The percentage of high-grade embryos was 49% for the women with antisperm antibodies versus 78% for the controls. These results suggest that antisperm antibodies within follicular fluid may not be completely eliminated

Table 5.2   *Effect of antisperm antibodies on* in vitro *fertilization rates in 32 men with autoimmunity to spermatozoa[a]*

	>80% IgA and IgG	>80% IgA	>80% IgG	>80% IgA and IgG
% of eggs fertilized	25%	30%	89%	73%
(no. of eggs				
inseminated)	(102)	(10)	(29)	(75)

Notes:
After DeAlmeida *et al.* (1989) and Clarke *et al.* (1985b).
[a] As determined by direct immunobead binding.

by washing and may impair fertilization or may be cytotoxic to the egg. However, despite these caveats, overall pregnancy rates remain relatively high.

In men with autoimmunity to sperm, the diminished number of antibody-coated sperm within cervical mucus after coitus markedly lowers the chances that the gametes will meet. IVF circumvents these problems of sperm transport. However, immunoglobulins bound to the sperm surface remain and cannot be removed during sperm capacitation following their recovery from semen. While antibodies present on the sperm tail do not play a significant role in preventing fertilization *in vitro*, sperm head-directed antibodies have the potential to alter the spermatozoan's egg penetrating ability (Aitkin *et al.*, 1987; Bronson *et al.*, 1989). Fortunately, these effects become important only when more than 80% of a sperm population used in IVF are coated with immunoglobulins (Clarke *et al.*, 1985b; DeAlmeida *et al.*, 1989) (Table 5.2). Using the hemizona assay as an indicator of sperm–zona interaction, variable inhibition of sperm binding has been demonstrated in the presence of head-directed antibodies (Mahoney *et al.*, 1991). Hence, even in the presence of saturating levels of antibody, the ability of sperm to fertilize may not be impaired once the gametes are placed together in culture.

As a laboratory technique to minimize the amount of antibody binding on sperm after ejaculation, it is good practice to produce the semen specimen directly at the laboratory, rather than transporting it from home during which time immunoglobulins may continue to accumulate on the sperm surface. The technique of ejaculating directly into a washing buffer with immediate processing thereafter appears to be most efficient in terms of both maximizing sperm recovery and minimizing the proportion of antibody-coated spermatozoa obtained. Use of Percoll centrifugation also appears to result in a more highly motile sperm preparation than do swim-up techniques. It should be noted, however, that these techniques will not completely eliminate antibodies from the sperm surface. Finally, the number of sperm placed in culture with eggs for IVF can be increased in an attempt to increase the likelihood of fertilization (Bronson, 1987). This normalization to a fixed number of motile, antibody-free sperm improves fertilization rates without substantially increasing the risk of polyspermy. In those other instances where sperm fertilizing ability is even more likely to be compromised, as in epididymal aspiration of spermatozoa, higher pregnancy rates have been obtained when more eggs are recovered.

Summary

The effects of autoimmunity to sperm on sperm function are complex and can be very heterogeneous. The additive effects of four loci of action (sperm transport, the kinetics of the acrosome reaction, interaction with the zona pellucida and the oolemma) must all be placed in a complex equation. Given the heterogeneity and complexity of the situation, the most practical clinical treatment approach would appear to be an empiric one. A first attempt should be made to bypass effects of antisperm antibodies on sperm transport by proceeding with a therapeutic trial of well-timed intrauterine insemination, in hormonally and sonographically monitored cycles. Antibody loading on sperm should be minimized by laboratory processing and/or cautious use of corticosteroids in well-counselled patients. Since gamete interactions leading to fertilization may be impaired by ASA, multiple follicular maturation with gonadotropins may be beneficial. If this approach does not succeed within a reasonable clinical trial period (four to six treatment cycles), fertilization *in vitro* of the maximum number of oocytes possible should be performed. This therapeutic procedure documents whether it is sperm attachment, penetration or fertilization that is impaired. If normal fertilization is documented, further attempts at *in vitro* fertilization or possibly gamete intrafallopian transfer would be reasonable. Conversely, a severely impaired fertilization rate is a possible indication for gamete micromanipulation and assisted fertilization. The effectiveness of these procedures as applied to immunologic infertility still needs to be clearly documented through future studies.

References

Aitkin, R.J., Hulme, M.J., Henderson, C.T., *et al.* (1987). Analysis of the surface labeling characteristics of human spermatozoa and the interaction with antisperm antibodies. *J. Reprod. Fertil.*, **80**, 473.

Alexander, N.J. & Andersen, D.J. (1979). Vasectomy: consequences of autoimmunity to sperm antigens. *Fertil. Steril.*, **32**, 253–9.

Allardyce, R.A. (1984). Effect of ingested sperm on fecundity in the rat. *J. Exp. Med.*, **159**, 1548–51.

Ayvaliotis, B., Bronson, R.A., Cooper, G.W. & Rosenfeld, D. (1985). Conception rates in couples where auto-immunity to sperm is detected. *Fertil. Steril.*, **43**, 739.

Bronson, R.A. (1987). Immunity in sperm and *in vitro* fertilization. *J. In Vitro Embryo Transfer*, **4**, 195.

Bronson, R.A. & Cooper, G.W. (1987). Effects of sperm-reactive monoclonal antibodies on the cervical mucus penetrating ability of human spermatozoa. *Am. J. Reprod. Immunol.*, **14**, 59.

Bronson, R.A., Cooper, G.W. & Rosenfeld, D.L. (1981). Membrane-bound sperm specific antibodies: their role in infertility. In *Bioregulators in Reproduction*, ed. H. Vogel & G. Jagiello, p. 526. New York: Academic Press.

Bronson, R.A., Cooper, G.W. & Rosenfeld, D.L. (1982). Correlation between regional specificity of antisperm antibodies to the spermatozoan surface and complement-mediated sperm immobilization. *Am. J. Reprod. Immunol.*, **2**, 222.

Bronson, R.A., Cooper, G.W., Rosenfeld, D.L., Gold, J., Kaplan, M. & Brody, N. (1983). Comparison of antisperm antibodies in homosexual and infertile men with autoimmunity to spermatozoa. Paper presented at Thirtieth Annual Meeting, Society for Gynecologic Investigation, 17–20 March, Washington, DC.

Bronson, R.A., Cooper, G.W. & Rosenfeld, D.L. (1984a). Sperm antibodies: their role in infertility. *Fertil. Steril.*, **42**, 271.

Bronson, R.A., Cooper, G.W. & Rosenfeld, D.L. (1984b). Auto-immunity to spermatozoa: effects on sperm penetration of cervical mucus as reflected by post-coital testing. *Fertil. Steril.*, **41**, 609.

Bronson, R.A., Cooper, G.W. & Phillips, D.M. (1989). Effects of antisperm antibodies on human sperm ultrastructure and function. *Hum. Reprod.*, **4**, 653.

Clarke, G.N., McBain, J.C., Lopata, A., *et al.* (1985a). *In vitro* fertilization: results for women with sperm antibodies in plasma and follicular fluid. *Am. J. Reprod. Immunol. Microbiol.*, **8**, 130.

Clarke, G.N., Lopata, A., McBain, J.C., *et al.* (1985b). Effect of sperm antibodies in males on human *in vitro* fertilization (IVF). *Am. J. Reprod. Immunol.*, **8**, 62.

Crago, S.S., Kutteh, W.H., Allansmith, M.R., Radl, J., Haaijman, J.J. & Mestecky, J. (1984). Distribution of IgA_1, IgA_2 and J chain containing cells in human tissue. *J. Immunol.*, **132**, 16–18.

D'Cruz, O.J., Haas, G.G., de La Rocha, R. & Lambert, H. (1991). Occurrence of serum antisperm antibodies in patients with cystic fibrosis. *Fertil. Steril.*, **56**, 519–27.

DeAlmeida, M. & Jouannet, P. (1981). Dexamethasone therapy in infertile men with auto-antibodies: immunological and sperm follow-up. *Clin. Exp. Immunol.*, **44**, 507.

DeAlmeida, M., Gazagne, I., Jeulin, C., *et al.* (1989). *In vitro* processing of sperm with autoantibodies and *in vitro* fertilization results. *Hum. Reprod.*, **4**, 49.

Delacroix, D.L., Elkon, K.B. & Vaerman, J.P. (1983). IgA size and IgA subclass distribution in serum and secretions. *Ann. NY Acad. Sci.*, **409**, 812–27.

Dodson, W.C., Whitesides, D.B., Hughes, C.L., *et al.* (1987). Superovulation with intrauterine insemination in the treatment of infertility: a possible alternative to gamete intrafallopian transfer and *in vitro* fertilization. *Fertil. Steril.*, **48**, 441.

Dym, M. (1973). The fine structure of the monkey (*Macaca*) sertoli cell and its role in maintaining the blood–testis barrier. *Anat. Rec.*, **175**, 639.

El-Demiry, M. & James, R. (1988). Lymphocyte subsets and macrophages in the male genital tract in health and disease. *Eur. J. Urol.*, **14**, 226.

Fowler, J.E. & Mariano, M. (1982). Immunologic response of the prostate to bacteria and bacterial prostatitis. II. Antigen specific immunoglobulin in prostatic fluid. *J. Urol.*, **128**, 105–15.

Franklin, R.R. & Dukes, C.D. (1964). Antispermatozoal antibody and unexplained infertility. *Am. J. Obstet. Gynecol.*, **89**, 6.

Freund, J., Lipton, M.M. & Thompson, G.E. (1979). Aspermatogenesis in the guinea pig induced by testicular tissue and adjuvants. *J. Exp. Med.*, **97**, 711.

Guazziero, S., Lembo, A., Ferro, G., Artibani, W., Merlo, F., Zanchetta, R. & Pagano, F. (1985). Sperm antibodies and infertility in patients with testicular cancer. *Urology*, **26**, 139–44.

Haensch, R. (1973). Spermatozoen-autoimmunphaenomehe bei Genitaltraumen und Verschlubbazzoospermie. *Andrologia*, **5**, 147–51.

Hellstrom, W.J.G., Overstreet, J.W., Samuels, S.J., *et al.* (1988). The relationship of circulating antisperm antibodies to sperm surface antibodies in infertile men. *J. Urol.*, **140**, 1039.

Hendry, W.F., Parslow, J., Stedronska, J. & Wallace, D.M.A. (1982). The diagnosis of unilateral testicular obstruction in subfertile males. *Br. J. Urol.*, **54**, 774–7.

Hendry, W.F., Treehuba, K., Hughes, L., *et al.* (1986). Cyclic prednisolone therapy for male infertility associated with auto-antibodies to spermatozoa. *Fertil. Steril.*, **45**, 249.

Hendry, W.F., Hughes, L., Scammeli, G., *et al.* (1990). Comparison of prednisolone and placebo in subfertile men with antibodies to spermatozoa. *Lancet*, **335**, 84.

Hjort, T. & Hansen, R.B. (1971). Immunofluorescent studies on human spermatozoa. I. The detection of different spermatozoal antibodies and their occurrence in normal and infertile women. *Clin. Exp. Immunol.*, **8**, 9.

Hjort, T., Husted, S. & Linnet-Jepsen, P. (1974). The effect of testis biopsy on autosensitization against spermatozoal antigens. *Clin. Exp. Immunol.*, **18**, 201–9.

Ishahakia, M.A. (1988). Characterization of baboon testicular antigens using monoclonal antisperm antibodies. *Biol. Reprod.*, **39**, 889.

Isogima, S., Li, T.S. & Ashitaka, Y. (1968). Immunologic analysis of sperm immobilizing factor found in sera of women with unexplained sterility. *Am. J. Obstet. Gynecol.*, **101**, 677.

Jager, S.S., Kremer, J. & Van Slochteren-Draaisma, T. (1978). A simple method of screening for antisperm antibodies in the human male: detection of spermatozoal surface IgG with the direct mixed agglutination reaction carried out in the untreated fresh human semen. *Int. J. Fertil.*, **23**, 12.

Jager, S., Kremer, J., Kuiken, J., *et al.* (1984a). The significance of the Fc part of antispermatozoal antibodies for the shaking phenomenon in the sperm–cervical mucus contact test. *Fertil. Steril.*, **36**,792.

Jager, S., Kremer, J., Kuiken, J., *et al.* (1984b). Induction of the shaking phenomenon by pretreatment of spermatozoa with sera containing antisperm antibodies. *Fertil. Steril.*, **36**, 784.

Jarow, J.P. & Sanzone, J.J. (1992). Risk factors for male partner antisperm antibodies. *J. Urol.*, **148**, 1805–7.

Kemmenn, E., Bohrer, M., Sheldon, R., *et al.* (1987). Active ovulation management increases the monthly probability of pregnancy occurrence in ovulatory women who receive intrauterine insemination. *Fertil. Steril.*, **48**, 916.

Kett, K., Brandtzaeg, D. & Radl, J. (1986). Different subclass distribution of IgA-producing cells in human lymphoid organs and various secretory tissues. *J. Immunol.*, **136**, 3631–5.

Kibrick, S., Belding, D.L. & Merrill, B. (1952). Methods for detection of antibodies against mammalian spermatozoa. II. A gelatin agglutination test. *Fertil. Steril.*, **3**, 430.

Korte, M.K. & Menge, A.C. (1990). Detection of agglutinating and immobilizing sperm antibodies. In *CRC Handbook of the Laboratory Diagnosis and Treatment of Infertility*, ed. B.A. Keel & B.W. Webster, pp. 167–75. Boston: CRC Press.

Landers, D.V., Bronson, R.A. & Pavia, C.S. (1990). Reproductive immunology. In *Basic Human Immunology*, ed. D.P. Site & A.L. Terr, pp. 200–16. Norwalk: Appleton and Lange.

Linnet, L., Hjort, T. & Fogh-Anderson, P. (1981). Association between failure to impregnate after vasovasostomy and sperm agglutinations in semen. *Lancet*, **I**, 117.

Lord, E.K., Senabaugh, G.F. & Stites, D.P. (1977). Immunosuppressive activity of human seminal plasma. I. Inhibition of *in vitro* lymphocyte activation. *J. Immunol.*, **118**, 1706.

Mahoney, M.C., Blakemore, P.F., Bronson, R.A. & Alexander, N.J. (1991). Inhibition of human sperm: zona pellucida tight binding in the presence of antisperm antibody positive polyclonal patient sera. *J. Reprod. Immunol.*, **19**, 287.

Mandelbaum, S.L., Diamond, M.P. & DeCherney, A.H. (1987). Relationship of antisperm antibodies to oocyte fertilization in *in vitro* fertilization–embryonic transfer. *Fertil Steril.*, **47**, 644.

Mastrogiacomo, I., Zanchetta, R., Graziotti, P., Betterle, C., Scrufari, P. & Lembo, A. (1982). Immunological and clinical study of patients after spermatic cord torsion. *Andrologia*, **14**, 25–9.

Meinhertz, H., Linnet, L., Fogh-Andersen, P. & Hjort, T. (1990). Antisperm antibodies and fertility after vasovasostomy; a follow-up study of 216 men. *Fertil. Steril.*, **54**, 315.

Meinhertz, H., Linnet, L., Fogh-Andersen, P. & Hjort, T. (1991). Antisperm antibodies on epididymal spermatozoa. *Am. J. Reprod. Immunol.*, **25**, 158–62.

Mestecky, J. & McGhee, J.R. (1987). Immunoglobulin A (IgA): molecular and cellular interactions involved in IgA biosynthesis and immune response. *Adv. Immunol.*, **40**, 153–245.

Ogra, P.L. & Ogra, S.S. (1973). Local antibody response to poliovaccine in the human female genital tract. *J. Immunol.*, **110**, 1307–11.

Parr, E.L. & Parr, M.B. (1990). A comparison of antibody titres in mouse uterus found after immunization by several routes, and the effect of the uterus on titres in vaginal fluid. *J. Reprod. Fertil.*, **89**, 619–25.

Parslow, J.M., Poulton, T.A., Bessee, G.M. & Hendry, W.F. (1985). The clinical relevance of classes of immunoglobulins on spermatozoa from infertile and vasovasotomized males. *Fertil. Steril.*, **43**, 621–5.

Price, R.J. & Boettcher, B. (1979). Presence of complement in cervical mucus and its possible relevance to infertility in women with complement-dependent sperm immobilizing antibodies. *Fertil. Steril.*, **31**, 61.

Primakoff, P., Lathrop, W. & Bronson, R.A. (1990). Identification of human sperm surface glycoproteins recognized by autoantisera from immune infertile men, women and vasectomized men. *Biol. Reprod.*, **42**, 929.

Quayle, A.J., Kelly, R.W., Hargreave, T.B., *et al.*, (1989). Immunosuppression by seminal prostaglandins. *Clin. Exp. Immunol.*, **75**, 387.

Richards, J.M., Bedford, J.M. & Witkin, S.S. (1984). Rectal insemination modifies immune responses in rabbits. *Science*, **224**, 390–2.

Rose, N.R., Hjort, T., Rumke, P., Harper, M.J.K. & Vyazov, O. (1976). Techniques for the detection of iso- and auto-antibodies to human spermatozoa. *Clin. Exp. Immunol.*, **23**, 175.

Rumke, P. (1974). Origin of immunoglobulin in semen. *Clin. Exp. Immunol.*, **12**, 287–97.

Rumke, P. & Hellinga, G. (1959). Auto-antibodies to spermatozoa in sterile men. *Am. J. Clin. Pathol.*, **32**, 357.

Shahmanesh, M., Stedronska, J. & Hendry, W.F. (1986). Antispermatozoal antibodies in men with urethritis. *Fertil. Steril.*, **46**, 308–11.

Shulman, J.F. & Shulman, S. (1982). Methylprednisolone treatment of immunologic infertility in the male. *Fertil. Steril.*, **38**, 591.

Shulman, S. (1976). Treatment of immune male infertility with methyl prednisolone. *Lancet*, **ii**, 1243.

Szymaniec, S., Quale, A.J., Hargreave, T.B., *et al.* (1987). Human seminal plasma suppresses lymphocyte responses *in vitro* in serum free medium. *J. Reprod. Immunol.*, **12**, 191.

Tung, K.S.K., Cooke, W.D. Jr, McCarthy, T.A., *et al.* (1976). Human sperm antigens and antisperm antibodies. *Clin. Exp. Immunol.*, **25**, 72.

Vasquez-Levin, M., Kaplan, P., Guzman, I., *et al.* (1991). The effect of female antisperm antibodies on *in vitro* fertilization, early embryonic development and pregnancy outcome. *Fertil. Steril.*, **56**, 84.

Wang, C., Baker, H.W.G., Jennings, M.G., *et al.* (1985). Interactions between cervical mucus and sperm surface antibodies. *Fertil. Steril.*, **44**, 484.

Wira, C.R. & Stern, J.E. (1990). Endocrine regulation of the mucosal immune system in the female reproductive tract: control of IgA, IgG and secretory component during the reproductive cycle, at implantation and throughout pregnancy. In *Hormones and Fetal Pathophysiology*, ed. J.R. Pasqualini & R. Scholler. New York: Marcel Dekker.

Witkin, S.S. (1988). Mechanisms of active suppression of the immune response to spermatozoa. *Am. J. Reprod. Immunol.*, **17**, 61.

Witkin, S.S. & Sonnabend, J. (1983). Immune response to spermatozoa in homosexual men. *Fertil. Steril.*, **39**, 337–42.

Witkin, S.S. & Toth, A. (1983). Relationship between genital tract infections, sperm antibodies in seminal fluid, and infertility. *Fertil. Steril.*, **40**, 805–8.

Wolff, H. & Schill, W.B. (1985). Antisperm antibodies in infertile and homosexual men: relationship to serologic and clinical findings. *Fertil. Steril.*, **44**, 673–7.

6

The sperm penetration assay

B. JANE ROGERS

Introduction

Since spermatozoa were first observed in the human ejaculate by Leeuwenhoek in the late seventeenth century, it has been believed that a threshold number of motile and morphologically normal spermatozoa is required to initiate a pregnancy. More recently it has been determined that the functional competence of these sperm is somewhat poorly reflected by the conventional semen analysis. Therefore, much work has been done to develop functional tests which may more accurately reflect fertility status. The sperm penetration assay (SPA) or zona-free hamster egg test is one such test which is designed to evaluate sperm functional competence or fertilizing potential. It is based on the phenomenon that a hamster egg, when rendered zona-free by proteolytic digestion of the zona pellucida, can be penetrated by spermatozoa from another species, such as the human. The cross-species 'fertilization' assay is correlated with true fertility and thus has diagnostic potential in human fertility problems. Much has been written about this assay since the presentation of our first human–hamster experiments in 1976 (Yanagimachi *et al.*, 1976). The purpose of this chapter is to focus on a few aspects of the assay, including a brief review of SPA methodology, comparison of the SPA with other semen tests, validity of the SPA in prediction of *in vivo* pregnancy, and predictive potential of the SPA for the success of *in vitro* fertilization (IVF).

SPA methodology

The original SPA methodology (Yanagimachi *et al.*, 1976) used washed sperm preincubated in BWW (Biggers, Whitten and Whittinghams's medium) for 2–7 hours. The first article, which provided fertile and infertile ranges for the assay (Rogers *et al.*, 1979), detailed a methodology incorporating an overnight incubation of 18–20 hours in BWW at 37°C in air, followed by a 2–3 hour co-incubation with zona-free hamster eggs. The examination of the eggs for the presence of swollen sperm heads was done on fresh or stained preparations (Fig. 6.1). Numerous modifications of this basic protocol have since been reported. The major variables have been sperm processing technique (e.g. TEST-yolk buffer, calcium ionophore A23187, follicular fluid), sperm prein-cubation time, sperm and egg co-incubation time, sperm concentration (e.g., microassay; Fig. 6.2), media and use of cryopreserved sperm and eggs. Details of these have been discussed previously (Rogers, 1985) and will not be repeated here.

Comparison of SPA with other semen tests

Routine semen parameters

Of the routine semen parameters, sperm motility and morphology appear to be most useful in predicting outcome of the zona-free hamster oocyte penetration assay (Rogers, 1985). If normozoospermic samples from a normal fertile group are evaluated, the SPA results do not appear to correlate with any conventional parameters of semen analysis. However, in oligozoospermic samples, statistically significant associations can be found between penetration rate and percent motility as well as percentage of normal forms (Rogers, 1985).

Since 1985 investigators have continued to attempt to establish a strong correlation between routine semen parameters and the SPA (Wang *et al.*, 1988, 1991; Kruger *et al.*, 1988; Holmgren *et al.*, 1989; Barg *et al.*, 1992). Wang *et al.* (1988) reported that they could predict the fertility of a group of patients with 70.4% accuracy by using a multivariate discriminant analysis of routine semen parameters. Kruger *et al.* (1988) reported a statistically significant relationship ($p=0.001$) between the percentage of sperm with normal morphology and penetration rate in the SPA. Holmgren *et al.* (1989) reported that all standard semen variables except volume were significantly correlated with penetration. Wang *et al.* (1991) reported 84% accuracy in predicting the outcome of the zona-free hamster occyte penetration test using the manually derived percentage of spermatozoa with normal and small heads. Barg *et al.* (1992) reported that over half their patients with pure teratozoospermia had significant impairment in sperm function. In their study Kruger's strict criteria for morphology were used together with the optimized SPA. Using these modified techniques for morphology and SPA, the original relationship between morphology and impaired sperm function reported in 1983 has been substantiated (Rogers *et al.*, 1983).

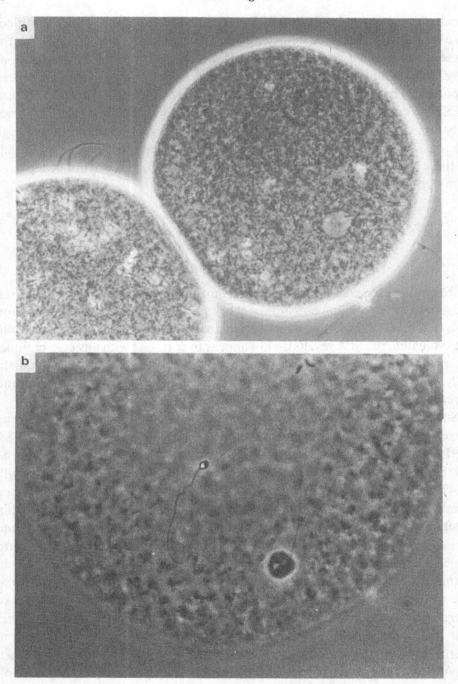

Fig. 6.1. Penetration of zona-free hamster eggs by human spermatozoa. (a) Unstained egg with a swollen sperm head and attached tail at about 4 o'clock; the swollen head appears as clear area. (b) Stained egg which was fixed and stained with acetolacmoid; the swollen head at about 5 o'clock is seen as a darkened sphere.

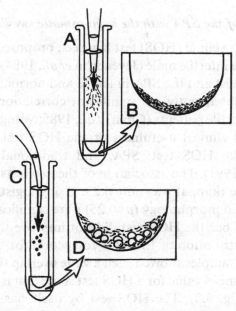

Fig. 6.2. Micro SPA. A: Preincubated human sperm are added to a microfuge tube. B: Sperm are concentrated at the bottom of the tube. C: Zona-free hamster eggs are added to the microfuge tube. D: Sperm and eggs are co-incubated for 3 hours at the bottom of the tube.

Computer-assisted semen analysis (CASA)

With the advent of computer-assisted semen analysis (CASA) attempts have been made to correlate more sophisticated motility parameters with fertilizing potential as assayed in the SPA. Discriminant analysis has been used to define a function that would classify SPA results as above or below a 10% penetration rate. Ginsburg *et al.* (1990) identified a significant function using the following variables: sperm concentration and motility in semen, and mean curvilinear velocity, linearity, and amplitude of lateral head displacement of washed sperm. The overall accuracy of this function for predicting SPA results was 72%. Similar results were reported by Fetterolf & Rogers (1990). Discriminant function analysis successfully classified 76% of patients with a positive SPA (using TEST-yolk buffer methodology) and 86% of nonpenetrators, on the basis of their computerized motility parameters. These studies demonstrate that computer-derived measurements of sperm movement may provide biologically useful diagnostic information.

Comparison of the SPA with the hypo-osmotic swelling (HOS) test

The hypo-osmotic swelling (HOS) test has been proposed as a useful assay in the diagnosis of the infertile male (Jeyendran *et al.*, 1984). A good correlation between the HOS test and the SPA in fertile and normal semen samples was initially found. Subsequently, no significant correlation was demonstrated with fertile and infertile patients (Chan *et al.*, 1985; Wang *et al.*, 1988). To validate the potential clinical usefulness of the HOS test, 92 ejaculates were evaluated using the HOS test, SPA, and traditional semen parameters (Rogers & Parker, 1991). The association of the two tests over and above that expected by chance (kappa) was only 0.23. Using logistic regression, sperm count ($p<0.001$) and morphology ($p<0.25$) were significant predictors of the SPA classification, but the HOS test did not improve the predictive results. Analysis of the distribution of the HOS test scores for 'fertile' (SPA>0) and 'infertile' (SPA=0) samples showed such a wide overlap that it was impossible to designate a threshold value for a HOS test score that is predictive of a positive SPA result (Fig. 6.3). The HOS test by itself has a modest ability to predict SPA.

Correlation of acrosome reaction and sperm performance in SPA

Attempts to measure acrosome reaction and relate this parameter to hamster ova penetration (Pilkian & Guerin, 1986) are equivocal, discouraging and sometimes confusing.

A study by van Kooij *et al.* (1986) monitored the acrosome reaction (AR) by the triple stain and related AR to incubation time and penetration of zona-free hamster eggs. They started out at 0 time with 11.6% AR and showed a peak of 35.9% at 5–7 hours of incubation. The comparisons of acrosome reaction to egg penetration are surprising. For example, one donor showed 60% AR but only 75% egg penetration. It is hard to understand why such a high AR percentage gave less than 100% penetration. Their percent acrosome reactions are much higher than those previously reported by Talbot & Chacon (1980) using fluorescein isothiocyanate (FITC)-RCA.

Other more recent work using two different acrosome reaction assays suggests that the acrosome reaction is not an accurate reflection of the fertilizing ability of the sperm. Using the triple stain technique, Yang *et al.* (1988) found that sperm from fertile donors and infertile patients displayed a similar capacity to undergo AR *in vitro*. Even though they did find a positive correlation between the incidence of AR and the penetration of hamster eggs, there was a high degree of individual variation. Using the FITC-labeled lectin

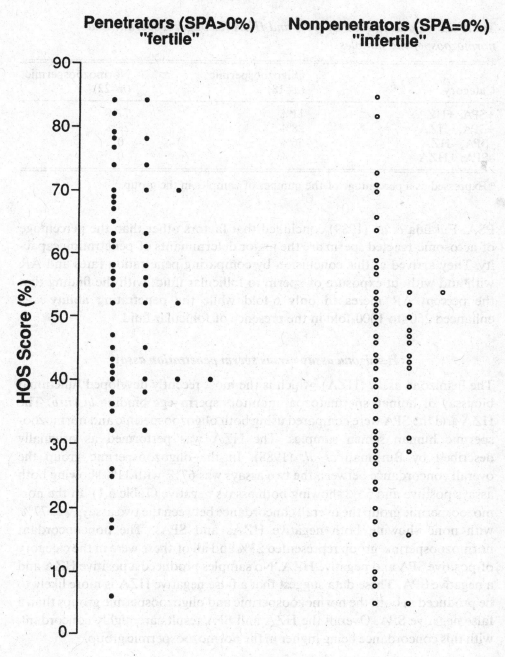

Fig. 6.3. Distribution of the percentage of swollen sperm (HOS score) from 'fertile' and 'infertile' ejaculates. Penetrators (*n* = 47) are defined as those who had a positive penetration rate (>0). Nonpenetrators (*n* = 45) are defined as those who had a negative penetration rate (0).

Table 6.1 *Concordance[a] of SPA and HZA for oligozoospermic and normozoospermic samples*

Category	Oligozoospermic (n=18)	Normozoospermic (n=22)
+SPA, +HZA	11%	77%
+SPA, –HZA	28%	23%
–SPA, –HZA	56%	0
–SPA, +HZA	5%	0

[a] Expressed as a percentage of the number of samples in the group.

PSA, Fukuda *et al.* (1989) concluded that factors other than the percentage of acrosome-reacted sperm are the major determinants of penetration capacity. They arrived at this conclusion by comparing penetration rates and AR with and without exposure of sperm to follicular fluid, with the finding that the percent AR increased only 6-fold while the penetrating ability was enhanced 250- to 1000-fold in the presence of follicular fluid.

Hemizona assay versus sperm penetration assay

The hemizona assay (HZA), which is the most recently developed functional bioassay of human spermatozoa, monitors sperm–egg binding *in vitro*. The HZA and the SPA were compared using both oligozoospermic and normozoospermic human semen samples. The HZA was performed as originally described by Burkman *et al.* (1988). In the oligozoospermic group the overall concordance between the two assays was 67%, with 11% showing both assays positive and 56% showing both assays negative (Table 6.1). In the normozoospermic group the overall concordance between the two assays was 77%, with none showing both negative HZAs and SPAs. The nonconcordant normozoospermic group represented 23% and all of these were in the category of positive SPA and negative HZA. No samples produced a positive HZA and a negative SPA. These data suggest that a false negative HZA is more likely to be produced in both the normozoospermic and oligozoospermic groups than a false negative SPA. Overall the HZA and SPA results are highly concordant, with this concordance being higher in the normozoospermic group.

Validity of SPA in prediction of pregnancy

Performance of the SPA is more complex and costly than a simple semen analysis, but it is of value in providing the clinician with an accurate assessment of the likely fertilizing ability of spermatozoa. Numerous investigators have published papers on the predictive potential of the assay using different approaches.

In 1985, Sutherland *et al.* concluded that the number of normal women spontaneously conceiving after their partner scored positive in the SPA was significantly higher than in their counterparts whose partners had negative SPA results (42% vs 11%). Furthermore, in 10 couples with long-standing infertility in which the woman was found to be normal and the man had two negative SPA results, 8 of the women conceived after donor insemination. Another approach was to perform the SPA on individual ejaculates that are used in a donor insemination program (Irvine & Aitken, 1986). Using a multivariate discriminant analysis, it was possible to distinguish successful from unsuccessful ejaculates with an accuracy of 81.25% ($p=0.019$), using data derived from the conventional semen profile, hamster oocyte penetration and the assessment of sperm movement.

Corson *et al.* (1988) looked at males from 227 infertile couples using the SPA and monitored pregnancy during a 30 month interval of follow-up. The monthly fecundity rate was twice as great for men with normal SPA values as for those with abnormal values. They concluded that the SPA had a legitimate role in the diagnosis of male infertility. The other positive study in 1988 included 74 men from infertile couples for whom a female infertility factor had been excluded. They were followed for up to 3 years after the SPA. At 156 weeks after a normal SPA the cumulative pregnancy rate was 68%, compared with only 27% for the group with an abnormal SPA (Shy *et al.*, 1988). Shy *et al.* concluded that when the SPA was performed on infertile men according to the standard protocol it helped predict future pregnancy potential. A report by Hargreave *et al.* (1988) detailed modified SPAs on samples from 111 men attending an infertility clinic. At the time of their initial assessment the men had poor routine semen parameters. The authors found that the hamster test results gave no additional prognostic information, a conclusion echoed by Mao & Grimes (1988).

Margalioth *et al.* (1989) followed 369 infertile couples with no evidence of female factors for from 2 to 5 years in an effort to determine the clinical long-term predictive value of the SPA. The percentage of men who impregnated their female partners was determined in relation to the SPA results. There was a significant difference in the fertility prognosis for those who had an SPA >19% compared with those with an SPA <20%. An SPA of >19% was predictive of higher pregnancy rates in both couples in which the man was oligozoospermic and in those with unexplained infertility. The specificity and positive predictive values of the SPA were higher than those of the semen analysis. Furthermore, other studies by Gwatkin *et al.* (1990) and Kremer & Jager (1990) confirm the ability of SPA scores above 20% to predict subsequent *in vivo* fertility.

Predictive potential of the SPA for IVF success

The diagnostic potential of the SPA for predicting success in IVF has been evaluated by numerous investigators using variable methodologies. The predictive potential of a modified SPA in accurately predicting outcome in IVF was evaluated by Bastias *et al.* (1987). The results suggested that a positive penetration in the SPA done using either a short or long capacitation time is predictive of successful fertilization of preovulatory oocytes *in vitro*. Furthermore, when the sperm suspension was incubated for an additional day in TEST-yolk buffer at 4°C and retested with hamster eggs, SPA results correlated 100% with successful or failed fertilization in IVF. The ability to use the SPA diagnostically is highly dependent on both methodology and expertise.

Margalioth *et al.* (1986) evaluated the SPA results in a study population of 134 couples undergoing IVF. For a tubal infertility group 94% of couples with positive SPA achieved fertilization *in vitro*. For those with unexplained infertility the result was 76%, and was 46% for those with male infertility. For the entire group the overall specificity of the SPA using this methodology was 85%. However, Margalioth *et al.* reported that in the 29 oligoasthenozoospermic men the SPA failed to predict IVF outcome. Corson *et al.* (1987) have also emphasized the usefulness of the SPA in predicting the percentage of human oocytes that can be expected to fertilize in an IVF cycle.

In 1987 Kuzan *et al.* reported that the SPA score was a poor indicator of sperm function in IVF, although out of 42 patients only 7 demonstrated a male factor, and there were only two failed fertilization cycles. No difference was found in fertilization results in IVF for the normal and low SPA groups. To evaluate the SPA's ability to predict fertilization failure it would be necessary to have a significant number of failures.

Recent modifications of the SPA have included 42 hour preincubation with TEST-yolk buffer (Lamb *et al.*, 1989) and incubation with human follicular fluid (McClure *et al.*, 1990), providing excellent correlation between the SPA results and *in vitro* fertilization.

An interesting use of epididymal aspirated sperm in the SPA and IVF reveals a good correlation (Rojas *et al.*, 1992). A positive SPA (>10%) was associated with positive IVF in 15 of 20 cases (75%). A negative (<10% penetration rate) SPA was associated with negative IVF in 10 of 11 cases (91%). The authors suggest that the SPA is an excellent bioassay to test laboratory experimental conditions for improving fertilizing capacity of human epididymal sperm.

Thus the SPA can be described as a powerful test even though its clinical significance in predicting male fertility is still disputed. The ability of the SPA to predict IVF success is not perfect, but appears to exceed by far that of any other current predictive semen parameter.

Rationale for and usefulness of SPA

What then is the rationale for performing an SPA in the clinical setting? Oligozoospermic males with normal FSH values constitute the largest portion of subfertile males. The traditional approach for treating such men has been to test for the presence of a varicocele and then proceed with medical therapy if one is not found. With the availability of the SPA, it is now possible to use the SPA as an initial evaluating mechanism before considering therapy. Even with a varicocele present, a positive SPA would suggest the lack of necessity of internal spermatic vein ligation. A positive SPA in an oligozoospermic man would suggest that medical therapy might not be required. In oligozoospermic situations the rationale for the SPA is to *establish fertilizing potential*. A negative (abnormal) SPA would suggest the necessity for surgery, medical therapy or intracytoplasmic sperm injection (ICSI). The SPA can be most effectively utilized, therefore, in establishing the presence or absence of fertilizing potential. If the sperm *do* demonstrate this functional ability, then post-ejaculatory sperm processing to assist the occurrence of fertilization can be attempted.

The SPA can be useful in both diagnosing and monitoring treatment in the subfertile male, but it is not intended as a routine screen for the investigation of every infertile couple. The test is most useful in cases of an equivocal semen analysis, moderate oligozoospermia or unexplained infertility. The subset of subfertile men who are not readily detectable, because of normal semen parameters, can be diagnosed with the SPA. Conversely, men with apparent abnormalities in the routine semen analysis can prove that their sperm can penetrate an oocyte in the SPA and subsequently initiate a pregnancy. The SPA can put a new perspective on sperm pathology, with the emphasis on functional abilities rather than the traditional evaluation of count, motility and morphology.

References

Barg, P., Novogrodsky, R., Barad, D. & Fisch, H. (1992). Sperm penetration assay (SPA) results in patients with abnormal sperm morphology. Eighteenth Annual Meeting of American Fertility Society, New Orleans, 2–5 November, Supplement, S116.

Barros, C., Gonzalez, J., Herrera, E. & Bustos-Obregon, E. (1979). Human sperm
   penetration into zona-free hamster oocytes as a test to evaluate the sperm
   fertilizing ability. *Andrologia*, **11**, 197–210.
Bastias, C. & Rogers, B.J. (1988). Enhancement of human sperm acrosome reaction
   and penetration ability by TEST-yolk buffer. Proceedings of the Forty-fourth
   Annual Meeting of the American Fertility Society, Atlanta, Georgia, p. 510.
Bastias, C., Wentz, A.C. & Rogers, B.J. (1987). Predictive potential of the modified
   SPA for IVF success. Fifth World Congress of In Vitro Fertilization and
   Embryo Transfer, Norfolk, Virginia 5–10 April.
Bielfield, P., Jeyendran, R.S., Holmgren, W.J. & Zaneveld, L.J.D. (1990). Effects of
   egg yolk medium on the acrosome reaction of human spermatozoa. *J. Androl.*,
   11, 260–9.
Burkman, L.J., Coddington, C.C., Franken, D.R., Kruger, T.F., Rosenwaks, Z. &
   Hodgen, G.D. (1988). The hemizona assay (HZA): development of a diagnostic
   test for the binding of human spermatozoa to the human hemizona pellucida to
   predict fertilization potential. *Fertil. Steril.*, **49**, 688–97.
Carrell, D.T., Bradshaw, W.S., Jones, K.P., Middleton, R.G., Peterson, C.M. & Urry,
   R.L. (1992). An evaluation of various treatments to increase sperm penetration
   capacity for potential use in an *in vitro* fertilization program. *Fertil. Steril.*, **57**,
   134–8.
Chan, S.Y.W., Fox, E.J., Chan, M.M.C., Tsoi, W., Tang, L.C.M., Tang, G.W.K. &
   Ho, P. (1985). The relationship between the human sperm hypoosmotic swelling
   test, routine semen analysis, and the human zona-free hamster ovum
   penetration test. *Fertil. Steril.*, **44**, 668–72.
Corson, S.L., Batzer, F.R., Go, K.J., Eisenberg, E., English, M.E., White, S.M.,
   Laberge, Y. & Goldman, N. (1987). Correlations between the human sperm–
   hamster egg penetration assay and *in vitro* fertilization results. *J. Reprod. Med.*,
   32, 879–87.
Corson, S.L., Batzer, F.R., Marmar, J. & Maislin, G. (1988). The human
   sperm–hamster egg assay: prognostic value. *Fertil. Steril.*, **49**, 328–34.
Fetterolf, P.M. & Rogers, B.J. (1988). Relationship of objective motion parameters to
   human sperm penetration ability. *Biol. Reprod.*, **38** (Suppl 1), 92.
Fetterolf, P.M. & Rogers, B.J. (1990). Prediction of human sperm penetrating ability
   using computerized motion parameters. *Mol. Reprod. Dev.*, **27**, 326–31.
Fujita, J.S., Van Campen, H. & Rogers, B.J. (1980). The effect of freezing on
   fertilizing capacity of human spermatozoa using zona-free eggs. *J. Androl.*, **1**,
   77a.
Fukuda, M., Cross, N.L., Cummings-Paulson, L. & Yee, B. (1989). Correlation of
   acrosomal status and sperm performance in the sperm penetration assay. *Fertil.
   Steril.*, **52**, 836–41.
Ginsburg, K.A., Sacco, A.G., Ager, J.W. & Moghissi, K.S. (1990). Variation of
   movement characteristics with washing and capacitation of spermatozoa. II.
   Multivariate statistical analysis and prediction of sperm penetrating ability.
   Fertil. Steril., **53**, 704–8.
Gwatkin, R.B.L., Collins, J.A., Jarrell, J.F., Kohut, J. & Milner, R.A. (1990). The
   value of semen analysis and sperm function assays in predicting pregnancy
   among infertile couples. *Fertil. Steril.*, **53**, 693–9.
Hargreave, T.B., Aitken, R.J. & Elton, R.A. (1988). Prognostic significance of the
   zona-free hamster egg test. *Br. J. Urol.*, **62**, 603–8.
Holmgren, W.J., Jeyendran, R.S., Nelf, M.R., Perez-Pelaez, M. & Zaneveld, L.J.D.

(1989). Preincubation of human spermatozoa in TEST-yolk medium: effect on penetration of zona-free hamster oocytes and correlation with other semen characteristics. *J. In Vitro Fert. Embryo Transfer*, **6**, 207–12.

Irvine, D.S. & Aitken, R.J. (1986). Predictive value of *in-vitro* sperm function tests in the context of an AID service. *Hum. Reprod.*, **1**, 539–45.

Jeyendran, R.S., van der Ven, H.H., Perez-Pelaez, M., Crabo, B.G. & Zaneveld, L.J.D. (1984). Development of an assay to assess the functional integrity of the human sperm membrane and its relationship to other semen characteristics. *J. Reprod. Fertil.*, **70**, 219–28.

Katayama, K.P., Stehlik, E., Roesler, M., Jeyendran, R.S., Holmgren, W.J. & Zaneveld, L.J.D. (1989). Treatment of human spermatozoa with an egg yolk medium can enhance the outcome of *in vitro* fertilization. *Fertil. Steril.*, **52**, 1077–9.

Kremer, J. & Jagar, S. (1990). The significance of the zona-free hamster oocyte test for the evaluation of male fertility. *Fertil. Steril.*, **54**, 509–12.

Kruger, T.F., Swanson, R.J., Hamilton, M., Simmons, K.F., Acosta, A.A., Matta, J.F., Oehninger, S. & Morshedi, M. (1988) Abnormal sperm morphology and other semen parameters related to the outcome of the hamster oocyte sperm penetration assay. *Int. J. Androl.*, **11**, 107–13.

Kuzan, F.B., Muller, C.H., Zarutskie, P.W., Dixon, L.L. & Soules, M.R. (1987). Human sperm penetration assay as an indicator of sperm function in human *in vitro* fertilization. *Fertil. Steril.*, **48**, 282–6.

Lamb, D.J., Johnson, A.R., Bassham, B.L. & Lipshultz, L.I. (1989). How the sperm penetration assay diagnoses infertility. *Contemp. Obstet. Gynecol.*, **31**, 108–14.

Laufer, N., Margalioth, E.J., Navot, D., Shemesh, A. & Schenker, J.G. (1985). Reduced penetration of zona-free hamster ova by cryopreserved human spermatozoa. *Archives of Andrology*, **14**, 217–22.

Mao, C. & Grimes, D.A. (1988). The sperm penetration assay: can it discriminate between fertile and infertile men? *Am. J. Obstet. Gynecol.*, **159**, 279–86.

Margalioth, E.J., Navot, D., Laufer, N., Lewin, A., Rabinowitz, R. & Schenker, J.G. (1986). Correlation between the zona-free hamster egg sperm penetration assay and human *in vitro* fertilization. *Fertil. Steril.*, **45**, 665–70.

Margalioth, E.J., Feinmesser, M., Navot, D., Mordel, N. & Bronson, R.A. (1989). The long-term predictive value of the zona-free hamster ova sperm penetration assay. *Fertil. Steril.*, **52**, 490–4.

Margalioth, E.J., Laufer, N., Navot, D., Voss, R. & Schenker, J.G. (1983). Reduced fertilization ability of zona-free hamster ova by spermatozoa from male partners of normal infertile couples. *Archives of Andrology*, **10**, 67–71.

McClure, R.D., Tom, R.A. & Dandekar, P.V. (1990). Optimizing the sperm penetration assay with human follicular fluid. *Fertil. Steril.*, **53**, 546–50.

Muller, C.H. & Zarutskie, P.W. (1992). Prediction and diagnosis of human *in vitro* fertilization success and failure by enhanced sperm penetration and sperm–zona binding assays. Forty-eighth Annual Meeting of American Fertility Society, New Orleans, 2–5 November, Supplement, S105.

Nahhras, F. & Blumefield, Z. (1989). Zona-free hamster egg penetration assay: prognostic indicator in an IVF program. *Arch. Androl.*, **23**, 33–7.

Pilikian, S. & Guerin, J.F. (1986). Acrosome-reacting capacity of frozen-thawed human semen: relation to hamster ova penetration. *Arch. Androl.*, **16**, 209–14.

Protocols for the zona-free hamster oocycte test (1993). Appendix XIX. In *World Health Organization Laboratory Manual for the Examination of Human Semen and Semen–Cervical Mucus Interaction*, 3rd edn, pp. 82–6. Cambridge: Cambridge University Press.

Rogers, B.J. (1985). The sperm penetration assay: its usefulness reevaluated. *Fertil. Steril.*, **43**, 821–40.

Rogers, B.J. (1986). The usefulness of the sperm penetration assay in predicting *in vitro* fertilization success. *J. In Vitro Fert. Embryo Transfer*, **3**, 209–11.

Rogers, B.J. (1988). Use of the SPA in assessing toxic effects on male fertilizing potential. *Reprod. Toxicol.*, **2**, 233–40.

Rogers, B.J. (1989*a*). Sperm penetration assay. In *Common Problems in Infertility and Impotence*, ed. J. Rajfer. Chicago: Yearbook Medical Publishers.

Rogers, B.J. (1989*b*). Examination of data from programs of *in vitro* fertilization in relation to sperm integrity and reproductive success. In *Sperm Measures and Reproductive Success*, ed. E.J. Burger, R.G. Tardiff, A.R. Scialli & H. Zenick, pp. 69–93. New York: Alan R. Liss.

Rogers, B.J., & Parker, R.A. (1991). Relationship between the human sperm hypo-osmotic swelling test and sperm penetration assay. *J. Androl.*, **12**, 152–8.

Rogers, B.J., Van Campen, H., Ueno, M., Lambert, H., Bronson, R. & Hale, R. (1979). Analysis of human spermatozoal fertilizing ability using zona-free ova. *Fertil. Steril.*, **32**, 664–70.

Rogers, B.J., Brentwood, B.J.H., Van Campen, H., Helmbrecht, G., Soderdahl, D. & Hale, R.W. (1983). Sperm morphology assessment as an indicator of human fertilizing capacity. *J. Androl.*, **4**, 119–25.

Rojas, F.J., La, A.T., Ord, T., Patrizio, P., Balmaceda, J.P., Silber, S.J. & Asch, R.H. (1992). Penetration of zona-free hamster oocytes using human sperm aspirated from the epididymis of men with congenital absence of the vas deferens: comparison with human *in vitro* fertilization. *Fertil. Steril.*, **58**, 1000–5.

Shy, K.K., Stenchever, M.A. & Muller, C.H. (1988). Sperm penetration assay and subsequent pregnancy: a prospective study of 74 infertile men. *Obstet. Gynecol.*, **71**, 685–90.

Soffer, Y., Golan, A., Herman, A., Pansky, M., Caspi, E. & Ron-El, R. (1992). Prediction of *in vitro* fertilization outcome by sperm penetration assay with TEST-yolk buffer preincubation. *Fertil. Steril.*, **58**, 556–62.

Sutherland, P.D., Matson, P.L., Moore, H.D.M., Goswamy, R., Parsons, J.H., Vaid, P. & Pryor, J.P. (1985). Clinical evaluation of the heterologous oocyte penetration (HOP) test. *Br. J. Urol.*, **57**, 233–6.

Talbot, P. & Chacon, R.S. (1980). A new procedure for rapidly scoring acrosome reactions of human sperm. *Gamete Res.*, **3**, 211–16.

Tesarik, J. (1985). Comparison of acrosome reaction-inducing activities of human cumulus oophorus, follicular fluid and ionophore A23187 in human sperm populations of proven fertilizing ability *in vitro*. *J. Reprod. Fertil.*, **74**, 383–8.

van Kooij, R.J., Balerna, M., Roatti, A. & Campana, A. (1986). Oocyte penetration and acrosome reactions of human spermatozoa. I. Influence of incubation time and medium composition. *Andrologia*, **18**, 152–60.

Wang, C., Chan, S.Y.W., Ng, M., So, W.W.K., Tsoi, W.S., Lo, T. & Leung, A. (1988) Diagnostic value of sperm function tests and routine semen analyses in fertile and infertile men. *J. Androl.*, **9**, 384–9.

Wang, C., Leung, A., Tsoi, W.L., Leung, J., Ng, V., Lee, K.F. & Chen, S.Y.W. (1991). Computer-assisted assessment of human sperm morphology: usefulness in predicting fertilizing capacity of human spermatozoa. *Fertil. Steril.*, **55**, 989–93.

Yanagimachi, R., Yanagimachi, H. & Rogers, B.J. (1976). The use of zona-free animal ova as a test system for the assessment of the fertilizing capacity of human spermatozoa. *Biol. Reprod.*, **15**, 471–6.

Yang, Y.S., Rojas, F.J. & Stone, S.C. (1988). Acrosome reaction of human spermatozoa in zona-free hamster egg penetration test. *Fertil. Steril.*, **50**, 954–9.

7

Intrauterine insemination for male factor

WILLIAM D. SCHLAFF and CALEB A. AWONIYI

Introduction

Earlier this century, Dr Robert L. Dickinson of New York City, during a symposium on infertility, described intrauterine insemination as follows: After the patient is positioned, 'the tenaculum steadies the cervix and serves to draw open the canal, which should rarely need to be wiped and on which no antiseptic should be used. The pipette is now very gently filled. The tip touches first the interior of the cervical canal as high as may be and is passed to near the fundus. Gentle, steady pressure is made on the bulb until "unwell feelings" are produced and are continued till there is consciousness of slight distress in the sides of the abdomen low down, at which time the fallopian tubes are presumed to have fluid in them.' (Dickinson, 1921). In his article, Dr Dickinson beautifully described all aspects of this procedure as a possible treatment of male factor infertility. Dr Edward Reynolds of Boston, in discussing Dr Dickinson's paper, commented that 'Washing semen through the tubes impresses me as unphysiologic. I should want to see a large number of successes before I was ready to use it. The use of artificial insemination promiscuously without careful isolation of the cases which are due largely to cervical obstacles, I believe to be thoroughly unscientific and not free from danger. It comes down, in short, to the general principle that routine adoption of any procedure for a condition which is a result of multiple and varying causes is poor practice' (Reynolds, 1921). Interestingly, this discussion took place at the Forty-fifth Annual Meeting of the American Gynecological Society in Chicago, Illinois, on 26 May 1920. This chapter will review the practice of intrauterine insemination for male factor infertility to help determine its place in contemporary therapy of the infertile male.

Table 7.1   *Indications for AIH in 1978*

	Indication	% cases
Oligozoospermia	(≤22 million/ml)	32.1
Hypozoospermia	(≤3.1 ml)	30.2
Hyperzoospermia	(≥4 ml)	26.4
Polyzoospermia	(≥100 million/ml)	9.4
Cervical factor		11.3
Retrograde ejaculation		3.8
Infrequent coitus		1.9
Patient's request		1.9

Notes:
Data abstracted from Nunley *et al.* (1978).
AIH, artificial insemination of husband's sperm.

Background and recent developments

Artificial insemination of husband's sperm (AIH) for male factor infertility has been advocated and practiced widely for many years. Until about 10 years ago, practitioners virtually always used a cervical cup or intracervical insemination (ICI) with or without a mechanical 'dam'. Historical indications were fairly broad (Table 7.1), and results were generally reported on the basis of crude pregnancy rates. No prospective, randomized trials of cervical cup or ICI for male factor infertility have been published. However, a review of six non-randomized studies of AIH reported an 18% crude pregnancy rate in treated cycles compared with a rate of 14% in nontreated cycles (Nachtigall *et al.*, 1979). Obviously, at least in this retrospective, non-controlled analysis, cervical cup insemination did not seem to provide a compelling benefit. Another interesting observation is that the reported crude pregnancy rate of 18% in the treated group is virtually identical to the observed crude pregnancy rates obtained with medical treatment of subfertile males (Schellen, 1982; Winters & Troen, 1982). Though not scientifically derived, these observations suggest that approximately 20% of couples will conceive with almost any therapy (and possibly with no therapy). This provides a historical control when considering the proposed benefit of intrauterine insemination (IUI) for male factor infertility.

IUI was reported sporadically as a potential treatment of male factor infertility beginning in the 1960s up to the early 1980s (Mastroianni *et al.*, 1957; Farris & Murphy, 1960; Cohen, 1962; Barwin, 1974; Glass & Ericcson, 1978; White & Glass, 1978; Kremer, 1979; Dmowski *et al.*, 1979; Harris *et al.* (1981) and summarized by Allen *et al.* in 1985. In general, indications for IUI were not confined to male factor infertility but also included antisperm antibodies and poor cervical mucus. A number of different techniques and instruments were described, all of which are similar to techniques in use now. In general, results were not very favorable particularly when the indication was male infertility. For example, in 1978 Glass & Ericsson reported 0 of 19 women conceived after a total of 67 cycles of IUI, while Dmowski *et al.* (1979) and Harris *et al.* (1981) reported fecundity rates (pregnancy rate per cycle) of 0.04 and 0.03, respectively. Crude pregnancy rates in both studies were only 15%. However, a study by Kerin and his collegues (1984) stimulated renewed interest in many centers for the use of IUI for male factor infertility. They reported 8 pregnancies in 39 IUI cycles compared with 0 in 38 cycles using LH-timed intercourse and 1 in 34 cycles using basal body temperature-timed intercourse. Successes occurred from specimens with initial sperm concentrations as low as 4 million/ml and motility as low as 12%. Furthermore, the post-insemination preparations averaged only 3.5 million/ml (with a range of 800 000 to 25 million), with a total motile sperm number ranging from 160 000 to 6.1 million. This report, coupled with several others in the early and mid 1980s (Davajan *et al.*, 1983; Goldfarb *et al.*, 1984; Huszar *et al.*, 1984; Sher *et al.*, 1984; Hewitt *et al.*, 1985; Wiltbank *et al.*, 1985; Hoing *et al.*, 1986), provided some impetus for the burgeoning use of this technique.

Rationale for IUI

Direct IUI of sperm cells is an attractive option for male factor infertility. When sperm are known to be either quantitatively or functionally suboptimal, it is on the one hand disturbing to anticipate the loss of good cells within the vagina and, on the other hand, reassuring to imagine that those most likely to initiate conception have the advantage of improved access to the site of fertilization. Additionally, the physician may be pressured to recommend IUI by a couple who report apparent loss of semen through vaginal leakage after intercourse.

On a more scientific basis, it is tempting to recommend IUI because of the possible enhancement of the specimen by the 'sperm washing' process. Specifically, sperm washing may be able to concentrate the sperm most likely to fertilize, remove acellular debris which may interfere with sperm movement, and eliminate leukocytes, prostaglandins, and other seminal factors which putatively interfere with sperm function and fertilizing ability. Techniques of sperm preparation are thoroughly discussed in Chapter 8. There is no place in contemporary medical practice for IUI of the whole ejaculate. Unwashed specimens contain seminal factors which may cause discomfort or cramping (Sahmay *et al.*, 1990), and are also more likely to be contaminated by microorganisms (Stone *et al.*, 1986). Furthermore, volumes greater than 0.5 ml are not recommended because the inseminate is likely to fill the uterus and be injected directly into the tubes and peritoneal cavity. This may theoretically result in flushing the oocyte out of the tube, reducing the chance of pregnancy (Franco *et al.*, 1992).

Indications and evaluation for IUI

Current proposed indications for IUI include cervical factor infertility, unexplained infertility, therapeutic donor insemination, ejaculatory abnormalities, oligo- or oligoasthenozoospermia, and sperm antibodies. This discussion will focus only on the last two indications. Prior to recommending IUI for any indication, a thorough evaluation of the male partner and, at least to some extent, the female partner is mandatory. Evaluation of the male should include careful medical and reproductive history focusing on pubertal development, history of previous pregnancies, injuries, surgery, and medications. A sensitive yet detailed sexual history should be obtained. A complete physical examination should be performed. Approximately 75–80% of men with male factor infertility will be found to have an abnormality directly attributable to the testes (Wong & Jones, 1983). Only about 10% will have a hormonal abnormality responsible for the sperm dysfunction, and a similar number will have a nontesticular, anatomic abnormality such as vasal agenesis or epididymal obstruction (Wong & Jones, 1983).

It is common for oligoasthenozoospermic men seeking infertility treatment to have female partners with concurrent reproductive problems. Previous studies have shown that up to 25% of men seeking vasectomy will have sperm concentrations less than 20 million/ml (Zukerman *et al.*, 1977). This and similar observations suggest that many oligozoospermic men may have apparently normal fertility if the female has uncompromised reproductive function, thereby reinforcing the recommendation that the partners of oligoasthenozoospermic men be evaluated prior to embarking on a treatment course of IUI. This evaluation should at least include a careful history and physical examination with special attention to possible ovulatory or anatomic abnormalities. Further evaluation including hormonal profiles, hysterosalpingography or laparoscopy may be considered depending on the clinical situation.

Once the evaluation has been completed, and prior to starting treatment, the physician should thoroughly review the diagnoses with the couple, and describe the process of IUI, including ovulatory monitoring relative to the time of insemination, risks and prognosis. When appropriate, couples should be encouraged to seek counseling with a therapist, usually a social worker or a psychologist. Generally, a course of 3–6 months of insemination is recommended. Frequently, IUI is performed by the staff at the center rather than the physician. It is highly recommended that the physician meet with the couple at least every 2–3 months to maximize patient compliance and satisfaction, and to ensure that the IUI process is optimal for conception to occur.

Timing and technique

Accurate timing is important in performing IUI for male factor infertility due to the presumed decreased functional capacity and survival of sperm from oligoasthenozoospermic males (Denil *et al.*, 1992). It has also been suggested that the intrauterine deposition of sperm may further reduce the survival or availability of sperm for fertilization, and thus may narrow the window of time when insemination is effective. The most common timing technique used for IUI is home urinary LH monitoring by monoclonal antibody kits. In general, these relatively convenient and inexpensive kits are as effective as frequent serum monitoring of LH in predicting the time of ovulation, and significantly more predictive than basal body temperature charting. Ovulation usually occurs within 24 hours of a colorimetric change in most monoclonal antibody assay kits. Therefore, we usually recommend insemination the day following detection of the LH surge. We often perform an ultrasound scan in conjunction with the insemination to ascertain whether ovulation has occurred. An irregular ovarian cyst with some degree of internal heterogeneity associated with a large amount of cul-de-sac fluid is suggestive of ovulation. Depending on logistical circumstances such as proximity, a follow-up ultrasound and insemination may be considered the following day if the follicle has not collapsed by the time of the first IUI.

At present, there is no clear agreement as to whether one or two inseminations per cycle should be recommended. A recent study evaluated the characteristics of semen samples obtained for IUI for male factor infertility on two consecutive days (Hornstein *et al.*, 1992). In oligozoospermic men, the data showed no difference in the post-wash motility or concentration on day 2 compared with day 1. In asthenozoospermic men, there was a slight decrease in concentration in the post-wash specimen on the second day, but there was no clinically significant decrease in post-wash motility. These results provide some reassurance that insemination on two consecutive days may well provide a stable population of sperm for insemination.

Techniques and instrumentation for IUI are fairly standard. A plastic catheter is usually used for the insemination (Fig. 7.1). Commonly used catheters include Tomcat (Sovereign, Sherwood Medical, St Louis, MO), Tef-

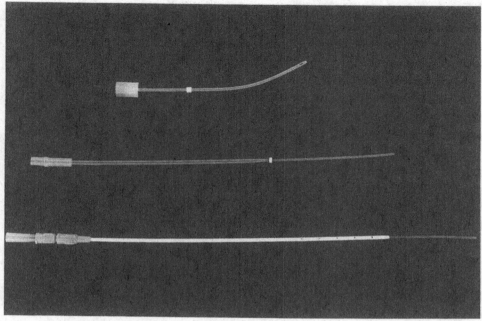

Fig. 7.1. Representative commercially available catheters for intrauterine insemination. At the top is shown the Modified Shepard Intrauterine Insemination Catheter (Cook OB/GYN, Spencer, IN), in the middle the Tefcat Intrauterine Insemination Catheter (Cook OB/GYN, Spencer, IN) and at the bottom the Edwards–Wallace Catheter (Wallace Limited, Essex, UK). The Edwards–Wallace Catheter, with its malleable inner catheter and less flexible outer sheath for traversing the cervical canal, was designed for embryo replacement during *in vitro* fertilization procedures; it has been successfully employed by some programs for intrauterine insemination as well.

Cat Catheter (Cook Ob-Gyn, Bloomington, IN), Makler IUI device (Sefi-Medical Instrument) or the Unimar intrauterine catheters (KDF-2.3 Unimar, Prodimed, Neuilly, France). These are all soft plastic or Teflon catheters that can be attached to a tuberculin syringe for insemination. Prior to performing the insemination, the plane of the uterus is determined by a digital examination. A speculum is then inserted, and the cervix is gently wiped with a large Q-tip or cotton ball. Neither antiseptic (Betadine) nor lubricant should be used during the process. Prior to drawing the inseminate into the catheter a volume of air, generally about 0.1 ml, should be drawn into the syringe. This 'bubble' will help to insure that all of the volume is inseminated. The catheter can be shaped or bent prior to insemination to try to accommodate the patient's particular uterine curvature. If the catheter is not easily inserted, a tenaculum may be required, particularly in the case of a uterus which is acutely ante- or retroflexed. The catheter still may not easily negotiate the internal os, particularly in the nulliparous patient. Should this be the case, a silver wire or lacrimal duct probe can be used to try to identify the proper angle into the uterine cavity. In uncommon circumstances, the plastic catheter cannot be successfully inserted into the intrauterine cavity at all. At these times, a metal catheter can be used. These are often associated with more cramping, discomfort, and bleeding, and we try to avoid them when possible. Once the catheter has been successfully passed through the internal os, it should be advanced to the level of the fundus. Once the patient is comfortable and has no further cramping the 0.3–0.4 ml volume is injected over approximately 1 minute. At the conclusion of the insemination, the catheter should be left in place for another minute, or until all cramping has stopped. The patient is made comfortable and asked to wait for up to 20 minutes prior to leaving. Physical activity need not be limited in any way following insemination.

Results

Reported crude pregnancy rates of IUI for oligoasthenozoospermia have ranged from 0 to 60%, with an average of 20–35%. A variety of different timing methods and insemination protocols have been reported, as have successes with a wide range of sperm concentration and motility characteristics. Unfortunately, the data are often difficult to interpret due to lack of uniformity in patient selection, insemination preparation and techniques and, above all, absence of a control group.

Table 7.2 summarizes data from studies of IUI for treatment of male factor infertility in spontaneous cycles. Several observations are apparent. Patient numbers are small, and only 6 of 21 studies have any type of control group. The composite crude pregnancy rate calculated from these studies is 19.9% (88 of 443 patients), a rate quite close to the historical control value of 18%. The average cycle fecundity based on a composite of these studies is 5.5% (87 pregnancies in 1593 cycles) compared with 2.5% (13 pregnancies in 518 cycles) for the various control groups. Apart from the two reports by Kerin (Kerin et al., 1984; Kerin & Quinn, 1987), the only other study showing any appreciable benefit had only 17 patients and 24 total cycles (Martinez et al., 1990). These data do not support any clear conclusion regarding the efficacy of IUI for male factor infertility in spontaneous cycles.

In later studies, it has been proposed that superovulation of the female partner may improve the success rate of IUI in male factor couples. Both clomiphene citrate alone and human menopausal gonadotropins (hMG) alone or in combination with clomiphene have been used. There are only four published studies where male factor couples were treated with clomiphene alone

Table 7.2 *Intrauterine insemination for male factor in unstimulated cycles*

	No. of patients	Pregnant/cycle Treated	Pregnant/cycle Control	IUI pregnancy rate (%)	IUI fecundity	Control fecundity
Barwin (1974)	12	8/NS	–	67	NS	–
Glass & Ericsson (1978)	19	0/67	–	0	0	–
Dmowski et al. (1979)	27	4/90	–	15	0.04	–
Kremer (1979)	6	1/NS	–	16	NS	–
Harris et al. (1981)	20	3/120	–	15	0.03	–
Marrs et al. (1983)	4	0/12	–	0	0	–
Kerin et al. (1984)	35	8/39	1/34[a]	NA	0.21	0.03
Toffle et al. (1985)	21	5/NS	–	24	NS	–
Wiltbank et al. (1985)	14	1/NS	–	7	NS	–
Confino et al. (1986)	27	0/NS	–	0	0	–
DiMarzo & Rakoff (1986)	9	2/NS	–	22	NS	–
Thomas et al. (1986)	10	0/32	3/14[a]	NA	0	0.21
Thomas et al. (1986)	10	0/32	0/31[b]	0	0	0
Hull et al. (1986)	8	0/20	–	0	0	–
Byrd et al. (1987)	15	8/36	–	53	0.22	–
Hughes et al. (1987)	20	0/32	–	0	0	–
Huszar & DeCherney (1987)	77	22/NS	–	29	NS	–
Kerin & Quinn (1987)	NS	26/296	6/213[a]	NA	0.09	0.03
Ho et al. (1989)	47	0/114	1/124[a]	0	0.01	–
te Velde et al. (1989)	30	3/112	2/90[a]	NA	0.03	0.02
Martinez et al. (1990)	17	2/12	0/12[a]	NA	0.16	0
Francavilla et al. (1990)	68	15/335	–	22	0.04	–
Galle et al. (1990)	15	1/NS	–	7	NS	–
Friedman et al. (1991b)	81	18/276	–	22	0.06	–

Notes:
Control groups: [a] spontaneous cycle+intercourse; [b] spontaneous cycle+intracervical insemination. –, no data.
NS, not stated; NA, not applicable.

and IUI. As can be seen from Table 7.3, there is insufficient information from these 95 patients to allow any conclusion regarding the effectiveness of clomiphene/IUI in the treatment of male factor infertility. There is more information regarding hMG/IUI, as shown in Table 7.4. The crude pregnancy rate calculated across these ten studies for treated women is 24.6% (32 pregnancies in 130 patients). Fortunately, many of these studies reported their data by fecundity rate and utilized control groups more commonly than the previous reports. Average fecundity in the treatment cycles is 9.3% (67 pregnancies in 723 cycles) compared with 2.4% in the various different control groups (12 pregnancies in 499 cycles). Due to the heterogeneity of control groups, it is impossible to evaluate statistical significance. It is perhaps most useful to focus on a single study to help draw a conclusion from these data. Chaffkin *et al.* (1991) randomized male factor patients to hMG/IUI versus spontaneous cycle plus IUI (i.e., IUI alone) or hMG plus intercourse (i.e., intercourse alone) and showed cycle fecundity of 0.15, 0.03, and 0.04 respectively. These controlled data, based on a fairly large sample size, are the most compelling available to suggest a benefit of hMG/IUI in the treatment of male factor infertility. It is to be hoped that any future studies on this subject will be equally well designed to provide additional information.

IUI has also been advocated for treatment of antisperm antibodies, largely since a report by Confino and his colleagues appeared in 1986 (Table 7.5). In this study, IUI was performed in 18 couples in whom 10 women and 8 men were found to have antisperm antibodies by a tray agglutination technique. Conception occurred with IUI in 4 of 10 women with antibodies, and in partners of 2 of 8 men with antibodies. The largest study was reported by Margalloth *et al.* (1988) and included 91 women demonstrated to have antisperm antibodies by immunobead assay. These women underwent 473 IUI cycles, 285 of which were spontaneous, 86 of which were clomiphene induced, and 102 of which were stimulated with hMG. Fecundity rates were 0.03, 0.07, and 0.11, respectively, suggesting that hMG/IUI had the highest success rates for these patients. There were no untreated controls in this study. Unfortunately, only one study of IUI for antisperm antibodies has had a control group, and there were no pregnancies in any patient in this report (Evans *et al.*, 1991). Overall, crude pregnancy rates range from 0 to 50%, and the heterogeneity of treatment protocols along with the absence of control groups makes it difficult to draw any conclusions regarding the efficacy of IUI in the treatment of male factor infertility due to antisperm antibodies. These data support the impression that antisperm antibodies in the female are more amenable to treatment by IUI than those in the male, but are not sufficient to allow a conclusive statement to be made.

Table 7.3 *Intrauterine insemination for male factor infertility in clomiphene-induced cycles*

	No. of patients	Pregnant/cycle Treated	Pregnant/cycle Control	IUI pregnancy rate (%)	IUI fecundity	Control fecundity
Hewitt et al. (1985)	36	3/64	–	8	0.05	–
Blumenfeld & Nahhas (1989)	13	5/43	–	38	0.12	–
Bolton et al. (1989)	29	5/158	–	17	0.03	–
Martinez et al. (1990)	17	2/12	0/12[a]	NA	0.16	0

Notes:
Control groups: [a] clomiphene+intercourse. –, no data.
NA, not applicable.

Table 7.4 *Intrauterine insemination for male factor infertility in hMG-induced cycles*

	No. of patients	Pregnant/cycle Treated	Pregnant/cycle Control	IUI pregnancy rate (%)	IUI fecundity	Control fecundity
Sher et al. (1984)	4	1/4	–	25	0.25	–
Cruz et al. (1986)	48	7/96	1/86[a]	NA	0.07	0.01
Kemman et al. (1987)	76	9/105	4/180[b]	20	0.02	0.08
Sunde et al. (1988)	40	8/56	–	20	0.15	–
Horvath et al. (1989b)	39	6/175	–	15	0.03	–
Blumenfeld & Nahhas (1989)	8	4/32	–	50	0.13	–
Dodson & Haney (1991)	39	13/85	–	33	0.15	–
Martinez et al. (1991)	16	2/28	0/28[c]	NA	0.07	0
Chaffkin et al. (1991)	NS	17/111	3/105[b]	NS	0.15	0.03
			3/68[d]	NS	0.15	0.04
Evans et al. (1991)	23	0/31	1/32[d]	NA	0	0.03

Notes:
Control groups: [a] hMG+intracervical insemination; [b] spontaneous cycle+IUI; [c] spontaneous cycle+intercourse; [d] hMG+intercourse. –, no data.
NS, not stated; NA, not applicable.

Table 7.5 *Intrauterine insemination for treatment of antisperm antibodies*

	No. of patients	Pregnant/cycle		IUI pregnancy rate (%)	IUI fecundity	Control fecundity
		Treated	Control			
Byrd et al. (1987)	4	0/12	—	0	0	—
Confino et al. (1986)	10 (female with antibodies)	4/NS	—	40	—	—
	8 (male with antibodies)	2/NS	—	25	—	—
Glass & Ericsson (1978)	1	0/NS	—	0	0	—
Kremer (1979)	20	4/NS	—	20	NS	—
Shulman et al. (1978)	7	1/NS	—	14	NS	—
Ulstein (1973)	4	2/NS	—	50	NS	—
Wiltbank et al. (1985)	8	2/NS	—	25	NS	—
Margalloth et al. (1988) (all female patients with antibodies)	67[a]	9/285	—	13	0.03	—
	20[b]	6/86	—	30	0.07	—
	28[c]	11/102	—	39	0.11	—
Toffle et al. (1985)	9	1/NS	—	11	NS	—
Galle et al. (1990)	5 (female with antibodies)	3/NS	—	60	NS	—
	1 (male with antibodies)	0/NS	—	0	0	—
	4 (both with antibodies)					
Evans et al. (1991)	14	1/NS	—	25	NS	—
		0/19[c]	0/22[c]	NA	0	0

Notes:
[a] Spontaneous cycle; [b] clomiphene-induced cycles; [c] hMG-induced cycles. −, no data.

The minimal number of sperm required to produce pregnancy with IUI is not established. There are a number of studies that have reported pregnancies with insemination of fewer than 1 million motile sperm (Kerin *et al.*, 1984; Hoing *et al.*, 1986; Byrd *et al.*, 1987; Kerin & Quinn, 1987). A review concluded that pregnancy is unlikely with insemination of fewer than 400 000 motile sperm (Kerin & Byrd, 1989). The authors further suggested that optimal pregnancy rates occurred with insemination of 15 million motile sperm, an observation supported by another large study (Horvath *et al.*, 1989*b*). Concentrations above 15 million motile cells, inherently unlikely in oligozoospermic men, did not seem to increase pregnancy rates any further (Kerin & Byrd, 1989). In fact, present data suggest that insemination of over 20 million motile sperm, at least in conjunction with hMG stimulated cycles, is associated with an increased rate of multiple gestation (Shelden *et al.*, 1988).

In every study analyzing the success of IUI for male factor infertility, most successes occur early in the treatment program: approximately 60–80% occur in the first two cycles, and over 90% occur within five or six cycles. Certainly this observation may, to some degree, reflect reticence on the part of the physician to recommend more than 6 months of treatment, as well as the patient's unwillingness to submit to more than six cycles.

Nevertheless, the uniformity of the data and life table analysis compel the conclusion that the majority of successes occur early, and that IUI for this indication should rarely be recommended beyond five or six cycles.

Risks

IUI is associated with very few significant medical risks. Allergic responses, including anaphylaxis, have been observed rarely (Sonenthal *et al.*, 1991; Smith *et al.*, 1992). Though microorganisms have been observed in the IUI specimens (Bolton *et al.* 1986; Stone *et al.*, 1986; Kuzan *et al.*, 1987), clinical infection is extremely uncommon (Horvath *et al.*, 1989*b*; Dodson & Haney, 1991). Given the rarity of this complication, routine use of prophylactic antibiotics cannot be recommended. Induction of antisperm antibodies by the antigenic load of sperm injected directly into the uterus is a theoretical risk of IUI, and supported at least by a small amount of preliminary data (Overstreet *et al.*, 1988; Friedman *et al.*, 1991*a*). However, at least two studies have shown no significant increase in the incidence of antibodies following IUI (Moretti-Rojas *et al.*, 1990; Horvath *et al.*, 1991*a*). If sperm antibodies are inducible with IUI, it appears to be relatively uncommon, and of uncertain clinical significance. While a theoretical concern, to our knowledge cervical or uterine perforation or significant anatomic injury has never been reported with standard IUI techniques.

Perhaps the greatest risk of IUI is prolonged ineffective treatment. This problem arises when there is inadequate monitoring of treatment or when there is no prospective therapeutic endpoint. As mentioned, IUI for male factor infertility should rarely be performed for more than a 6 month period. If pregnancy does not occur by this time, strong consideration should be given to other forms of assisted reproductive technology, donor insemination, or social options such as adoption.

Conclusions

Intrauterine insemination for male factor infertility, though widespread, has not been thoroughly studied or conclusively proven to be effective. Several questions such as the minimal number of motile sperm required and the reasonable length of a therapeutic trial have been answered. Present practitioners of IUI should adhere to the guidelines supported by the data summarized in this chapter, but should also strive to develop the large, multi-center trials necessary to understand fully the role of IUI in the treatment of male factor infertility.

References

Allen, N.C., Herbert, C.M. III, Maxson, W.S., *et al.* (1985). Intrauterine insemination: a critical review. *Fertil. Steril.*, **44**, 569–80.

Barwin, B.N. (1974). Intrauterine insemination of husband's sperm. *J. Reprod. Fertil.*, **36**, 101–6.

Blumenfeld, Z. & Nahhas, F. (1989). Pretreatment of sperm with human follicular fluid for borderline male infertility. *Fertil. Steril.*, **51**, 863–8.

Bolton, V.N., Warren, R.E. & Braude, P.R. (1986). Removal of bacterial contaminants from semen for *in vitro* fertilization or artificial insemination by the use of buoyant density centrifugation. *Fertil. Steril.*, **46**, 1128–72.

Bolton, V.N., Braude, P.R., Ockenden, K., *et al.* (1989). An evaluation of semen analysis and *in vitro* tests of sperm function in the prediction of the outcome of intrauterine AIH. *Hum. Reprod.*, **4**, 674–9.

Byrd, W., Ackerman, G.E., Carr, B.R., *et al.* (1987). Treatment of refractory infertility by transcervical intrauterine insemination of washed spermatozoa. *Fertil. Steril.*, **48**, 921–7.

Chaffkin, L.M., Nulsen, J.C., Luciano, A.A., *et al.* (1991). A comparative analysis of cycle fecundity rates associated with combined human menopausal gonadotropin (hMG) and intrauterine insemination (IUI) versus either hMG or IUI alone. *Fertil. Steril.*, **55**, 252–7.

Cohen, M.R. (1962). Intrauterine insemination. *Int. J. Fertil.*, **7**, 235–40.

Confino, E., Friberg, J., Dudkiewicz, A.B. & Gleicher, N. (1986). Intrauterine inseminations with washed human spermatozoa. *Fertil. Steril.*, **46**, 55–60.

Cruz, R.I., Kemman, E., Brandeis, V.T., Becker, K.A., Beck, M., Beardsley, L. & Shelton, R. (1986). A prospective study of intrauterine insemination of processed sperm from men with oligoasthenospermia in superovulated women. *Fertil. Steril.*, **46**, 673–7.

Davajan, V., Vargyas, J.M., Kletzky, O.A., *et al.* (1983). Intrauterine insemination with washed sperm to treat infertility (abstract). *Fertil. Steril.*, **40**, 419.

Denil, J., Ohl, D.A., Hurd, W.W., Menge, A.C. & Hiner, M.R. (1992). Motility longevity of sperm samples processed for intrauterine insemination. *Fertil. Steril.*, **58**, 436–8.

Dickinson, R.L. (1921). Artificial impregnation: essays in tubal insemination. *Am. J. Obstet. Gynecol.*, **1**, 255–61.

DiMarzo, S.J. & Rakoff, J.S. (1986). Intrauterine insemination with husband's washed sperm. *Fertil. Steril.*, **46**, 470–5.

Dmowski, W.P., Gaynor, L., Lawrence, M., *et al.* (1979). Artificial insemination homologous with oligospermic semen separated on albumin columns. *Fertil. Steril.*, **31**, 58–62.

Dodson, W.C. & Haney, A.F. (1991). Controlled ovarian hyperstimulation and intrauterine insemination for treatment of infertility. *Fertil. Steril.*, **55**, 457–67.

Evans, J., Wells, C., Gregory, L., *et al.* (1991). A comparison of intrauterine insemination, intraperitoneal insemination, and natural intercourse with superovulated women. *Fertil. Steril.*, **56**, 1183–7.

Farris, E.J. & Murphy, D.P. (1960). The characteristics of the two parts of the partitioned ejaculation and the advantages of its use for intrauterine insemination. *Fertil. Steril.*, **11**, 465–9.

Francavilla, F., Romano, R., Santucci, R., *et al.* (1990). Effect of sperm morphology and motile sperm count on outcome of intrauterine insemination in oligozoospermia and/or asthenozoospermia. *Fertil. Steril.*, **53**, 892–7.

Franco, J.G. Jr, Baruff, R.L.R., Mauri, A.L., *et al.* (1992). Radiologic evaluation of incremental intrauterine instillation of contrast material. *Fertil. Steril.*, **58**, 1065–7.

Friedman, A.J., Juneau-Norcross, M. & Sedensky, B. (1991*a*). Antisperm antibody production following intrauterine insemination. *Hum. Reprod.*, **6**, 1125–8.

Friedman, A.J., Juneau-Norcross, M., Sedensky, B., *et al.* (1991*b*). Life table analysis of intrauterine pregnancy success rates for couples with cervical factor, male factor, and idiopathic infertility. *Fertil Steril.*, **55**, 1005–7.

Galle, P.C., McRae, M.A., Colliver, J.A., *et al.* (1990). Sperm washing and intrauterine insemination for cervical factor, oligospermia, immunologic infertility and unexplained infertility. *J. Reprod. Med.*, **35**, 116–22.

Glass, R.N. & Ericcson, R.J. (1978). Intrauterine insemination of isolated motile sperm. *Fertil. Steril.*, **29**, 535–8.

Goldfarb, J.M., Sheean, L.A. & Utian, W.H. (1984). Intrauterine insemination: reappraisal with a new method (abstract). *Fertil. Steril.*, **41**, 108–9S.

Harris, S.J., Milligan, M.P., Masson, G.M., *et al.* (1981). Improved separation of motile sperm in asthenospermia and its application to artificial insemination homologous. *Fertil. Steril.*, **36**, 219–21.

Hewitt, J., Cohen, J., Krishnaswamy, V., *et al.* (1985). Treatment of idiopathic infertility, cervical mucus hostility, and male infertility: artificial insemination with husband's semen or *in vitro* fertilization? *Fertil. Steril.*, **44**, 350–5.

Ho, P.-C., Poon, I.M.L., Chan, S.Y.W., *et al.* (1989). Intrauterine insemination is not useful in oligoasthenospermia. *Fertil. Steril.*, **51**, 682–4.

Hoing, L.M., Devroey, P. & Van Steirteghem, A.C. (1986). Treatment of infertility because of oligoasthenoteratospermia by transcervical intrauterine insemination of motile spermatozoa. *Fertil. Steril.*, **45**, 388–91.

Hornstein, M.D., Cohen, J.N., Thomas, P.P., Gleason, R.E., Friedman, A.J. &

Mutter, G.L. (1992). The effect of consecutive day inseminations on semen characteristics in an intrauterine insemination program. *Fertil. Steril.*, **58**, 433–5.

Horvath, P.M., Beck, M., Bohrer, M.K., *et al.* (1989*a*). A prospective study on the lack of development of antisperm antibodies in women undergoing intrauterine insemination. *Am. J. Obstet. Gynecol.*, **160**, 631–7.

Horvath, P.M., Bohrer, M., Shelden, R.M., *et al.* (1989*b*). The relationship of sperm parameters to cycle fecundity in superovulated women undergoing intrauterine insemination. *Fertil. Steril.*, **52**, 288–94.

Hughes, E.G., Collins, J.P. & Garner, P.R. (1987). Homologous artificial insemination for oligoasthenospermia: a randomized controlled study comparing intracervical and intrauterine techniques. *Fertil. Steril.*, **48**, 278–81.

Hull, M.E., Vasquez, J.M., Magyar, D.M., *et al.* (1986). Experience with intrauterine insemination for cervical factor and oligospermia. *Am. J. Obstet. Gynecol.*, **154**, 1333–8.

Huszar, G. & DeCherney, A. (1987). The role of intrauterine insemination in the treatment of infertile couples: the Yale experience. *Semin. Reprod. Endocrinol.*, **5**, 11–21.

Huszar, G., Makler, A., Murrillo, O., *et al.* (1984). The efficacy of intrauterine insemination (abstract). *Fertil. Steril.*, **41**, 1085.

Kemman, E., Bohrer, M., Shelden, R., *et al.* (1987). Active ovulation management increases the monthly probability of pregnancy occurrence in ovulatory women who receive intrauterine insemination. *Fertil. Steril.*, **48**, 916–20.

Kerin, J. & Byrd, W. (1989). Supracervical placement of spermatozoa. In *Controversies in Reproductive Endocrinology and Infertility*, ed. M.R. Soules, pp. 183–204. New York: Elsevier.

Kerin, J. & Quinn, P. (1987). Washed intrauterine insemination in the treatment of oligospermic infertility. *Semin. Reprod. Endocrinol.*, **5**, 23–33.

Kerin, J.F.P., Peek, J., Warnes, G.M., *et al.* (1984). Improved conception rate after intrauterine insemination of washed spermatozoa from men with poor quality semen. *Lancet.*, **1**, 553–5.

Kremer, J. (1979). A new technique for intrauterine insemination. *Int. J. Fertil.*, **24**, 53–6.

Kuzan, F.B., Hillier, S.C. & Zarutskie, P.W. (1987). Comparison of three wash techniques for the removal of microorganisms from semen. *Obstet. Gynecol.*, **70**, 836–9.

Margalloth, E.J., Sauter, E., Bronson, R.A., *et al.* (1988). Intrauterine insemination as a treatment for antisperm antibodies in the female. *Fertil. Steril.*, **50**, 441–6.

Marrs, R.P., Vargyas, J.M., Saito, H., Gibbons, W.E., Berger, T. & Mishell, D.R. Jr (1983). Clinical applications of techniques used in human *in vitro* fertilization research. *Am. J. Obstet. Gynecol.*, **146**, 477–81.

Martinez, A.R., Bernardus, R.E., Voorhorst, F.J., *et al.* (1990). Intrauterine insemination does and clomiphene citrate does not improve fecundity in couples with infertility due to male or idiopathic factors: a prospective, randomized, controlled study. *Fertil. Steril.*, **53**, 847–53.

Martinez, A.R., Bernardus, R.E., Voorhorst, F.J., *et al.* (1991). Pregnancy rates after timed intercourse or intrauterine insemination after human menopausal gonadotropin stimulation of normal ovulatory cycles; a controlled study. *Fertil. Steril.*, **55**, 258–5.

Mastroianni, L. Jr, Laberge, J.L. & Rock, L. (1957). Appraisal of the efficacy of artificial insemination with husband's sperm and evaluation of insemination technique. *Fertil. Steril.*, **8**, 260–6.

Moretti-Rojas, I., Rojas, F.J., Leisure, M., *et al.* (1990). Intrauterine insemination with washed human spermatozoa does not induce formation of antisperm antibodies. *Fertil. Steril.*, **53**, 180–2.

Nachtigall, R.D., Faure, N. & Glass, R.H. (1979). Artificial insemination of husband's sperm. *Fertil. Steril.*, **32**, 141–7.

Nunley, W.C., Kitchin,J.D. III & Thiagarajah, S. (1978). Homologous insemination. *Fertil. Steril.*, **30**, 510–15.

Overstreet, J.W., Hanson, F.W., Brazil, C., *et al.* (1988). Antisperm antibodies in women receiving intrauterine insemination (abstract 138). Thirty-fifth Annual Meeting of the Society for Gynecologic Investigation, March 1988, Baltimore, MD.

Reynolds, E. (1921). Discussion. Artificial impregnation: essays in tubal insemination. *Am. J. Obstet. Gynecol.*, **1**, 306.

Sahmay, S., Atasu, T. & Karacan, I. (1990). The effect of intrauterine insemination on uterine activity. *Int. J. Fertil.*, **35**, 310–14.

Schellen, A.M.C.M. (1982). Clomiphene citrate in the treatment of male infertility. In *Treatment of Male Infertility*, ed. J. Bain, W.-B. Schill & L. Schwarzstein, pp. 33–44. New York: Springer.

Shelden, R., Kemman, E., Bohrer, M., *et al.* (1988). Multiple gestation is associated with the use of high sperm numbers in the intrauterine insemination specimen in women undergoing gonadotropin stimulation. *Fertil. Steril.*, **49**, 607–10.

Sher, G., Knutzen, V.K., Stratton, C.J., *et al.* (1984). *In vitro* sperm capacitation and transcervical intrauterine insemination for the treatment of refractory infertility: phase I. *Fertil. Steril.*, **41**, 260–4.

Shulman, S., Harlin, B., Davis, P., *et al.* (1978). Immune infertility and new approaches to treatment. *Fertil. Steril.*, **29**, 309–13.

Smith, Y.R., Hurd, W.W., Menge, A.C., *et al.* (1992). Allergic reactions to penicillin during *in vitro* fertilization and intrauterine insemination. *Fertil. Steril.*, **58**, 847–9.

Sonenthal, K.R., McKnight, T., Shaughnessy, M.A., *et al.* (1991). Anaphylaxis during intrauterine insemination secondary to bovine serum albumin. *Fertil. Steril.*, **56**, 1188–91.

Stone, S.C., de la Maza, L.M. & Peterson, E.M. (1986). Recovery of microorganisms from the pelvic cavity after intracervical or intrauterine artificial insemination. *Fertil. Steril.*, **46**, 61–5.

Sunde, A., Kahn, J. & Molne, K. (1988). Intrauterine insemination. *Hum. Reprod.*, **3**, 97–9.

te Velde, E.R., vanKooy, R.J. & Waterreus, J.J.H. (1989). Intrauterine insemination of washed husband's spermatozoa: a controlled study. *Fertil. Steril.*, **51**, 182–5.

Thomas, E.J., McTighe, L., King, H., Lenton, E.A., Harper, R. & Cooke, I.D. (1986). Failure of high intrauterine insemination of husband's semen. *Lancet*, **2**, 693–4.

Toffle, R.C., Nagel, T.C., Tagatz, G.E., *et al.*, (1985). Intrauterine insemination: the University of Minnesota experience. *Fertil. Steril.*, **43**, 743–7.

Ulstein, M. (1973). Fertility of husbands at homologous insemination. *Acta Obstet. Gynecol. Scand.*, **52**, 5–8.

White, F.M. & Glass, F.H. (1978). Intrauterine insemination with husband's semen. *Obstet. Gynecol.*, **47**, 119–21.

Wiltbank, M.C., Kosasa, S. & Rogers, B. (1985). Treatment of infertile patients by intrauterine insemination of washed spermatozoa. *Andrologia*, **17**, 22–30.

Winters, S.J. & Troen, P. (1982). Gonadotropin therapy in male infertility. In *Treatment of Male Infertility*, ed. J. Bain, W.-B. Schill & L. Schwarzstein, pp. 85–101. New York: Springer.

Wong, T.-W. & Jones, T.M. (1983). Evaluation of testicular biopsy in male infertility studies. In *Infertility in the Male*, ed. L.I. Lipshultz & S.S. Howards, pp. 217–48. New York: Churchill Livingstone.

Zukerman, Z., Rodriguez-Rigau, L.J., Smith, K.D., *et al.* (1977). Frequency distribution of sperm counts in fertile and infertile males. *Fertil. Steril.*, **28**, 1310–13.

8

Processing human semen for insemination: comparison of methods

WILLIAM BYRD

Introduction

The introduction of *in vitro* fertilization and other assisted reproductive technologies (ART) has provided the catalyst for the further development of techniques which -isolate motile sperm. The goal of these sperm isolation procedures is the accumulation of a highly motile population of morphologically normal cells in a relatively small volume of medium. This sperm mixture can then be used for a number of different ART procedures. One such procedure, the most widely utilized in ART, is insemination using either the male partner's or donor sperm. The type of insemination performed is defined by the source of sperm, whether from partner or donor, and the site in the reproductive tract where the sperm are deposited. Other possible uses of washed sperm are insemination of oocytes *in vitro*. This procedure is usually used for patients who cannot or do not benefit from partner or donor insemination.

Intracervical insemination (ICI) has been one of the most widely used treatments for infertile patients. The indications for ICI are restricted to conditions where normal deposition of sperm cannot take place, such as hypospadias, impotence, or sexual dysfunction (vaginismus or dyspareunia), or donor insemination. Studies using fresh donor sperm have shown that couples undergoing ICI should experience pregnancy rates of 8–17% per ICI treatment cycle and approximately 60% of all couples should conceive after 6 months of treatment (Bradshaw *et al.*, 1987).

ICI is performed intravaginally using either an unprocessed ejaculate or washed sperm. If the sperm are introduced at any point superior to the internal os of the cervix, it is considered intrauterine insemination (IUI). The main indications for IUI include male factor infertility, female cervical factor, transport problems where the sperm cannot reach the egg, unexplained infertility, and endometriosis (see Chapters 7, 10 and 12). Sperm deposition directly into the fallopian tubes via the cervix is referred to as transuterotubal insemination

(TUTI), while sperm injection directly into the peritoneal cavity is referred to as direct intraperitoneal insemination (DIPI). The choice of technique or where the sperm will be deposited depends largely upon the clinical indication(s) for infertility.

IUI, DIPI, and TUTI have the same function as gamete intrafallopian transfer (GIFT) or *in vitro* fertilization (IVF), that is, increasing the number of gametes at or near the site of fertilization and thus improving the chance of fertilization. During normal coitus, cervical mucus serves as a mechanical–immunological filtering device which facilitates the separation of sperm from the seminal plasma. The loose network of glycoprotein fibers in cervical mucus limits the passage of sperm. Only highly motile sperm are able to traverse the limited interstitial spaces between the mucin fibers while non-motile cells, debris and seminal plasma are excluded. The extent of this filtering is evidenced in studies by Settlage *et al.* (1973), in which only 0.1% of sperm placed in the upper vagina were found in the cervical canal 1 hour after insemination. Other investigators have demonstrated a reduction in sperm numbers along the reproductive tract of 5–6 orders of magnitude (Mortimer & Templeton, 1982). Direct deposition of motile sperm into the reproductive tract can reverse this situation and thus increase the chances for successful fertilization.

While ICI may be performed using the ejaculate or processed sperm, other types of insemination require some form of sperm processing. There are three major reasons to process sperm: (1) to isolate sperm from the seminal plasma, (2) to initiate capacitation, and (3) to concentrate a motile population of cells in a small volume of medium. Removal of the seminal plasma has several important functions. First, it removes the factors which block capacitation or maturation of human sperm (Kanawar *et al.*, 1979). Also, prolonged exposure to seminal plasma can decrease sperm fertilizing ability (Wolf & Sokoloski, 1982). Prostaglandins in the seminal plasma induce cramping when introduced into the uterine cavity. Allen *et al.* (1985) reported severe cramps in 6–17% of patients who underwent IUI with unwashed specimens. Isolating sperm from the seminal plasma and reducing the volume of the insemination sample to less than 0.5 ml decreases this problem. Microorganism contamination can commonly be found in semen and it is possible that the microorganisms, if left in the specimen, could contribute to a decrease in the fertilization rate (Busolo *et al.*, 1983; Hewitt *et al.*, 1985; Bolton *et al.*, 1986). In a review of 38 studies, Sacks & Simon (1991) found only 6 infections in over 3267 women, an incidence of 1.83 per 1000. This rate was not altered by semen washing with antibiotics or the administration of prophylactic antibiotics to the women. With this in mind, this review will examine the most commonly used sperm preparation techniques.

Preparation of sperm

The human ejaculate is a mixture of motile, nonmotile and dead sperm as well as different types of seminal components such as debris, prostaglandins, and microorganisms. Initial attempts at AIH–IUI utilized unwashed semen in which the sperm was concentrated by centrifugation (Mastroianni *et al.*, 1957). Of the 29 patients receiving IUI in Mastroianni's study, 1 conceived and 5 patients complained of abdominal cramping. When cervical or vaginal inseminations were performed with non-treated sperm there was a pregnancy rate of 6.4–9.7%. The authors concluded that AIH–IUI for male factor couples was fruitless and that vaginal insemination with nontreated sperm was the most successful procedure. In 1976, Dixon *et al.* treated with cervical cap or intra-cervical insemination a series of 158 patients who suffered from male factor, immunologic or unexplained infertility. They noted a 9.5% pregnancy rate following treatment compared with an 18% pregnancy rate in nontreatment cycles. Although these reports discouraged the use of insemination for male factor infertility, there was renewed interest in sperm preparations and washing with the advent of ART programs.

Separation techniques

When the cervical barrier is bypassed with IUI, or insemination is performed *in vitro*, a sperm preparation composed of viable, motile sperm free of seminal plasma and debris is required. A variety of methods have been developed to separate motile sperm from semen, each with advantages and disadvantages. The most commonly used sperm isolation techniques described here involve washing and centrifugation, which may directly or indirectly result in some damage to the sperm (Aitken & Clarkson, 1987; Kerin & Byrd, 1989; Tarlatzia *et al.*, 1991). A recent concern expressed by Mortimer (1991) is that the more traditional sperm washing method for preparation of sperm will cause iatrogenic damage to sperm. Aitken & Clarkson (1987) have shown that the centrifugal force generated during washing generates reactive oxygen species (ROS). Since sperm are particularly high in polyunsaturated fatty acids and lack repair mechanisms to protect from oxidation, they are particularly sensitive to lipid peroxidation membrane damage induced by ROS. The source of ROS could be either the sperm or the white blood cells in the ejaculate.

A variety of different media have been used successfully for IUI preparations. Media used for sperm preparations are generally isotonic saline solutions that are buffered to a pH favorable to sperm and are usually supplemented with serum or albumin. Ideally the sperm isolation technique using such media would be rapid, inexpensive and would concentrate the motile sperm without damaging them.

Collection and processing of retrograde ejaculates

In males with uncorrectable retrograde ejaculation, it may be necessary to collect the sperm from the urine before it can be processed for insemination. There are several factors that must be considered including the acidity and osmolarity of the urine, excessive dilution and urine contamination of the sperm (Zavos & Wilson, 1984). An alkaline urine is required for this technique since acidification of the sperm in the urine will cause immobilization. The man takes 300–500 mg of sodium bicarbonate orally four times a day for 2 days, to ensure alkalinization of the urine. Approximately 1 hour before insemination, the bladder is emptied, followed by masturbation and urination. This sample can be mixed with medium and the sperm collected by centrifugation. Alternatively, the bladder can be cannulated and 250–500 ml of HEPES-buffered isotonic medium can be introduced into the bladder. The man masturbates, voids, and the urine sample is centrifuged in sterile-capped 50 ml tissue grade centrifuge tubes for 20–30 minutes to collect the sperm. The prolonged centrifugation time is required to pellet the sperm from the urine. The urine is discarded and the pellet containing sperm, nonmotile cells, and debris can then be processed using one of the following procedures. Due to the large amount of debris found in such circumstances, Percoll density centrifugation method or Sephadex column filtration methods are recommended.

Simple washing

The simplest and one of the most widely used techniques for preparing sperm is dilution of the semen with buffered saline or culture media followed by centrifugation at 300–800*g* to concentrate sperm. This simple wash was first described by Hanson & Rock (1951). While this technique eliminates or dilutes the effect of the seminal plasma, the resultant pellet will contain motile and non-motile sperm, cellular and particulate matter; bacteria may also be included in the material to be inseminated. There is a moderately good yield of motile cells compared with other techniques which will be discussed (Table 8.1). Disadvantages of this preparation technique are the generation of ROS, failure to remove unwanted semen constituents, and inclusion of nonmotile sperm cells, in response to centrifugation. Hence this preparation should be avoided when there is a high percentage of immotile sperm, excess cellular contamination, or debris in the ejaculate.

Table 8.1   *The efficiency of different sperm isolation procedures with fresh and frozen sperm*

Technique	% motile cells recovered
Simple wash	3–68
Swim-up	4–58
Percoll gradients	9–70
Albumin gradients	13–60
Glass wool filtration	46–71
Hyaluronic acid swim-up	12–18
Sephadex columns	5–50

'Swim-up' method

The earliest method, and still one of the most widely used, for separating motile from nonmotile sperm and cellular debris is the sperm-rise technique of Drevius (1971) or the swim-up of Lopata *et al.* (1976). The swim-up technique involves the layering of medium directly over semen samples, and the subsequent migration of motile sperm into the overlying culture medium following 30–90 minutes of incubation. This layer is then removed and motile cells recovered from it. The presence of small amounts of seminal plasma generally requires a centrifugation and resuspension step at this point. Variations on this technique include a preliminary wash followed by the incubation as above. To enhance sperm recovery it is also possible to layer the sperm directly over medium or serum and collect the 'swim-down' sperm (Gonzales & Pella, 1993). One problem with the swim-up technique is that the sperm have to migrate against gravitational force resulting in a low percentage recovery (Lopata *et al.*, 1976; Russell & Rogers, 1987; Table 8.1). The percentage of morphologically normal forms increases from 53% normal in washed samples to 80.8% normal forms following swim-up (Russell & Rogers, 1987).

Glass-wool filtration

Separation of motile sperm from other seminal plasma components on glass wool columns was first described by Paulson *et al.* (1979). The liquified specimen is placed on a column consisting of 5-inch glass Pasture pipette filled with loosely packed glass-wool fibers. This procedure is relatively fast, only requiring about 10 minutes for filtration. However, there is some evidence of structural damage to sperm (Sherman *et al.*, 1981) and glass fibers may contaminate the inseminating mixture. Since seminal plasma is still present, a washing step may be required. The recovery of motile sperm using this technique is high in comparison with others (Table 8.1). Using a modified technique, Jeyendran *et al.* (1986) demonstrated that sperm recovered from the column retain the functional integrity of their membranes after filtration. The sperm population recovered after glass-wool filtration is functionally superior to the original ejaculate in terms of zona-free hamster oocyte penetration (Rana *et al.*, 1989) and the technique appears to work well with asthenozoospermic samples (Rhemrev *et al.*, 1989) and those with high viscosity. Katayama *et al.* (1989) found that filtration of sperm resulted in a higher percentage of fertilization than did the swim-up procedure in a human IVF program. Due to the possible presence of glass-wool fibers in the inseminating mixture, care must be taken to ensure that the specimen is free of contamination before it is used for insemination.

Albumin columns

Ericsson *et al.* (1973) described the use of human serum albumin columns to separate progressively motile sperm from nonmotile forms and debris. A small volume of semen (0.5 ml) is diluted with 10% human serum and placed on a small column containing medium supplemented with 7.5–15% albumin on a discontinuous gradient. The mixture is then incubated for 60–120 minutes after which motile sperm can be recovered from the bottom of the column.

Glass & Ericsson (1978) first reported using this procedure for a case of sperm agglutinating antibodies; however, no pregnancy was achieved. Dmowski and colleagues (1979) introduced a modification of this technique in which semen was diluted (1:1 with medium), centrifuged, the sperm pellet resuspended and then motile sperm isolated on two-step albumin gradients. While albumin gradients have a good yield of sperm (Table 8.1), their use currently appears to be limited to sperm gender selection techniques.

Discontinuous or continuous gradient systems

A modified colloidal silica medium for density gradient separation of cells was developed in 1977 by Pertoft *et al.* (1977). Gorus & Pipeleers (1981) separated human sperm on the basis of their progressive motility by centrifuging fresh semen samples on these continuous Percoll (Pharmacia AB, Uppsala, Sweden) gradients. Percoll is diluted with culture medium to make solutions in the 40–90% Percoll range. These solutions are then layered on top of each other to form either discontinuous or continuous gradients, and then the semen sample is layered on top of the Percoll and centrifuged. Following centrifugation, the more progressively motile sperm are found distributed in the higher-density Percoll fractions in the bottom of the tube. One drawback to such an application is that it requires a final wash in Percoll-free physiological medium to remove colloidal silica particles from the sample. There is also the possibility of endotoxin contamination from the Percoll. The separation of sperm on Percoll has been shown to reduce bacterial contamination of the specimen (Bolton *et al.*, 1986).

While this method has proven efficacy in selecting motile sperm for insemination (Pousette *et al.*, 1986; Lalich *et al.*, 1988; Tanphaichitr *et al.*, 1988; Pardo & Bancells, 1989), recovery of motile sperm is rather low (Table 8.1). The factors regulating the recovery of sperm are the density of the sperm, sperm motility, the centrifugal force used, and the final volume of Percoll gradients (Velez, 1991). The use of Percoll gradients helps select for morphologically normal forms (Pousette *et al.*, 1986).

Other density gradient materials used for sperm isolation include Nycodenz (Nycomed Diagnostics, Oslo, Norway), an iodinated organic molecule dissolved in Tris buffer. One recent study (Gellert-Mortimer *et al.*, 1988) showed that Nycodenz gradients can be used effectively to isolate motile sperm from oligoasthenozoospermic males.

Both these density gradient techniques have been shown to improve sperm function as measured by the zona-free hamster egg bioassay (Berger *et al.*, 1985; Serafini *et al.*, 1990).

Sperm migration separation techniques

Several separation techniques utilizing physical barriers or gradients to isolate sperm on the basis of their motility are available. One such technique is a modification of the swim-up technique, in which the semen sample is overlaid with hyaluronate (Sperm Select, Pharmacia AB, Uppsala, Sweden) as described by Wikland *et al.* (1987). Hyaluronate is a linear polysaccharide (molecular weight approximately 4×10^6) that can be found in both hard and soft connective tissue. This technique creates an interface that only actively motile sperm can swim across. The advantage to Sperm Select is that it mimics cervical mucus (a linear hydrophobic glycoprotein) in composition. Sperm selected in this fashion may have decreased oxidative damage. Moreover, the sperm that are recovered can be directly inseminated, without additional processing.

Another approach combines the physical separation of sperm using a glass tube (Wang tube) that allows motile sperm migration (Wang *et al.*, 1992). The motility of the sperm swimming through the tubes can be viewed in real time by placing the device on a microscope stage. Following migration, the more motile sperm can be removed from the device and used for insemination.

Another technique which isolates sperm from seminal plasma without the initial use of centrifugation has been termed migration-sedimentation (Tea *et al.*, 1983). In this procedure, liquefied semen is layered around the outer of two concentrically arranged tubes which are then filled with medium. Motile sperm migrate up the medium column, over the lip of the inner tube and are then collected from the inner tube medium following 60 minutes of incubation. This technique seems to be particularly effective in eliminating sperm with midpiece and tail defects. Its drawback is the need to use several tubes for oligozoo-spermic or oligoasthenozoospermic samples since only a small fraction (0.3 ml) of the ejaculate can be processed in each tube.

Sephadex columns

Sephadex columns have been used to separate motile cells from semen (Graham *et al.*, 1976; Drobnis *et al.*, 1991; Zavos & Centola, 1991). Raw ejaculates are applied to the top of a hydrated column of Sephadex beads and medium. The mixture is allowed to run through the column by hydrostatic pressure, separating the motile sperm which pass through the column from immotile cells and debris which are trapped. The advantages of Sephadex column separation are its rapid separation of motile sperm and a very high recovery of motile cells, usually requiring about 15 minutes. The only apparent drawbacks to this system are the lower number of morphologically normal cells recovered when compared with swim-up preparations (Zavos & Centola, 1991; Byrd *et al.*, 1994*a*). Since seminal plasma components are still mixed with the sperm, a subsequent centrifugation step is still required. Viscous samples also tend to clog up the system.

Membrane separation of sperm from semen

While other separation systems have used gradients to block or impede non-motile sperm migration, the L4 membrane technique relies on the physical separation of sperm from semen on semipermeable membranes (Agarwal *et al.*, 1991). The L4 membrane is a fibrous polyester sheet approved for blood transfusion, and has previously been used to separate white blood cells from human serum. While the sheet does absorb white blood cells, sperm pass through freely.

To isolate sperm using this method the semen sample is first diluted with medium and then placed in a tube such as a syringe containing two L4 membranes on the bottom of the tube. The mixture is then allowed to flow through the membranes by gravity. Filtered specimens containing motile sperm are collected by centrifugation, the pellets resuspended and the resulting mixture used for insemination.

Summary

A comparison of sperm recovery using different isolation techniques for both male factor and non-male factor patients is seen in Fig. 8.1. The mean recovery rates appear better for both simple washing and Percoll density

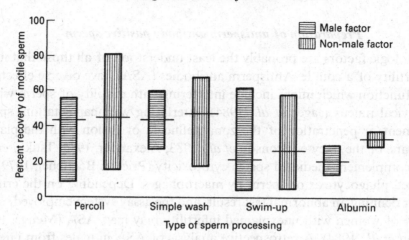

Fig. 8.1. The percent recovery of motile sperm in male factor and non-male factor patients using different sperm isolation procedures (Percoll, simple wash, swim-up, albumin) as taken from different reports in the literature. The mean percent recovery is indicated by the horizontal line through the bar; other values represent the highest and lowest recorded percent recoveries for each procedure.

centrifugation methods. There appears to be little difference in the average percentage recovery from male factor compared with nonmale factor patients. Indeed, in each case, the mean percentage motile sperm recovery was higher, although not significantly, for specimens obtained from male factor patients.

Sex selection techniques

There are several methods for enriching an inseminating fraction for X- or Y-bearing sperm (Gledhill, 1988). One of the most widely used of these has been the albumin separation technique developed by Ericsson *et al.* (1973). In one report, a male birth rate of 73% was reported using this technique in several centers (Beernink & Ericsson, 1982). However, this study and others have been criticized in the past for lack of controls, small numbers in the study groups, and the lack of prospective randomized trials (Gledhill, 1988). Despite the difficulties experienced, controlling the gender of offspring, particularly in the presence of X-linked diseases, is of considerable therapeutic interest. With the development of newer technologies, perhaps the achievement of separated sperm fractions will be feasible. In a recent report the successful separation of X- and Y-bearing human sperm was reported (Johnson *et al.*, 1993). This report demonstrated a separation of sperm with greater than 80% purity for X sperm and 75% purity for Y sperm.

Preparation of antisperm antibody positive sperm

Immunologic factors are probably the least understood of all those that influence fertility of a couple. Antisperm antibodies (ASA) have diverse effects on sperm function which might include interfering with motility of sperm within the cervical mucus (Jager *et al.*, 1984); interfering with capacitation, sperm attachment or penetration of the zona pellucida or fusion with the plasma membrane of the oocyte (Bronson *et al.*, 1983; Alexander, 1984; Tsukui *et al.*, 1986); complement-mediated sperm cytotoxicity (Price & Boettcher, 1979); or enhanced phagocytosis of sperm by macrophages. Depending on the criteria used for defining an abnormal test result, and the assay system employed, up to 10–20% of women with unexplained infertility may have ASA (Menge, 1980; Bronson *et al.*, 1984). A retrospective analysis of ASA in males from infertile couples (*n*=793) has demonstrated that 20% had significant levels of serum IgG, 11% had significant levels of serum IgA, and over 10% had significant levels of IgA and IgG on the surface of their sperm using the Immunobead test (Kutteh *et al.*, 1992). It should be noted that a large proportion of these patients had been referred with a dignosis of male factor. The degree of infertility seems to be influenced by the isotype or class of antibody as well as the site of binding of the ASA on the sperm surface (Bronson *et al.*, 1984) (see Chapter 5).

Preparation of antisperm antibody positive sperm

Several different treatments have been suggested to treat men with ASA, including corticosteroids (Haas & Maganiello, 1987) and IVF (Junk *et al.*, 1986; Clarke *et al.*, 1988). Data from studies on immunologic infertility and intrauterine insemination (IUI) suggest that pregnancy rates per cycle of between 0 and 18.5% may be achieved with male immunologic infertility (Toffle *et al.*, 1985; Confino *et al.*, 1986; Byrd *et al.*, 1987; Margalloth *et al.*, 1988; Yovich & Matson, 1988; Byrd *et al.*, 1994*b*). The wide variation in pregnancy rates may be due to the type of ASA present, their localization, and the number of sperm that are coated with ASA. It would appear from the larger study by Margalloth *et al.* (1988) that superovulation improves the chances of pregnancy in a couple with ASA.

Other methods have been suggested to remove ASA on the sperm surface prior to IUI or IVF. These include elution of antibodies from the sperm surface by washing and centrifugation (Haas *et al.*, 1988), treatment with low pH or high ionic strength media (Haas *et al.*, 1988), absorption of ASA with Immunobeads (Jeulin *et al.*, 1989), absorption with protein A (Clarke *et al.*, 1988), immune absorption of ASA (Kiser *et al.*, 1987), absorption of ASA from the seminal plasma by collection of the ejaculate into medium with a high serum concentration (Byrd *et al.*, 1994*b*), protease digestion of sperm-bound ASA (Kutteh *et al.*, 1994), and isolation of immunodepleted sperm using Percoll density centrifugation (Almagor *et al.*, 1992). Unfortunately, with most of these studies there is little information regarding the subsequent fertility of couples following these treatments. One report has prospectively analyzed the influence of exposing sperm with significant IgA or IgG surface binding to a serum-containing medium (Byrd *et al.*, 1994*b*). While serum exposure significantly reduced the levels of IgA and IgG bound to the sperm surface, there was no statistical difference in the pregnancy rates following IUI when comparing untreated with treated samples.

Development of antisperm antibodies

One question raised about the safety of placement of large numbers of sperm into the uterine cavity is whether such therapy can lead to the development of ASA (Kremer, 1979; Bronson *et al.*, 1984). Several factors are thought to prevent the formation of an immune response in these women, including the cervical filtration of sperm, phagocytosis of sperm, and the presence of immunosuppressive substances in the seminal fluid. The induction of immunity to sperm in women who have measurable antibody titers or those who have not been previously sensitized to sperm has been examined (Kremer, 1979; Sunde *et al.*, 1988; Goldberg *et al.*, 1990; Moretti-Rojas *et al.*, 1990; Friedman *et al.*, 1991). Studies have focused on measuring ASA levels in women following several cycles of IUI (Sunde *et al.*, 1988; Goldberg *et al.*, 1990). Such studies find little or no evidence to support the hypothesis that sperm antibody levels as measured by indirect Immunobead testing increase after IUI. Furthermore, Friedman *et al.* (1991) found that the presence of ASA in the male partner or the number of IUI cycles did not increase the risk of a woman developing ASA following IUI. It should be noted that it is difficult to correlate the presence of a 'positive' sperm antibody assay and clinical outcome, because of varying criteria in different laboratories. In the absence of control groups not undergoing IUI and long-term follow-up of antibody levels, more data are required before a final conclusion can be drawn.

Preparation of fresh and frozen sperm

While the quarantine and testing of donors has blocked the potential spread of sexually transmitted diseases, it has caused new concerns. Several studies have demonstrated that cryopreservation of sperm results in reduced motility and viability when compared with fresh samples (Graczykowski & Siegel, 1991). These frozen–thawed sperm suffer from a time-related decrease in fertilizing

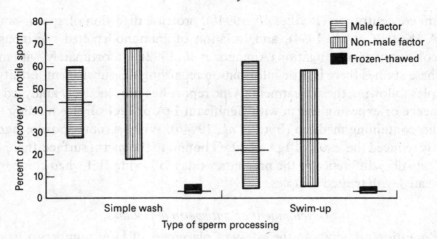

Fig. 8.2. The percent recovery of fresh and frozen–thawed sperm in male factor and non-male factor patients using two different isolation procedures (simple wash and swim-up). The mean percent recovery of motile sperm is indicated by the horizontal line through the bar; other values represent the highest and lowest recorded percent recoveries for each procedure.

capacity after washing and resuspension (Critser *et al.*, 1987; Graczykowski & Siegel, 1991). Cryopreservation significantly decreases the yield following simple washing (Graczykowski & Siegel, 1991). Cryopreserved sperm has also been reported to be less effective than freshly ejaculated sperm when comparing several different donors (Brown *et al.*, 1988). These differences between fresh and frozen sperm are probably related to the susceptibility of the sperm membranes to cryodamage.

Due to overt or latent sperm cryoinjury following freeze–thawing, different approaches have been recommended to improve fertilization potential. Prospective studies have demonstrated that utilizing IUI results in a statistically significant increase in the pregnancy rate when compared with ICI (Byrd *et al.*, 1990; Patton *et al.*, 1990). All the sperm preparation techniques listed above can be used to isolate frozen–thawed sperm. A comparison of recovery rates for fresh and frozen–thawed sperm is shown in Fig. 8.2. Only two sperm preparations are compared due to the lack of reported studies using the other techniques. However, it is clear from these data that the mean percent recovery of sperm following cryopreservation, thawing and sperm processing using either simple wash or swim-up is approximately 5% – considerably lower than the recovery rates reported for fresh sperm. There has been one prospective randomized study which has compared simple wash, Percoll density isolation, and isolation on Sephadex columns (Byrd *et al.*, 1994*a*). There were no statistical differences in the pregnancy rates using these three different preparation techniques. Isolation of motile sperm on Percoll density gradients resulted in lower pregnancy rates when compared with the other two methods.

Sperm numbers and timing of insemination

IVF, GIFT and micromanipulation techniques require only a few hundred thousand sperm, while successful pregnancies have occurred following IUI with fewer than 500 000 motile sperm (Kerin *et al.*, 1984; Byrd *et al.*, 1987; Karlstrom *et al.*, 1991). However, a review suggests that the pregnancy rate following IUI with fewer than 1 million motile sperm is quite low (Kerin & Byrd, 1989; Tucker *et al.*, 1990). In general, there is an increase in the pregnancy rate with increasing numbers of motile sperm inseminated (Shelden *et al.*, 1988; Horvath *et al.*, 1989), but no apparent advantage to insemination of more than 20 million motile cells from either fresh or frozen–thawed specimens. If fewer than 5 million motile sperm are inseminated there is a decrease in the pregnancy rate per cycle. In the case of women stimulated with hMG, however, there are two studies suggesting different results. Shelden *et al.* (1988) found that there was a significant increase in the pregnancy rate when more than 20 million motile cells were used, while Horvath *et al.* (1989) could not demonstrate a difference in the pregnancy rate in these women when from 1 million to 100 million motile sperm were used for insemination.

In the case of severe male factor, the possibility of pooling sequential ejaculates should be considered. A report by Tur-Kaspa *et al.* (1990) suggested that there is no significant difference between the quality of two sequential ejaculates. By collecting two samples within 4 hours, these may be pooled and utilized for IUI.

The timing of insemination is important, particularly with frozen sperm which has limited viability. Sperm placed in the uterus normally migrate rapidly into the fallopian tubes and peritoneal cavity (Mortimer & Templeton, 1982). There is no reservoir of sperm as seen with vaginal or intracervical sperm placement. As the survival time of sperm is not precisely known, insemination should be performed as close as possible to the anticipated time of ovulation. The most commonly used methods for timing during natural or spontaneous cycles are basal body temperature (BBT) charts, cervical mucus scores, quantitative and qualitative urinary LH concentrations and ultrasound (US) monitoring.

The detection of LH in urine or serum has been aided by the development of rapid LH kits. Urinary LH assays based on monoclonal antibodies have been used effectively to monitor ovulatory cycles. On the basis of previous published studies (Kerin & Byrd, 1989; Byrd *et al.*, 1990) the optimal time for insemination is the day after LH rise (15.8 ± 2.6 hours after the LH peak or about 30–33 hours after the LH rise in urine).

Conclusion

At present it is difficult to determine *a priori* which sperm separation method or technique to employ in a given situation. The literature has failed to resolve this issue, with some reports favoring Percoll density gradient centrifugation (Berger *et al.*, 1985; Guerin *et al.*, 1989; McClure *et al.*, 1989; Van Der Zwalmen *et al.*, 1991) and others simple swim-up techniques (Tanphaichitr *et al.*, 1988; Morales *et al.*, 1991; Englert *et al.*, 1992; Ng *et al.*, 1992). The discrepancies in these studies may be due in part to the lack of standardization in sperm preparation techniques, and to intrinsic differences in sperm populations both between and among patients. The occurrence of pregnancies that are independent of treatment, and lack of properly controlled studies, add to the confusion.

While there are still many questions regarding 'the best' sperm preparation to use, these techniques have now been firmly established in ART programs. The best suggestion is to individualize each patient's sperm preparation based on his semen analysis, the ART procedure contemplated and the results of a trial employing different isolation procedures. These evolving techniques should continue to offer motile sperm preparations that can be used to treat infertility in couples trying to achieve pregnancy.

References

Agarwal, A., Manglona, A. & Loughlin, K.R. (1991). Filtration of spermatozoa through L membrane: a new method. *Fertil. Steril.*, **56**, 1162–7.

Aitken, R.J. & Clarkson, J.S. (1987). Cellular basis of defective sperm function and its association with the genesis of reactive oxygen species by human spermatozoa. *J. Reprod. and Fertil.*, **81**, 459–69.

Alexander, N.J. (1984). Antibodies to human spermatozoa impede sperm penetration of cervical mucus or hamster eggs. *Fertil. Steril.*, **41**, 433–9.

Allen, N.C., Herbert, C.M., Maxson, W.S., Rogers, B.J., Diamond, M.P. & Wentz, A.C. (1985). Intrauterine insemination: a critical review. *Fertil. Steril.*, **44**, 569–80.

Almagor, M., Margalioth, E.J. & Yaffe, H. (1992). Density differences between spermatozoa with antisperm autoantibodies and spermatozoa covered with antisperm antibodies from serum. *Hum. Reprod.*, **7**, 959–61.

Beernink, F.J. & Ericsson, R.J. (1982). Male sex preselection through sperm isolation. *Fertil. Steril.*, **38**, 493–5.

Berger, T., Marrs, R.P. & Moyer, D.L. (1985). Comparison of techniques for selection of motile spermatozoa. *Fertil. Steril.*, **43**, 268–73.

Bolton, V.N., Warren, R.E. & Braude, P.R. (1986). Removal of bacterial contaminants from semen for *in vitro* fertilization or artificial insemination by the use of buoyant density centrifugation. *Fertil. Steril.*, **46**, 1128–32.

Bradshaw, K.D., Guzick, D.S., Grun, B., Johnson, N. & Ackerman, G. (1987). Cumulative pregnancy rates for donor insemination according to ovulatory function and tubal status. *Fertil. Steril.*, **48**, 1051–4.

Bronson, R.A., Cooper, G.W. & Rosenfeld, D.L. (1983). Complement-mediated effects of sperm head-directed human antibodies on the ability of human spermatozoa to penetrate zona-free hamster eggs. *Fertil. Steril.*, **40**, 91–5.

Bronson, R.A., Cooper, G.W. & Rosenfeld, D.L. (1984). Sperm antibodies: their role in infertility. *Fertil. Steril.*, **42**, 171–83.

Brown, C.A., Boone, W.R. & Shapiro, S.S. (1988). Improved cryopreserved semen fecundability in an alternating fresh-frozen artificial insemination program. *Fertil. Steril.*, **50**, 825–7.

Busolo, F., Zanchet, R., Lanzone, E. & Cuinato, R. (1983). Microbial flora in semen of asymptomatic infertile men. *Andrologia*, **16**, 269–75.

Byrd, W., Ackerman, G.E., Carr, B.R., Edman, C.D., Guzick, D.S. & McConnell, J.D. (1987). Treatment of refractory infertility by transcervical intrauterine insemination of washed spermatozoa. *Fertil. Steril.*, **48**, 921–7.

Byrd, W., Bradshaw, K., Carr, B., Edman, C., Odom, J. & Ackerman, G. (1990). A prospective randomized study of pregnancy rates following intrauterine and intracervical insemination using frozen donor sperm. *Fertil. Steril.*, **53**, 521–7.

Byrd, W., Drobnis, E.Z., Kutteh, W.H., Marshburn, P. & Carr, B.R. (1994a). Intrauterine insemination with frozen donor sperm: a prospective randomized trial comparing three different sperm preparation techniques. *Fertil. Steril.*, **62**, 850–6.

Byrd, W., Kutteh, W.H. & Carr, B.R. (1994b). Treatment of antibody-associated sperm with media containing high serum content: a prospective trial of fertility following intrauterine insemination in men with high sperm antibodies. *Am. J. Reprod. Immunol.*, **31**, 84–90.

Clarke, G.N., Hyne, R.W., Du Plessis, Y. & Johnston, W.I.H. (1988). Sperm antibodies and human *in vitro* fertilization. *Fertil. Steril.*, **49**, 1018–25.

Confino, E., Friberg, J., Dudkiewicz, A.B. & Gleicher, N. (1986). Intrauterine inseminations with washed human spermatozoa. *Fertil. Steril.*, **46**, 55–60.

Crister, J.K., Arneson, B.W., Aaker, D.V., Huse-Benda, A.R. & Ball, B.D. (1987). Cryopreservation of human spermatozoa. II. Postthaw chronology of motility and of zona-free hamster ova penetration. *Fertil. Steril.*, **47**, 980–4.

Dixon, R.E., Buttram, V.C. Jr & Schum, C.W. (1976). Artificial insemination using homologous semen: a review of 158 cases. *Fertil. Steril.*, **27**, 647–54.

Dmowski, W.P., Gaynor, L., Lawrence, M., Rao, R. & Scommegna, A. (1979). Artificial insemination homologous with oligospermic semen separated on albumin columns. *Fertil. Steril.*, **31**, 58–62.

Drevius, L.-O. (1971). The 'sperm-rise' test. *J. Reprod. Fertil.*, **24**, 427–9.

Drobnis, E.Z., Zhong, C.Q. & Overstreet, J.W. (1991). Separation of cryopreserved human semen using Sephadex columns, washing or Percoll gradients. *J. Androl.*, **12**, 201–8.

Englert, Y., Van den Bergh, M., Rodesch, C., Bertrand, E., Biramane, R. & Legreve, A. (1992). Comparative auto-controlled study between swim-up and Percoll preparation of fresh semen samples for *in-vitro* fertilization. *Hum. Reprod.*, **7**, 399–402.

Ericsson, R.J., Langevin, C.N. & Nishino, M. (1973). Isolation of fraction rich in human Y sperm. *Nature*, **246**, 421–4.

Friedman, A.J., Juneau-Norcross, M. & Sedensky, B. (1991). Antisperm antibody production following intrauterine insemination. *Hum. Reprod.*, **6**, 1125–8.

Gellert-Mortimer, S.T., Clark, G.N., Baker, H.W.G., Hyne, R.V. & Johnston, W.I.H. (1988). Evaluation of Nycodenz and Percoll density gradients for the selection of motile human spermatozoa. *Fertil. Steril.*, **49**, 335–41.

Glass, R.H. & Ericsson, R.J. (1978). Intrauterine insemination of isolated motile sperm. *Fertil. Steril.*, **29**, 535–9.

Gledhill, B.L. (1988). Selection and separation of X- and Y-chromosome-bearing mammalian sperm. *Gamete Res.*, **20**, 377–95.

Goldberg, J.M., Haering, P.L., Friedman, C.I., Dodds, W.G. & Kim, M.H. (1990). Antisperm antibodies in women undergoing intrauterine insemination. *Am. J. Obstet. Gynecol.*, **163**, 65–8.

Gonzales, F.G. & Pella, R.E. (1993). Swim-down: a rapid and easy method to select motile spermatozoa. *Arch. Androl.*, **30**, 29–34.

Gorus, F.K. & Pipeleers, D.G. (1981). A rapid method for the fractionation of human spermatozoa according to their progressive motility. *Fertil. Steril.*, **35**, 662–5.

Graczykowski, J.W. & Siegel, M.S. (1991). Influence of sperm processing on the fertilizing capacity and recovery of motile sperm from thawed human semen. *J. Androl.*, **26**, 155–61.

Graham, E.F., Vasquez, I.A., Schmehl, M.K.L. & Evensen, B.K. (1976). An assay of semen quality by use of Sephadex filtration. *International Congress of Animal Reproduction and Artificial Insemination*, **8**, 896–9.

Guerin, J.F., Mathieu, C., Lornage, J., Pinatel, M.C. & Boulieu, D. (1989). Improvement of survival and fertilizing capacity of human spermatozoa in an IVF program by selection on discontinuous Percoll gradients. *Hum. Reprod.*, **4**, 798–804.

Haas, G.G. Jr & Maganiello, P. (1987). A double-blind, placebo-controlled study of the use of methylprednisolone in infertile men with sperm-associated immunoglobulins. *Fertil. Steril.*, **47**, 295–301.

Haas, G.G. Jr, D'Cruz, O.J. & Denum, B. (1988). Effect of repeated washing on sperm bound immunoglobulin G. *J. Androl.*, **9**, 190–6.

Hanson, F.M. & Rock, J. (1951). Artificial insemination with husband's sperm. *Fertil. Steril.*, **2**, 162–74.

Hewitt, J., Cohen, J., Gehilly, C.B., Roland, G., Steptoe, P., Webster, J., Edwards, R.G. & Fishell, S.B. (1985). Seminal bacterial pathogens and *in vitro* fertilization. *J. In Vitro Fert. Embryo Transf.*, **41**, 260–4.

Horvath, P., Bohrer, M., Shelden, R. & Kemmann, E. (1989). The relationship of sperm parameters to cycle fecundity in superovulated women undergoing intrauterine insemination. *Fertil. Steril.*, **52**, 288–94.

Jager, S., Kremer, J. & de Wilde-Janssen, I.W. (1984). Are sperm immobilizing antibodies in cervical mucus an explanation for a poor post-coital test? *Am. J. Reprod. Immunol.*, **5**, 56–61.

Jeulin, C., Soumah, A., Da Silva, G. & De Almeida, M. (1989). *In vitro* processing of sperm with autoantibodies: analysis of sperm populations. *Hum. Reprod.*, **4**, 44–8.

Jeyendran, R.S., Perez-Pelaez, M. & Crabo, B.G. (1986). Concentration of viable spermatozoa for artificial insemination. *Fertil. Steril.*, **45**, 132–4.

Johnson, L.A., Welch, G.R., Keyvanfar, K., Dorfmann, A., Fugger, E.F. & Schulman, J.D. (1993). Gender preselection in humans? Flow cytometric separation of X and Y spermatozoa for the prevention of X-linked diseases. *Hum. Reprod.*, **8**, 1733–9.

Junk, S.M., Matson, P.L., Yovich, J.M., Bootsma, B. & Yovich, J.L. (1986). The fertilization of human oocytes by spermatozoa from men with antispermatozoal antibodies in semen. *J. In Vitro Fertil. Embryo Transf.*, **3**, 350–3.

Kanawar, K.C., Yanagimachi, R. & Lopata, A. (1979). Effects of human seminal plasma on the fertilizing capacity of human spermatozoa. *Fertil. Steril.*, **31**, 321–7.

Karlstrom, P.O., Bakos, O., Bergh, T. & Lundkvist, O. (1991). Intrauterine insemination and comparison of two methods of sperm preparation. *Hum. Reprod.*, **6**, 390–5.

Katayama, K.P., Stehlik, E. & Jeyendran, R.S. (1989). *In vitro* fertilization outcome: glass wool-filtered sperm versus swim-up sperm. *Fertil. Steril.*, **52**, 670–2.

Kerin, J. & Byrd, W. (1989). Supracervical placement of spermatozoa: utility of intrauterine and tubal insemination. In *Controversies in Reproductive Endocrinology and Infertility*, ed. M.R. Soules, pp. 183–204. New York: Elsevier.

Kerin, J.F.P., Peek, J., Warnes, G.M., Kirby, C., Jeffrey, R., Matthews, C.D. & Cox, L.W. (1984). Improved conception rate after intrauterine insemination of washed spermatozoa from men with poor quality semen. *Lancet*, **i**, 533–5.

Kiser, G.C., Alexander, J.J., Fuchs, E.F. & Fulgham, D.L. (1987). *In vitro* immune absorption of antisperm antibodies with immunobeadrise, immunomagnetic, and immunocolumn separation techniques. *Fertil. Steril.*, **47**, 466–74.

Kremer, J. (1979). A new technique for intrauterine insemination. *Int. J. Fertil.*, **24**, 53–6.

Kutteh, W.H., McAllister, D., Byrd, W. & Mestecky, J. (1992). Antisperm antibodies: current knowledge and new horizons. *Mol. Androl.*, **4**, 183–93.

Lalich, R.A., Marut, E.L., Prins, G.S. & Scommegna, A. (1988). Life table analysis of intrauterine insemination pregnancy rates. *Am. J. Obstet. Gynecol.*, **158**, 980–4.

Lopata, A., Patullo, M.J., Chang, A. & James, B. (1976). A method for collecting motile spermatozoa from human semen. *Fertil. Steril.*, **27**, 677–84.

Margalloth, E.J., Sauter, E., Bronson, R.A., Rosenfeld, D.L., School, G.M. & Cooper, G.W. (1988). Intrauterine insemination as treatment for antisperm antibodies in the female. *Fertil. Steril.*, **50**, 441–6.

Mastroianni, L. Jr, Laberge, J.L. & Rock, J. (1957). Appraisal of the efficacy of artificial insemination with husband's sperm and evaluation of insemination techniques. *Fertil. Steril.*, **8**, 260–6.

McClure, R.D., Nunes, L. & Tom, R. (1989). Semen manipulation: improved sperm recovery and function with a two-layer Percoll gradient. *Fertil. Steril.*, **51**, 874–7.

Menge, A.C. (1980). Clinical immunologic infertility: diagnostic measures, incidence of antisperm antibodies. In *Immunologic Aspects of Infertility and Fertility*, ed. D.S. Dhindsa & G.F.B. Schumacher, p. 205. New York: Elsevier.

Morales, P., Vantman, D., Barros, C. & Vigil, P. (1991). Human spermatozoa selected by Percoll gradient or swim-up are equally capable of binding to the human zona pellucida and undergoing the acrosome reaction. *Fertil. Steril.*, **6**, 401–4.

Moretti-Rojas, I., Rojas, F.J., Leisure, M., Stone, S.C. & Asch, R.H. (1990). Intrauterine inseminations with washed human spermatozoa does not induce formation of antisperm antibodies. *Fertil. Steril.*, **53**, 180–2.

Mortimer, D. (1991). Sperm preparation techniques and iatrogenic failures of *in-vitro* fertilization. *Hum. Reprod.*, **6**, 173–6.

Mortimer, D. & Templeton, A.A. (1982). Sperm transport in the human female reproductive tract in relation to semen analysis characteristics and time of ovulation. *J. Reprod. Fertil.*, **64**, 401–8.

Ng, F.L.H., Liu, D.L. & Baker, H.W.G. (1992). Comparison of Percoll, mini-Percoll and swim-up methods for sperm preparation from abnormal semen samples. *Hum. Reprod.*, **7**, 261–6.

Pardo, M. & Bancells, N. (1989). Artificial insemination with husband's sperm (AIH): techniques for sperm selection. *Arch. Androl.*, **22**, 15–27.

Patton, P.E., Burry, K.A., Novy, M.J. & Wolf, D.P. (1990). A comparative evaluation of intracervical and intrauterine routes in donor therapeutic insemination. *Hum. Reprod.*, **5**, 263–5.

Paulson, J.D., Polakoski, K. & Leto, S. (1979). Further characterization of glass wool column filtration of human semen. *Fertil. Steril.*, **32**, 125–6.

Pertoft, H.C. & Laurent, T.C. (1977). Isopycnic separation of cells and cell organelles on centrifugation in modified colloidal silica gradients. In *Methods of Cell Separation*, vol. 1, ed. N. Catsimpoolas. pp. 25–32. New York: Plenum Press.

Pousette, A., Akerlof, E., Rosenborg, L. & Fredricsson, B. (1986). Increase in progressive motility and improved morphology of human spermatozoa following their migration through Percoll gradients. *Int. J. Androl.*, **9**, 1–13.

Price, R.J. & Boettcher, B. (1979). The presence of complement in human cervical mucus and its possible relevance to infertility in women with complement-dependent sperm-immobilizing antibodies. *Fertil. Steril.*, **32**, 61–4.

Rana, N., Jeyendran, R.S., Holmgren, W.J., Rotman, C. & Zaneveld, L.J.D. (1989). Glass wool-filtered spermatozoa and their oocyte penetrating capacity. *J. In Vitro Fertil. Embryo Transf.*, **6**, 280–4.

Rhemrev, J., Jeyendran, R.S., Vermeiden, J.P.W.& Zaneveld, L.J.D. (1989). Human sperm separation by glass wool filtration and two-layer, discontinuous Percoll gradient centrifugation. *Fertil. Steril.*, **51**, 685–90.

Russell, L.D. & Rogers, B.J. (1987). Improvement in the quality and fertilization potential of a human sperm population using the rise technique. *J. Androl.*, **8**, 25–33.

Sacks, P.C. & Simon, J.A. (1991). Infectious complications of intrauterine insemination: a case report and literature review. *Int. J. Fertil.*, **36**, 331–9.

Serafini, P., Blank, W., Tran, C., Mansourian, M., Tan, T. & Batzofin, J. (1990). Enhanced penetration of zona-free hamster ova by sperm prepared by Nycodenz and Percoll gradient centrifugation. *Fertil. Steril.*, **53**, 551–5.

Settlage, D.S.F., Motoshima, M. & Tredway, D.R. (1973). Sperm transport from the external cervical os to the fallopian tubes in women: a time and quantitation study. *Fertil. Steril.*, **24**, 655–61.

Shelden, R., Kemmann, E., Bohrer, M. & Pasquale, S. (1988). Multiple gestation is associated with the use of high sperm numbers in the intrauterine insemination specimen in women undergoing gonadotropin stimulation. *Fertil. Steril.*, **49**, 607–10.

Sherman, J.K., Paulson, J.D. & Liu, K.C. (1981). Effect of glass wool filtration on ultrastructure of human spermatozoa. *Fertil. Steril.*, **36**, 643–7.

Sunde, A., Kahn, J. & Molne, K. (1988). Intrauterine Insemination. *Hum. Reprod.*, **193**, 97–9.

Tanphaichitr, N., Agulnick, A., Seibel, M. & Taymor, M. (1988). Comparison of the *in vitro* fertilization rate by human sperm capacitated by multi-tube swim-up and Percoll gradient centrifugation. *J. In Vitro Fert. Embryo Transf.*, **5**, 119–22.

Tarlatzia, B.C., Bontis, J., Kolibianakis, E.M., Sanopoulou, T., Papadimas, J., Lagos, S. & Mantalenakis, S. (1991). Evaluation of intrauterine insemination with washed spermatozoa from the husband in the treatment of infertility. *Hum. Reprod.*, **6**, 1241–6.

Tea, N.T., Jondet, M. & Scholler, R. (1983). Oricede d'isolement de spermatozoides mobiles du sperme humain par la methode de migration-sedimentation. *Pathol. Biol.*, **31**,688–93.

Toffle, R.C., Nagel, T.C., Tagatz, G.E., Phansey, S.A., Okagaki, T. & Wavrin, C.A. (1985). Intrauterine insemination: the University of Minnesota experience. *Fertil. Steril.*, **43**, 743–7.

Tsukui, S., Noda, Y., Yano, J., Fukuda, A. & Moti, T. (1986). Inhibition of sperm penetration through human zona pellucida by antisperm antibodies. *Fertil. Steril.*, **46**, 92–6.

Tucker, M.J., Wong, C.J.Y., Chang, Y.M., Leong, K.H. & Leung, C.K.M. (1990). Intrauterine insemination as frontline treatment for non-tubal infertility. *Asia Oceania, J. Obst. Gynecol.*, **16**, 137–43.

Tur-Kaspa, I., Dudkiewicz, A., Confino, E. & Gleicher, R. (1990). Pooled sequential ejaculates: a way to increase the total number of motile sperm from oligospermic men. *Fertil. Steril.*, **54**, 906–9.

Van Der Zwalmen, P., Bertin-Segal, G., Geerts, L., Debauche, C. & Schoysman, R. (1991). Sperm morphology and IVF pregnancy rate: comparison between Percoll gradient centrifugation and swim-up procedures. *Hum. Reprod.*, **6**, 581–8.

Velez de la Calle, J.F. (1991). Human spermatozoa selection in improved discontinuous Percoll gradients. *Fertil. Steril.*, **56**, 737–42.

Wang, F.N., Lin, C.T., Hong, C.Y., Hsiung, C.H., Su, T.P. & Tsai, H.D. (1992). Modification of the Wang Tube to improve *in vitro* semen manipulation. *Arch. Androl.*, **29**, 267–9.

Wikland, M., Wik, O., Steen, Y., Qvist, K., Soderlund, B. & Janson, P.O. (1987). A self-migration method for preparation of sperm for *in-vitro* fertilization. *Hum. Reprod.*, **3**, 191–5.

Wolf, D.P. & Soksloski, J.E. (1982). Characterization of the sperm penetration assay. *J. Androl.*, **3**, 445–51.

Yovich, J.L. & Matson, P.L. (1988). The treatment of infertility by the high intrauterine insemination of husband's washed spermatozoa. *Hum. Reprod.*, **3**, 939–43.

Zavos, P.M. & Centola, G.M. (1991). Selection of sperm from oligozoospermic men for ARTA: comparisons between swim-up and Spermprep filtration. *ARTA*, **1**, 338–45.

Zavos, P.M. & Wilson, E.A. (1984). Retrograde ejaculation: etiology and treatment via the use of a new noninvasive method. *Fertil. Steril.*, **42**, 627–632.

9

New assays for evaluating sperm function

LANI J. BURKMAN

Introduction: Functional assays versus cell markers

Physicians and scientists dealing with the practical aspects of male infertility are driven towards the goal of identifying *why* the spermatozoa from a particular man have not achieved fertilization (diagnostic) and *whether* the sperm from a particular man have the capacity to fertilize an egg (prognostic). Furthermore, the information gathered will, it is hoped, lead to a *therapeutic* strategy for correcting or bypassing spermatozoal defects. The information at these three levels (diagnostic/prognostic/therapeutic) must come from quantitative and qualitative analysis of either cell *markers* or assays of *sperm function*. Cell markers differ from sperm functional assays, particularly in their contribution to clinical decision-making.

Evaluation of sperm markers gives information about the presence of a cellular factor, anatomic feature or cell response. The test yields a yes/no answer, or quantitates the level or concentration of the marker. These data allow the investigator to conclude that the patient is similar to fertile men or, conversely, similar to subfertile populations with respect to the marker. Today, examples of cell or fertility markers include: sperm viability, sperm density, percent motility, morphology, grade of progression (on a scale of 1 to 4), mean velocity, mean head amplitude (ALH), hyperosmotic swelling of the flagellar membrane (HOS), intracellular ATP concentration, level of creatine phosphokinase and presence of intact acrosomes. Acceptable levels of these markers have a direct or indirect relationship to necessary sperm functions. For some of these cell markers, it is obvious that its complete absence precludes normal fertilization (e.g. lack of motility or complete absence of acrosomes). More importantly, however, a normal level for *all* of the markers listed above does not lead one to the conclusion that the sperm population is assuredly fertile (Calvo *et al.*, 1989).

In contrast to sperm markers, assays of sperm function could be defined as measuring the ability of sperm to complete a physiologic process which is clas-

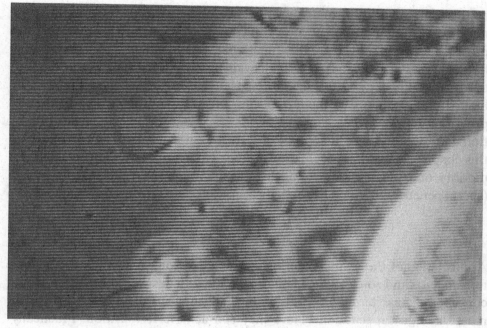

Fig. 9.1. Videomicrograph of human hyperactivated sperm attached to surface of non-living human zona pellucida (× 600).

sically viewed as *requisite* for fertilization *in vivo*. A mammalian spermatozoon must complete each of the following processes in order to achieve fertilization by natural means: penetrate the cervical mucus, arrive at the ampulla of the oviduct (by effective flagellar motion and interaction with the female reproductive tract), penetrate the cumulus oophorus, bind to the zona pellucida, complete the acrosome reaction, penetrate the zona pellucida (by chemical release and vigorous sperm motility; see Fig. 9.1), bind to the oolemma, and provide a nucleus which can decondense and interact with the maternal chromosomes (Yanagimachi, 1988). Some infertility clinics have even viewed human *in vitro* fertilization (IVF) as the ultimate functional test; however, if this test fails, one has not necessarily gained useful information concerning which physiologic process in fertilization was deficient.

Our current understanding of sperm capacitation and the fertilization process is somewhat rudimentary. This is reflected in the fact that virtually all the functional assays used today rely on gross visual assessment. Examples include scoring hamster egg penetrations (decondensed sperm heads and presence of tails in the ooplasm; Rogers, 1985), acrosome reactions (staining or fluorescence over the sperm head) and binding of sperm to the zona pellucida (counting of sperm on the zona surface: Burkman *et al.*, 1988*a*). One exception to this is the detection of hyperactivated sperm patterns by computerized motility analysis (Burkman, 1991). Just as with some of the cell markers, proven failure in *any* of these functional assays would preclude normal fertilization. An excellent result in all available functional tests would support the prediction of good fertilization capacity. However, in view of our still limited understanding of the fertilization process, these same data could not prove that fertilization will occur. It is also true that reliance on any one functional assay cannot give assurance of fertilization potential. The remainder of this chapter will address evaluation of the acrosome reaction, hyperactivated motility and, finally, assays utilizing the human zona pellucida. The SPA (sperm penetration assay) has already been considered in depth in chapter 6.

Sperm capacitation

Appreciation of these three functional topics (acrosome reaction, hyperactivation analysis and zona pellucida binding) requires a basic understanding of the concept of 'capacitation.' In 1951, both Chang and Austin reported that sperm must undergo capacitation before they can achieve fertilization. Practically speaking, this means that freshly ejaculated sperm (from the human or any other mammal) are not yet capable of fertilizing an egg (see Yanagimachi, 1988). After separation from the seminal plasma, these sperm require a period of residence within the female reproductive tract (or incubation with an appropriate fertilization medium). During this capacitation period, the spermatozoon is altered (Yanagimachi, 1988; Katz *et al.*, 1989) in a number of ways, including changes in the outer sperm membrane structure (fluidity, lipid content, loss of certain proteins, exposure of other proteins), altered metabolism and increased vigor of swimming. There has been some debate (Bedford, 1983; Chang, 1984) on the precise endpoint that defines the completion of the capacitation process. One such definition refers to a series of physiologic changes in sperm that render the spermatozoa capable of fertilizing eggs (Austin, 1952). The most popular position, however, is that a sperm which has begun to exhibit hyperactivated movements and is ready to initiate the acrosome reaction has become 'fully capacitated' (Katz *et al.*, 1989).

Assays of the human acrosome reaction

The mammalian sperm acrosome is a specialized cap or double-membraned compartment which covers the anterior portion of the sperm head (Fig. 9.2). This structure contains a number of enzymes, including acrosin and hyaluronidase, which were packaged then applied to the surface of the sperm

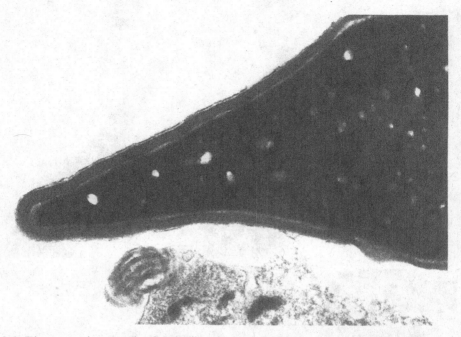

Fig. 9.2. Electron micrograph of a section through a human sperm with the acrosome intact (× 45 000).

nucleus as the cell developed in the testis (Yanagimachi, 1988). After ejaculation (or special handling of cauda epididymal sperm) and appropriate washing and incubation, the acrosome reaction (AR) can be initiated *in vitro*. Onset of the acrosome reaction can be triggered physiologically by interaction with the egg and its vestments, occur spontaneously in culture medium alone, or be artificially stimulated by chemicals added to the incubation medium (see below).

The origins of an acrosome 'assay' are related to the early fertilization work in small rodents. Not only did mice, hamsters, guinea pigs and rats provide the earliest observations of sperm–egg interaction, these species also had spermatozoa with large acrosomes, easily studied at the light microscopic level (Yanagimachi, 1988). Compared with these laboratory animals, where the progress of sperm capacitation could be monitored by directly observing the swelling and shedding of the acrosomal cap, the acrosome of the human spermatozoon is small and difficult to visualize. Until recently, evaluation of the human acrosome reaction (Fig. 9.3) was limited principally to electron microscopic studies (Talbot & Chacon, 1980). Hence, the development of more practical assays of acrosome reaction potential in the human has been a major goal. A short introduction to the more popular methods for acrosomal assessment

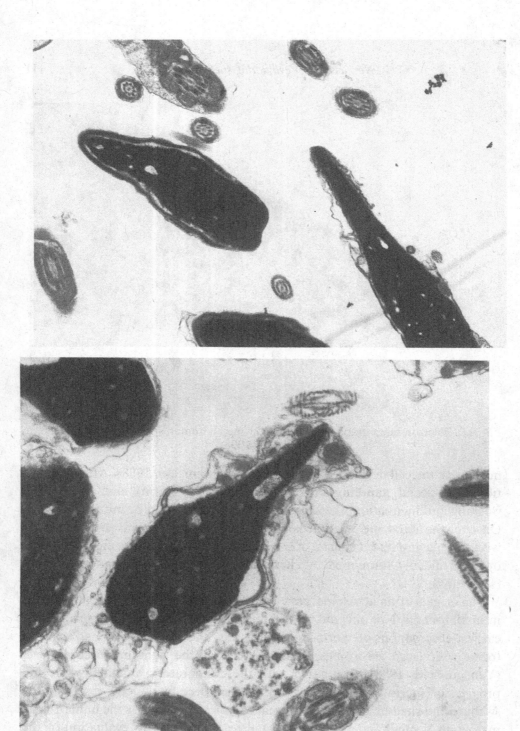

Fig. 9.3. Two electron micrographs of sections through human sperm. Top: sperm on the left has an intact acrosome; the acrosome of the sperm at the right has reacted and is partially shed. Bottom: Human sperm with acrosome reaction nearly completed. Note the vesicles as well as the expanded and ruffled outer acrosomal membrane.

will be followed by a discussion of their relative advantages and clinical interpretation.

A simple, tri-color staining method to evaluate acrosomes was published in 1981 by Talbot and Chacon. A washed sperm sample is first incubated with trypan blue to distinguish dead cells, smeared on slides, then exposed to the stains rose bengal and bismarck brown. If the procedures are followed for careful preparation of the staining solutions, temperature control and correct timing of exposure (Talbot & Dudenhausen, 1981), these slides give very good differentiation of viability (dead cells are stained purple), presence of an intact acrosome (rose color over the apical, acrosomal region) or loss of the acrosome (acrosome reaction; gold and white color over the entire sperm head). This triple-stain assay requires little equipment and has been used in a number of publications by many laboratories.

Fluorescence microscopy, coupled with the development of appropriate 'probes' of the human acrosome, has provided several options for assessing either the internal compartment of the human acrosome or the outer acrosomal surface (Cross & Meizel, 1989, for review and excellent figures). If sperm smeared on a slide are permeabilized with methanol, then certain plant lectins or specific antibodies can detect intracellular material in the acrosomal region. These probes include the HS21 antibody (Wolf et al., 1985), monoclonal antibodies (Humagen, Virginia; Laboratoire Theramex (GB24) Monaco), and fluorescein isothiocyanate (FITC) labelled lectins conjugated with concanavalin A, Pisum sativum agglutinin from the pea or PNA from peanuts. When these probes are taken up by acrosome-intact cells (see Cross & Meizel, 1989) the acrosome is brightly fluorescent, while acrosome-reacted cells show either no fluorescence or have a bright band at the equatorial region (see also Tesarik et al., 1993). Secondly, acrosomal status can be examined by fluorescent methods which utilize other probes directed to the external surface of the sperm acrosome. In addition to monoclonal antibodies (Saling & Lakoski, 1985), sperm labelled with the antibiotic chlortetracycline (CTC) will exhibit specific fluorescent patterns before finally completing the acrosome reaction (Ward & Storey, 1984; Lee et al., 1987). The acrosomal method chosen by individual laboratories will depend on: (1) the availability of a fluorescence microscope, (2) the labor to be invested (with CTC as the fastest, triple-stain intermediate, and other probes requiring the most labor), and (3) desired stability of the preparation (CTC least, 1–2 days for other fluorescent probes, and years for triple-stain).

The principal issues in considering an assay of acrosome function may relate to assay reliability and relevance of the information to clinical decision-making. According to several studies, different methodologies can give very similar results (Talbot & Chacon, 1980, 1981; Kallajoki et al., 1986). If one first considers spontaneous acrosomal loss in freshly prepared samples (less than 1 hour of capacitation), then the acrosome reaction (AR) rate is typically 5–10% (Byrd *et al.*, 1989). If human sperm are incubated for several hours in common fertilization media, the maximal rate of spontaneous AR is of the order of 25–35% of the total sperm population. Many investigators argue that this spontaneous AR rate is not meaningful (Cummins *et al.*, 1991), since dying sperm can shed their acrosome, and the event is occurring in the absence of a physiological stimulus such as zona pellucida or the follicular fluid. Evidence exists that sperm from some subfertile men spontaneously lose their acrosomes faster than fertile men. Therefore, fresh samples which reflect a 15% or 20% AR have a reduced fertilization potential due to this acrosomal instability.

In contrast to spontaneous AR, some clinics are evaluating subfertile men by means of a new category of acrosome reaction tests described as 'induced' or 'stimulated' AR assays. Here the sperm are briefly incubated with factors which induce an AR, such as follicular fluid, calcium ionophores or phosphodiesterase inhibitors. Following incubation, the sperm acrosomes are examined according to the triple-stain method or with fluorescent probes (Calvo *et al.*, 1989; Anderson *et al.*, 1992). In general, these stimulated protocols demonstrate overall AR rates of up to 50–80% of all sperm for proven fertile samples. One study evaluated the AR response of sperm samples proven infertile during human IVF (Pampiglione *et al.*, 1993). When stimulated with calcium ionophore A23187, such samples had a mean AR rate of 34%, significantly lower than the mean of 64% seen with men proven fertile with IVF. This study suggested that an AR result <31% was predictive of IVF failure. As the AR is a required step in the fertilization process, evaluations of initial acrosomal status and/or the potential for normal levels of AR can provide unique information on patient prognosis.

Assays of sperm hyperactivation potential

Hyperactivation (HA) is a distinctive, vigorous type of movement observed during sperm capacitation and is closely associated with ovulation and fertilization (Yanagimachi, 1988). Sperm HA is apparently required for zona pellucida penetration (Fraser, 1981; Fleming & Yanagimachi, 1982) and perhaps also for effective oviductal sperm transport and penetration of the cumulus oophorus (Katz *et al.*, 1989; Tesarik *et al.*, 1990). During the past decade, successful *in vitro* therapy for human fertilization has provided the critical milieu for observing human sperm movements in the context of proven fertilization (Burkman, 1984; Mortimer *et al.*, 1984). For further discussion on the early investigations of HA motility and its physiology, the reader is referred to the 1990 review by Burkman. When compared with the common protocols

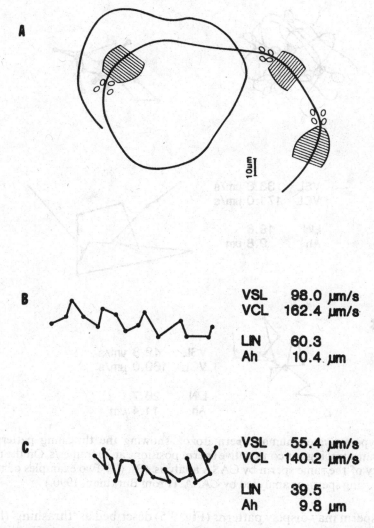

Fig. 9.4. Hyperactivated human spermatozoa showing the circling, high-curvature pattern. (A) Circling sperm as seen directly at the microscope. (B), (C) Two examples of the track and movement data from CASA analysis (30 frames; velocity, linearity, ALH). (From Burkman, 1990.)

for hamster egg penetration (Chapter 6) and acrosome reactions, evaluation of human sperm HA is relatively recent and still evolving.

In contrast to sperm movement in semen, the individual HA sperm in a washed preparation have a very non-linear path, that is, they swim with less 'forward progression.' Sperm expressing the most common HA pattern (Fig. 9.4) have a quasi-circular path (about 50–200 µm in diameter) with vigorous side-to-side head movements (the amplitude of the head displacement, ALH, is large).

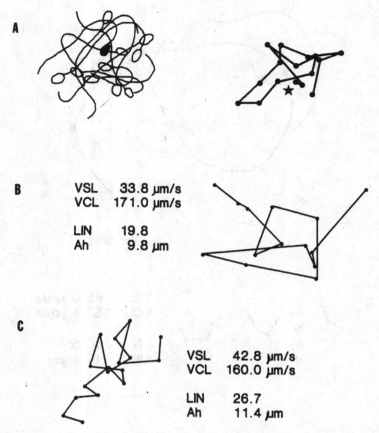

Fig. 9.5. Hyperactivated human spermatozoa showing the thrashing pattern. (A) Frame-by-frame tracings of consecutive sperm positions at 30 frames/s. On the right is the trajectory of the same sperm by CASA analysis. (B), (C) Two examples of thrashing sperm as analyzed by CASA. (From Burkman, 1990.)

Other HA sperm may display patterns (Fig. 9.5) described as 'thrashing' (having an extremely erratic trajectory), 'helical' or 'star-spin' (spinning in place and sometimes stuck to the glass: see figures in Burkman, 1990). In the human, multiphasic HA spermatozoa may switch from one pattern to another (Burkman, 1990). When HA motility is studied over 24 hours, the observer will note that in human sperm, HA is not a well-synchronized phenomenon. In other words, among the sperm which acquire HA, one subpopulation will show HA early in capacitation, while other HA populations will appear later (see Burkman, 1990).

Since the initial publications in 1984, a number of techniques have been applied to the study of human HA: direct visualization, slow-motion analysis of videotapes, multiple-exposure photography (MEP), or computer-assisted analysis using digitized images (CASA). Burkman (1991) and Mortimer &

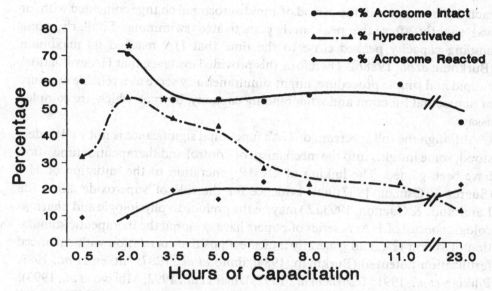

Fig. 9.6. Simultaneous monitoring of sperm acrosomal status (by monoclonal antibody) and changes in hyperactivated motility over 23 hours. Data were pooled over four experiments, using synchronized sperm populations from four fertile men. (See Burkman *et al.*, 1988*b*, Burkman, 1990, for more detail.)

Mortimer (1990) arrived at similar threshold criteria for the automatic identification of classic sperm hyperactivation by CASA methods. The criteria published by Pilikian *et al.* (1991) and Mbizvo *et al.* (1993) are somewhat more lenient. In contrast, the first group to publish CASA studies of hyperactivation (Robertson *et al.*, 1988; Mack *et al.*, 1988) espoused a definition which accepts only a fraction of the HA sperm identified by the other laboratories (i.e. only thrash, star, and a portion of the helical sperm) (see Burkman, 1990).

Early studies on human HA have suggested that it might serve as a visually accessible marker reflecting both acrosomal status and egg binding capacity, thus indicating that an HA assay could have value. In 1987, Jinno *et al.* showed that sperm populations having high levels of HA penetrated hamster ova at a high rate and, conversely, sperm which exhibited low HA showed significantly less egg penetration. Since the hamster assay outcome is an indirect measure of completed acrosome reactions (Zaneveld & Jeyendran, 1988), the data of Jinno *et al.* implied that sperm samples showing high levels of HA are also undergoing the acrosome reaction at a relatively high rate. Thus, assessment of the peak incidence of HA may be indicative of the potential for completing the functional acrosomal reaction. Secondly, a study on the kinetics of capacitation and egg interaction confirmed the physiologic link between HA and acrosome reactions as well as zona binding (Fig. 9.6; Burkman *et al.*, 1988*b*). For each donor examined, the period of rapid acrosomal change coincided with, or was slightly after, the peak in hyperactivated swimming. Similarly, zona binding capacity peaked close to the time that HA reached its maximum (Burkman *et al.*, 1988*b*). Therefore, this provided evidence that HA evaluation, a rapid and simple procedure, might simultaneously serve as a reliable measure of acrosomal function and zona binding capacity, both of which are complex assays.

Although the full spectrum of HA's functional significance is not well understood, some insights into the mechanism of control and therapeutic stimulation have been gained. The linking of cAMP generation to the initiation of HA (Suarez & Osman, 1987) and evidence for the role of superoxide anion (de Lamirande & Gagnon, 1993*a,b*) may be the prelude to physiologic and pharmacologic control of HA. A series of papers have explored the therapeutic stimulation of sperm HA, and generally indicate a positive correlation with enhanced fertilization potential (Burkman, 1984; Jinno *et al.*, 1987; Aitken *et al.*, 1986; Pilikian *et al.*, 1991; Tesarik *et al.*, 1992; Uhler *et al.*, 1992; Mbizvo *et al.*, 1993).

Confidence in the clinical use of an HA assay rests on its repeatability as well as the degree to which it can predict poor fertilization. The correlation of HA with good fertilizing potential was first evident in 1984 (Burkman, 1984) when investigating the mean incidence of HA in sperm from men requesting IVF therapy: the mean %HA for subfertile men (8%) was significantly less than the mean for a group of men proven fertile during IVF (20%; semi-objective video-analysis). In a second study, seven men proven infertile during IVF were compared with a proven fertile group: the mean %HA for the infertile group was only half that of the fertile group ($p<0.05$; Coddington *et al.*, 1991). This latter study also showed that the HA capacity was statistically and positively correlated with sperm zona binding potential and sperm morphology.

The repeatability of HA assay results within a given man was confirmed in a later report (Burkman & Samrock, 1992). This study of 18 donors and patients examined paired HA assays (i.e. each assay compared with the *subsequent* test for that man). For these assay pairs, peak %HA was consistent 89% of the time. In other words, a man with low %HA on the first test again showed low %HA on the subsequent test. Likewise, men whose first assay yielded a high %HA would show a high HA value for the subsequent test. These results indicate that a diagnostic, prescreening HA test may reliably predict the HA potential of another semen sample obtained on the day of the therapeutic procedure (intra-uterine insemination or IVF).

Computer-assisted identification of HA has also demonstrated that its careful assessment could be predictive of fertilization success during IVF. Karande *et al.* (1990, 1996) reported that 89% of the IVF cases with excellent fertilization rates could be predicted using two HA endpoints (see below). The automated SORT option in a Hamilton Thorne Motility Analyzer was used to detect classic HA patterns based on three criteria: curvilinear velocity ≥ 100 μm/s, ALH ≥ 7.5 μm and, simultaneously, linearity ≤ 65 (Burkman, 1991). Since men vary as to the capacitation time required to support peak HA (Burkman, 1986), motility was evaluated at both 2 hours and 4 hours of capacitation. Analysis of the data indicated that the relative *change* in %HA between the two timepoints, and the *lowest* HA percentage for that patient, would help predict subnormal fertilization rates in IVF. Specifically, two negative HA conditions were identified for the 38 cases studied: (1) when the *lower* of the two HA values was $\leq 15\%$, and (2) when the slope between the two HA values was flat. When the sperm population exhibited only one or neither of these conditions ($n=27$), 89% of cases showed a good fertilization rate ($\geq 75\%$). When neither problem existed, all the cases had a good fertilization rate (5/5). However, when both negative conditions existed ($n=11$), only half the cases had a good fertilization rate despite very high IVF insemination concentrations (Karande *et al.*, 1990, 1996). These data are a key indication that prescreening of IVF patients (or potential intrauterine insemination cases) may provide substantial guidance as to their fertilization potential and the specialized handling by the laboratory personnel.

As individual laboratories and clinics explore the feasibility of an HA assay, attention must be given to the impact of changing medium, protein supplement, chamber depth or other assay parameters. The incidence of HA will be considerably lower in certain simple media when compared with common IVF media (i.e. BWW versus Ham's F10 or HTF); in samples held at room temperature versus 37°C; in media supplemented with bovine serum albumin in contrast to human serum albumin or human serum; or in media buffered to lower pH values (7.0–7.4). For better standardization of conditions, use of Ham's F10 and 3 mg/ml human serum albumin is the recommendation whenever data will be compared between laboratories. To avoid spatial limitations on the vigorously moving flagellum, the sperm should be examined in a chamber with a depth exceeding 30 μm, since the flagellar beat envelope can exceed 25 μm (Burkman, 1984). If the concentration of sperm in each viewing field is excessive, error can be introduced, whether HA is analyzed visually or by CASA. Therefore, the number of motile sperm swimming within the field of view should be limited to approximately 20–30. The final values should be based on analysis of the movements of at least 200 motile sperm. If CASA systems are used to identify HA automatically, the user must be cognizant of the threshold criteria which underlie this detection and their impact on the data interpretation (see Chapter 4).

The maximal HA values reported recently by various laboratories are dependent on the choice of CASA set up parameters. Relatively low HA values, varying approximately from 0 to 10%, are evident in the papers by Grunert *et al.* (1990), Wang *et al.* (1991) and Pearlstone *et al.* (1993), reflecting their use of the Robertson/Mack guidelines. In contrast, Tesarik *et al.* (1992), Murad *et al.* (1992), and de Lamirande & Gagnon (1993*a,b*) found HA values as high as 30% when using the criteria of Mortimer & Mortimer (1990) or Burkman (1991). Interestingly, Wang *et al.* (1993) analyzed their HA data twice, using different HA criteria. The expected differences in HA magnitude were confirmed, but the results from the two systems were highly correlated ($r=0.85$, $p<0.001$). These conclusions remind us that an increase or decrease in *any* HA swimming pattern (star, helical, circling, etc.), or the sum *total* of these patterns, is a true measure of change in sperm function. These changes in HA reflect sperm responsiveness to capacitating conditions, exposure to toxins, or stimulatory factors.

This sensitivity of HA to the immediate conditions leads to one additional practical use of HA in the laboratory: monitoring of human sperm HA as a highly efficient quality control assay. In contrast to other sperm functional changes such as the acrosome reaction, HA is a unique mode in motility which may be acquired for a short while and is then eventually *lost* by the individual sperm. Therefore, poor culture conditions may suppress acquisition of HA or may curtail the duration of the HA state in a given sperm. Burkman (1994) has reported the use of HA analysis in media quality control.

Functional assays utilizing the zona pellucida

The most persuasive test conditions for predicting fertilization potential have relied on the physiology of the egg or the zona pellucida, since these functions epitomize normal fertilization. Despite the advances made in animal fertilization research in the 1960s and early 1970s (Yanagimachi, 1981), the sperm–zona specificity encountered in mammalian species frustrated attempts to use surrogate intact eggs for human fertilization research. The pioneers of the 1970s took bold steps to isolate human oocytes for direct but controversial examination of sperm fertilization potential (see Edwards, 1974). In 1976, two new functional assays were introduced which permitted surrogate, *in vitro* testing of human sperm competence. The zona-free hamster ovum penetration assay (Yanagimachi *et al.*, 1976; see Chapter 6) and the non-living human zona penetration test (Overstreet & Hembree, 1976) served as catalysts for a new wave of clinically relevant research on human sperm capacitation and motility.

As IVF became an established therapy in infertility clinics worldwide, increased access to non-viable oocytes spurred interest in zona-based functional assays. Overstreet & Hembree (1976) dissected post-morten ovarian tissue to recover zona-intact human oocytes. The fresh or DMSO-stored oocytes were coincubated with washed human spermatozoa for up to 24 hours, then gently rolled under a coverslip for identification of sperm which had penetrated into the zona pellucida or perivitelline space. Overstreet and colleagues have exploited the assay's unique capabilities to demonstrate prediction of fertilizing potential (Overstreet *et al.*, 1980*a*), development of an *in vitro* capacitation system (Overstreet *et al.*, 1980*b*), and new findings on the kinetics of sperm–egg binding (Singer *et al.*, 1985). A second group of investigators (Liu *et al.*, 1989) has recently confirmed the power of this zona-intact sperm assay in predicting subsequent IVF outcome. Their use of competitive zona binding by fluorescently labelled sperm is a revised application of previous protocols (Overstreet & Hembree, 1976; Blazak *et al.*, 1982). If the oocytes are available, whole-zona assays require relatively simple equipment, can be completed within several hours, and demonstrate a very good correlation with the patient's fertilization capacity.

The most recent concept in sperm–zona fertilization tests is the hemizona assay (HZA; Burkman *et al.* 1988*a*), which merges the old zona penetration assay with newer micromanipulation approaches. In 1986, our interest with a gamete interaction assay had turned towards investigation of hyperactivated sperm as they approached and attached to the human zona pellucida (see Fig. 9.1; Burkman & Coddington, 1986). By carefully cutting a zona pellucida in half, it was theoretically possible to test two different sperm populations on each half of the same zona (internal control). The availability of matching zona halves (hemizonae) would solve the problematic inter-egg variation in oocyte fertilization capacity which was apparent from IVF studies (Franken *et al.*, 1991; Overstreet *et al.*, 1980*a*). In addition to studies of sperm physiology (Burkman *et al.*, 1988*b*), early trials showed promise for comparing the zona binding of sperm from infertile men versus sperm from prospective IVF patients.

The initial validation of the HZA addressed a dozen critical questions. Individual studies (Burkman *et al.*, 1988*a*) demonstrated that the zona could be reliably cut into equal halves (Fig. 9.7), cutting did not impair binding capacity, the matching halves had equivalent potentials for binding and maximal sperm binding occurred after 4–5 hours of coincubation. Using spermatozoa from infertile men and donors, subsequent reports from several laboratories have further concluded that sperm HA was significantly correlated with hemizona binding and sperm morphology, frozen-thawed sperm exhibited a 30% loss in

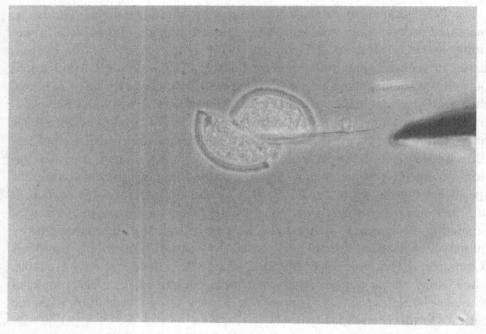

Fig. 9.7. Two matching hemizonae created by bisecting a non-living human oocyte. The tip of the cutting blade is seen at the right edge (× 200).

hemizona binding capacity compared with fresh sperm (Coddington *et al.*, 1991), the control hemizona must bind ≥20 sperm in order to define a valid assay (Franken *et al.*, 1991) and most of these tightly bound sperm are acrosome-reacted (Fulgham *et al.*, 1992). Among other topics, the influence of zona maturation (Oehninger *et al.*, 1991), sperm immobilizing antibodies (Shibahara *et al.*, 1991) and sperm stimulants (Kaskar *et al.*, 1993) have been investigated in relation to hemizona binding. Significantly, independent laboratories (Hammitt *et al.*, 1993; Lessing *et al.*, 1994) have also utilized the HZA with positive results. The details on methods for the standard HZA (see Fig. 9.8) and additional supporting studies can be reviewed in Burkman *et al.* (1990) and Oehninger (1992).

When considering use of the HZA for clinical diagnosis, one must address several issues. Is the HZA predictive of fertilization outcome? What is the rate of false positive results? How can HZA results guide therapy? Judging by the volume of HZA publications since 1988, it is likely that the parameters and validation of the HZA have been more carefully scrutinized than those of any other fertilization assay introduced in the past decade. Current HZA data demonstrate that interassay variation is 10%, with a correct predictive power of 80–85% (Oehninger *et al.*, 1992). Utilizing a Hemizona

The Hemizona Assay (HZA)

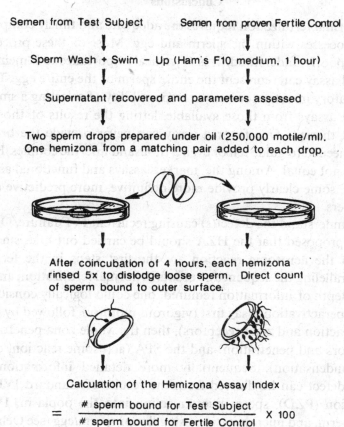

Semen from Test Subject   Semen from proven Fertile Control

↓   ↓

Sperm Wash + Swim – Up (Ham's F10 medium, 1 hour)

↓   ↓

Supernatant recovered and parameters assessed

↓   ↓

Two sperm drops prepared under oil (250,000 motile/ml).
One hemizona from a matching pair added to each drop.

After coincubation of 4 hours, each hemizona
rinsed 5x to dislodge loose sperm. Direct count
of sperm bound to outer surface.

Calculation of the Hemizona Assay Index

$$= \frac{\text{\# sperm bound for Test Subject}}{\text{\# sperm bound for Fertile Control}} \times 100$$

Fig. 9.8. Protocol for the hemizona assay showing matching zona halves, incubation droplet, and the appearance of each hemizona when tightly bound sperm are counted at the end of the assay. Definition of the Hemizona Index (HZI) is given at the bottom.

Index (HZI; see Fig. 9.8) cut-off of 35%, Oehninger *et al*. reiterate earlier conclusions that the chances of good fertilization (defined as ≥65% of eggs fertilized) are 81% when HZI >35, and the chances of poor fertilization are 100% when HZI <35. Similar statistics were derived by Franken *et al*. (1993) using a conservative definition of male factor in IVF. With an HZI cut-off of 30% and 'good' IVF fertilization taken as ≥55%, their HZA sensitivity and specificity were 75%, with a positive predictive value of 81% and a negative predictive value of 68% (Franken *et al*., 1993). In all these studies it is emphasized that the HZA, like other functional tests, cannot detect every class of fertilization defects.

Conclusions

Achieving normal fertilization requires the adequate and timely completion of dozens of processes within the sperm and egg. Most of these processes are unknown or poorly understood. It is of critical importance to remember that no functional assay can represent the entire sperm or the entire egg. The clinician or laboratory investigator has the responsibility of selecting a small array of functional assays from those available, letting the results of those assays guide patient therapy. One favored assay can never provide the breadth of information needed to guide ten or even a thousand infertile couples. However, all assays are not equal. Among the 'marker' assays and functional assays discussed above, some clearly provide more definitive, more predictive information than others.

To better understand the defect(s) causing recurrent IVF failure, Oehninger *et al.* (1992) proposed that the HZA should be carried out first, since sperm binding with the acrosome reaction are the first steps in the fertilization sequence. Paralleling the sequence of events in normal fertilization, and dependent on the depth of information required, one could logically consider doing the sperm hyperactivation assay first (vigorous motility), followed by the HZA (acrosome reaction and zona receptors), then the whole zona penetration test (zona receptors and penetration) and the SPA (acrosome reaction, oolemma fusion, decondensation). Sequentially more detailed information on the fertilization defect can be derived from the results of standard IVF, partial zona dissection (PZD), sperm microinjection into the ooplasm, IVF using donor egg/sperm, and microinjection using donor sperm/egg (see Oehninger *et al.*, 1992).

References

Aitken, R., Mattei, A. & Irvine, S. (1986). Paradoxical stimulation of human sperm motility by 2-deoxyadenosine. *J. Reprod. Fertil.*, **78**, 515–27.

Anderson, R.A. *et al.* (1992). Facilitative effect of pulsed addition of dibutyryl cAMP on the acrosome reaction of noncapacitated human spermatozoa. *J. Androl.*, **13**, 398–408.

Austin, C.R. (1951). Observations on the penetration of the sperm into the mammalian egg. *Aust. J. Sci. Res. B*, **4**, 581–96.

Austin, C.R. (1952). The 'capacitation' of the mammalian sperm. *Nature*, **170**, 326–7.

Bedford, J.M. (1983). Significance of the need for sperm capacitation before fertilization in eutherian mammals. *Biol. Reprod.*, **28**, 108–20.

Blazak, W.F., Overstreet, J.W., Katz, D.F. & Hanson, F.W. (1982). A competitive *in vitro* assay of human sperm fertilizing ability utilizing contrasting fluorescent sperm markers. *J. Androl.*, **3**, 165–71.

Burkman, L.J. (1984). Characterization of hyperactivated motility by human spermatozoa during capacitation: comparison of fertile and oligozoospermic sperm populations. *Arch. Androl.*, **13**, 153–65.

Burkman, L. (1986). Temporal pattern of hyperactivation-like motility in human spermatozoa. *Biol. Reprod.*, **34** (Suppl. 1), 226.

Burkman, L.J. (1990). Hyperactivated motility of human spermatozoa during *in vitro* capacitation. In *Controls of Sperm Motility*, ed. C. Gagnon, pp. 304–29. Boca Raton: CRC Press.

Burkman, L.J. (1991). Discrimination between nonhyperactivated and classical hyperactivated motility patterns in human spermatozoa using computerized analysis. *Fertil. Steril.*, **55**, 363–71.

Burkman, L. (1994). Human sperm hyperactivation and CASA analysis as a quick QC/toxicity assay (abstract). *Fertil. Steril.* (Program suppl.), S174.

Burkman, L. & Coddington, C.C. (1986). Interaction of hyperactivated-like human spermatozoa with the human zona pellucida (abstract). *Fertil. Steril.* (Program Suppl.), p. 129.

Burkman, L. & Samrock, R. (1992). Sperm hyperactivation (HA) assay: values are repeatable within individual men (abstract). *Fertil. Steril.* (Program Suppl.), p. 186.

Burkman, L., Coddington, C., Franken, C., Kruger, T., Rosenwaks, Z. & Hodgen, G. (1988a). The Hemizona Assay (HZA): development of a diagnostic test for the binding of human spermatozoa to human hemizona pellucida to predict fertilization potential. *Fertil. Steril.* **49**, 688–97.

Burkman, L., Johnson, D., Fulgham, D., Alexander, N. & Hodgen, G. (1988b). Temporal relationships between zona binding, hyperactivated motion (HA) and acrosome reactions (AR) in sperm from fertile men (abstract). Presented at the Serono Symposium on Gamete Physiology, Newport Beach, 6–10 November.

Burkman, L., Coddington, C., Franken, D., Oehninger, S. & Hodgen, G. (1990). The hemizona assay (HZA): assessment of fertilizing potential by means of human sperm binding to the human zona pellucida. In *Laboratory Diagnosis and Treatment of Infertility*, ed. B. Keel & B. Webster, pp. 213–28. Boca Raton: CRC Press.

Burkman, L., Rogers, B., Kiessling, A. & Epstein, D. (1991). Comparing three reproductive assays for their quality control (QC) potential (abstract). *Fertil. Steril.* (Program Suppl.), S145.

Byrd, W., Tsu, J. & Wolf, D.P. (1989). Kinetics of spontaneous and induced acrosomal loss in human sperm incubated under capacitating and noncapacitating conditions. *Gamete Res.*, **22**, 109–22.

Calvo, L. *et al.* (1989). Follicular fluid-induced acrosome reaction distinguishes a subgroup of men with unexplained infertility not indentified by semen analysis. *Fertil. Steril.*, **52**, 1048–54.

Chang, M.C. (1951). Fertilizing capacity of spermatozoa deposited into Fallopian tubes. *Nature*, **168**, 697–8.

Chang, M.C. (1984). The meaning of sperm capacitation; a historical perspective. *J. Androl.*, **5**, 45–50.

Coddington, C., Franken, D., Burkman, L., Oosthuizen, W., Kruger, T. & Hodgen, G. (1991). Functional aspects of human sperm binding to the zona pellucida using the hemizona assay. *J. Androl.*, **12**, 1–8.

Cross, N.L. & Meizel, S. (1989). Methods for evaluating the acrosomal status of mammalian sperm. *Biol. Reprod.*, **4**, 635–41.

Cummins, J.M., Pember, S.M., Jequier, A.M., Yoviċh, J.L. & Hartmann, P.E. (1991). A test of the human sperm acrosome reaction following ionophore challenge. *J. Androl.*, **12**, 98–103.

de Lamirande, E. & Gagnon, C. (1993*a*). Human sperm hyperactivation in whole semen and its association with low superoxide scavenging capacity in seminal plasma. *Fertil. Steril.*, **59**, 1291–5.

de Lamirande, E. & Gagnon, C. (1993*b*). Human sperm hyperactivation and capacitation as parts of an oxidative process. *Free Rádical Biol.*, **14**, 157–66.

Edwards, R.G. (1974). Control of human ovulation, fertilization and implantation. *Proc. R. Soc. Med.*, **67**, 932–6.

Fleming, A. & Yanagimachi, R. (1982). Fertile life of acrosome-reacted guinea pig spermatozoa. *J. Exp. Zool.*, **220**, 109–15.

Franken, D.R., Coddington, C.C., Burkman, L.J., Oosthuiżen, W.T., Oehinger, S.C., Kruger, T.F. & Hodgen, G.D. (1991). Defining the valid hemizona assay: accounting for binding variability within zonae pellucidae and within semen samples from fertile males. *Fertil. Steril.*, **56**, 1156–61.

Franken, D.R., Acosta, A.A., Kruger, T.F. Lombard, C.J., Oehninger, S. & Hodgen, G.D. (1993). The hemizona assay: its role in identifying male factor infertility in assisted reproduction. *Fertil. Steril.*, **59**, 1075–80.

Fraser, L. (1981). Dibutyryl cyclic AMP decreases capacitation time *in vitro* in mouse spermatozoa. *J. Reprod. Fertil.* **62**, 63–72.

Fulgham, D.L., Coddington, C., Johnson, D., Herr, J., Alexander, N. & Hodgen, G.D. (1992). Human sperm acrosome reaction on zona pellucida: a time course study. *ARTA*, **3**, 25–34.

Grunert, J.-H., De Geyter, C. & Nieschlag, E. (1990). Objective identification of hyperactivated human spermatozoa by computerized sperm motion analysis with the Hamilton–Thorn sperm motility analyser. *Hum. Reprod.*, **5**, 593–9.

Hammitt, D.G., Syrop, C.H., Walker, D.L. & Bennett, M.R. (1993). Conditions of oocyte storage and use of noninseminated as compared with inseminated, nonfertilized oocytes for the hemizona assay. *Fertil. Steril.*, **60**, 131–6.

Jinno, M., Burkman, L. & Coddington, C. (1987). Human sperm hyperactivated motility (HA) and egg penetration (abstract). *Biol. Reprod.*, **36**, 53.

Kallajoki, M., Virtanen, I. & Suominen, J. (1986). The fate of acrosomal staining during the acrosome reaction of human spermatozoa as revealed by a monoclonal antibody and PNA-lectin. *Int. J. Androl.*, **9**, 181–94.

Karande, V., Mbizvo, M., Burkman, L., Veeck, L. & Alexander, N. (1990). Hyperactivation (HA) of human sperm is a prognostic indicator of fertilization during IVF (abstract). *J. Androl.* (Program Suppl.), 28P.

Karande, V., Burkman, L., Mbizvo, M., Veeck, L. & Alexander, N. (1996). Hyperactivated motility (HA) of human spermatozoa may be a prognostic indicator of fertilization during IVF. *Fertil. Steril.*, in review.

Kaskar, K., Franken, D.R., Van Der Horst, G., Kruger, T.F., Oehninger, S. & Hodgen, G.D. (1993). Motility/zona pellucida binding of human sperm. II. Effect of caffeine on sperm normo- and teratozoospermic men. *ARTA*, **4**, 295–308.

Katz, D., Drobnis, E. & Overstreet, J. (1989). Factors regulating mammalian sperm migration through the female reproductive tract and oocyte vestments. *Gamete Res.*, **22**, 443.

Lee, M.A., Trucco, G.S., Bechtol, K.B., Wummer, N., Kopf, G.S., Blasco, L. & Storey, B.T. (1987). Capacitation and acrosome reactions in human spermatozoa monitored by a chlortetracycline fluorescence assay. *Fertil. Steril.*, **48**, 649–58.

Lessing, J.B., Yogev, L., Gamzu, R., Amit, A., Homonnai, Z.T., Barak, Y., Yavetz, H. & Paz, G. (1994). Hemizona assay (HZA) coupled with sperm motility for prediction of *in vitro* fertilization (IVF) outcome (abstract). *Fertil. Steril.* (Program Suppl.), S118.

Liu, D., Clark, G., Lopata, A. & Johnston, W. (1989). A sperm–zona pellucida binding test and *in vitro* fertilization. *Fertil. Steril.*, **52**, 281–7.

Mack, S. Wolf, D. & Tash, J. (1988). Quantitation of specific parameters of motility in large numbers of human sperm by digital image processing. *Biol. Reprod.*, **38**, 270–81.

Mbizvo, M., Johnston, R. & Baker, G. (1993). The effect of the motility stimulants, caffeine, pentoxifylline, and 2-deoxyadenosine on hyperactivation of cryopreserved human sperm. *Fertil. Steril.*, **59**, 1112–17.

Menkveld, R., Franken, D.R., Kruger, T.F., Oehninger, S. & Hodgen, G.D. (1991). Sperm selection capacity of the human zona pellucida. *Mol. Reprod. Dev.* **30**, 346–52.

Morales, P., Overstreet, J. & Katz, D. (1988). Changes in human sperm motion during capacitation *in vitro*. *J. Reprod. Fertil.*, **83**, 119–28.

Mortimer, D., Courtot, A., Giovangrandi, Y., Jeulin, C. & David, G. (1984). Human sperm motility after migration into, and incubation in, synthetic media. *Gamete Res.*, **9**, 131–44.

Mortimer, S. & Mortimer, D. (1990). Kinematics of human spermatozoa incubated under capacitating conditions. *J. Androl.*, **11**, 195–203.

Murad, C., De Lamirande, E. & Gagnon, C. (1992). Hyperactivated motility is coupled with interdependent modifications at axonemal and cytosolic levels of human spermatozoa. *J. Androl.*, **13**, 323–31.

Oehninger, S. (1992). Diagnostic significance of sperm–zona pellucida interaction. *Reprod. Med. Rev.* **1**, 57–81.

Oehninger, S., Veeck, L., Franken, D., Kruger, T.F., Acosta, A.A. & Hodgen, G.D. (1991). Human preovulatory oocytes have a higher sperm-binding ability than immature oocytes under hemizona assay conditions: evidence supporting the concept of 'zona maturation'. *Fertil. Steril.*, **55**, 1165–70.

Oehninger, S., Franken, D., Alexander, N. & Hodgen, G.D. (1992). Hemizona assay and its impact on the identification and treatment of human sperm dysfunctions. *Andrologia*, **24**, 307–21.

Overstreet, J.W. & Hembree, W.C. (1976). Penetration of the zona pellucida of nonliving human oocytes by human spermatozoa *in vitro*. *Fertil. Steril.*, **27**, 815–31.

Overstreet, J.W., Yanagimachi, R., Katz, D., Hiyashi, K. & Hanson, F. (1980a). Penetration of human spermatozoa into the human zona pellucida and the zona-free hamster egg: a study of fertile donors and infertile patients. *Fertil. Steril.* **33**, 534–42.

Overstreet, J.W., Gould, J.E., Katz, D.F. & Hanson, F.W. (1980b). *In vitro* capacitation of human spermatozoa after passage through a column of cervical mucus. *Fertil. Steril.*, **34**, 604–6.

Pampiglione, J.S., Tan, S.-L. & Campbell, S. (1993). The use of the stimulated acrosome reaction test as a test of fertilizing ability in human spermatozoa. *Fertil. Steril.*, **59**, 1280–4.

Pearlstone, A., Chan, S., Tucker, M., Wiker, S. & Wang, C. (1993). The effects of Vero (Green monkey kidney) cell coculture on the motility patterns of cryopreserved human spermatozoa. *Fertil. Steril.*, **59**, 1105–11.

Pilikian, S., Adeleine, P., Czyba, J., Ecochard, R., Guerin, J. & Mimouni, P. (1991).

Hyperactivated motility of sperm from fertile donors and asthenozoospermic patients before and after treatment with ionophore. *Int. J. Androl.*, **14**, 167–73.

Robertson, L., Wolf, D. & Tash, J. (1988). Temporal changes in motility parameters related to acrosomal status: identification and characterization of populations of hyperactivated sperm. *Biol. Reprod.*, **39**, 797–805.

Rogers, B.J. (1985). The sperm penetration assay: its usefulness re-evaluated. *Fertil. Steril.*, **43**, 821–9.

Saling, P.M. & Lakoski, K.A. (1985). Mouse sperm antigens that participate in fertilization. II. Inhibition of sperm penetration through the zona pellucida using monoclonal antibodies. *Biol. Reprod.*, **33**, 527–36.

Shibahara, H., Shigeta, M., Koyama, K., Burkman, L.J., Alexander, N.J. & Isojima, S. (1991). Inhibition of sperm–zona pellucida tight binding by sperm immobilizing antibodies as assessed by the hemizona assay (HZA). *Acta Obstet. Gynaecol. Japoni.*, **43**, 237–8.

Singer, S.L., Lambert, H., Overstreet, J.W., Hanson, F.W. & Yanagimachi, R. (1985). The kinetics of human sperm binding to the human zona pellucida and zona-free hamster oocytes *in vitro. Gamete Res.*, **12**, 29–39.

Suarez, S. & Osman, R. (1987). Initiation of hyperactivated flagellar bending in mouse sperm within the female reprodutive tract. *Biol. Reprod.*, **36**, 1191–8.

Talbot, P. & Chacon, R. (1980). A new procedure for rapidly scoring acrosome reaction of human sperm. *Gamete Res.*, **3**, 211–16.

Talbot, P. & Chacon, R. (1981). A triple-stain technique for evaluating normal acrosome reactions of human sperm. *J. Exp. Zool.*, **215**, 201–8.

Talbot, P. & Dudenhausen, E. (1981). Factors affecting triple staining of human sperm. *Stain Technol.*, **56**, 307–9.

Tesarik, J., Mendoza, C. & Testart, J. (1990). Effect of human cumulus oophorus on movement characteristics of human capacitated spermatozoa. *J. Reprod. Fertil.*, **88**, 665–75.

Tesarik, J., Thebault, A. & Testart, J. (1992). Effect of pentoxifylline on sperm movement characteristics in normozoospermic and asthenozoospermic specimens. *Hum. Reprod.*, **7**, 1257–63.

Tesarik, J., Mendoza, C. & Carreras, A. (1993). Fast acrosome reaction measure: a highly sensitive method for evaluating stimulus-induced acrosome reaction. *Fertil. Steril.*, **59**, 424–30.

Uhler, M., Leung, A., Chan, S. & Wang, C. (1992). Direct effects of progesterone and antiprogesterone on human sperm hyperactivated motility and acrosome reaction. *Fertil. Steril.*, **58**, 1191–8.

Wang, C., Leung, A., Tsoi, W.-L., Leung, J., Ng, V., Lee, K.-F. & Chan, S. (1991). Evaluation of human sperm hyperactivated motility and its relationship with the zona-free hamster oocyte sperm penetration assay. *J. Androl.*, **12**, 253–7.

Wang, C., Lee, G., Leung, A., Surrey, E. & Chan, S. (1993). Human sperm hyperactivation and acrosome reaction and their relationships to human *in vitro* fertilization. *Fertil. Steril.*, **59**, 1221–7.

Ward, C.R. & Storey, B.T. (1984). Determination of the time course of capacitation in mouse spermatozoa using a chlortetracycline fluorescence assay. *Dev. Biol.*, **104**, 287–296.

Wolf, D.P., *et al.* (1985). Acrosomal status evaluation in human ejaculated sperm with monoclonal antibodies. *Biol. Reprod.*, **32**, 1157–62.

Yanagimachi, R. (1981). Mammalian fertilization. In *The Physiology of*

Reproduction, ed. L. Mastroianni & J.B. Biggers, pp. 81–182. New York: Plenum Press.

Yanagimachi, R. (1988). Mammalian fertilization. In *The Physiology of Reproduction*, ed. E. Knobil, pp. 135–55. New York: Raven Press.

Yanagimachi, R., Yanagimachi, H. & Rogers, B.J. (1976). The use of zona-free animal ova as a test system for the assessment of the fertilizing capacity of human spermatozoa. *Biol. Reprod.*, **15**, 471–6.

Zaneveld, L. & Jeyendran, R. (1988). Modern assessment of semen for diagnostic purposes. *Semin. Reprod. Endocr.*, **4**, 323–37.

10

Assisted reproductive technology for male factor infertility

WILLIAM R. PHIPPS

Introduction

The standard *in vitro* fertilization (IVF) procedure was originally developed to treat infertility secondary to irreparable tubal factor. It soon became clear, however, that couples with infertility on the basis of other factors, including those with an apparent male factor, might benefit from IVF (Mahadevan *et al.*, 1983; Battin *et al.*, 1985; Cohen *et al.*, 1985) or other assisted reproductive technology (ART) procedures requiring oocyte retrieval such as gamete intra-fallopian transfer (GIFT) (Matson *et al.*, 1987). This chapter provides an overview of the use of ART for male factor infertility. The emphasis will be on IVF. Many of the topics covered are reviewed in greater detail in other chapters, and in particular the assisted fertilization techniques are described in Chapter 11.

Current application of ART to male factor infertility

The term ART in its broader sense encompasses a large number of fertility-enhancing processes, including not only techniques requiring oocyte retrieval but also less involved techniques such as intrauterine insemination (IUI) (Brown & Lavy, 1992). All these have been applied to cases of male factor infertility. They differ substantially in terms of their overall complexity, laboratory requirements, invasiveness and cost.

Often ART techniques can be applied to cases of male factor infertility even when the precise nature of the underlying problem is not understood. ART techniques have also been increasingly applied to less common male factor cases such as obstructive azoospermia secondary to failed vasovasostomy or congenital absence of the vas deferens (Silber *et al.*, 1988; Bennett, 1990), and ejaculatory failure secondary to spinal cord injury, diabetes mellitus or other conditions (Bennett, 1990; Rainsbury, 1992). ART techniques using donor semen have also been used very successfully in apparently normal women following failed trials of therapeutic donor insemination (Cefalu *et al.*, 1988; Robinson *et al.*, 1993).

Specific ART techniques

The standard IVF procedure generally involves treatment of the female partner with an ovarian stimulation regimen designed to achieve multiple follicular development. Currently follicular aspiration is carried out using an ultrasound-guided, transvaginal approach, without the need for laparoscopy or general anesthesia. The oocytes retrieved are inseminated *in vitro*, generally 4–6 hours following retrieval, and then assessed for fertilization 12–18 hours later. Assuming fertilization occurs, embryo transfer into the uterus is carried out 2–3 days following retrieval. In 1991, for ART centers in the United States and Canada submitting their results to the Society for Assisted Reproductive Technology (SART), 22% of nearly 24 000 initiated standard IVF cycles included a diagnosis of a male factor on the basis of an abnormal semen analysis (Society for Assisted Reproductive Technology, 1993).

The standard GIFT procedure also requires oocyte retrieval after ovarian stimulation, but, as generally performed, additionally involves a laparoscopy at the time of oocyte retrieval so that both oocytes and spermatozoa can be transferred into the fallopian tube. Transcervical tubal transfer techniques, obviating the need for laparoscopy or general anesthesia, have been used (Jansen & Anderson, 1987; Bustillo *et al.*, 1988), but not on a widespread basis. With GIFT, fertilization presumably occurs in the tube prior to the embryo entering the uterine cavity. Accordingly, candidates for GIFT must have at least one normal functioning tube. In the presence of a male factor, an increased number of sperm are generally transferred as compared with cases without a male factor (Matson *et al.*, 1987; van der Merwe *et al.*, 1990; Brinsden & Asch, 1992). In 1991, for centers reporting to SART, 19% of nearly 5500 intended GIFT cycles included a diagnosis of a male factor.

Two variants of the standard IVF procedure – zygote intrafallopian transfer (ZIFT) (Devroey *et al.*, 1989) and tubal embryo transfer (TET) (Balmaceda *et al.*, 1988) – were developed to combine apparent advantages of both IVF and GIFT. With both ZIFT and TET, insemination is carried out *in vitro* following oocyte retrieval. With ZIFT, tubal transfer of zygotes with two pronuclei is performed 1 day after retrieval. With TET, transfer at the 2- to 8-cell embryo stage is carried out 2 days after retrieval. Compared with the standard IVF procedure, both ZIFT and TET may provide an increased chance of fertilization as compared with GIFT, while allowing for documentation of fertilization in

those cases in which no pregnancy occurs. As with GIFT, both ZIFT and TET
allow for the theoretical advantage of the embryo entering the uterine cavity
from the tube in a more physiologic manner as compared with IVF. Both procedures of course require at least one normal functioning tube, and both have
the significant disadvantage of requiring two separate operative procedures on
subsequent days, including a laparoscopy for the transfer. As is the case for
GIFT, a transcervical approach for the embryo transfer has been used
(Scholtes *et al.*, 1990). In 1991, about 2100 ZIFT or TET cycles were performed
at centers reporting to SART, and it is likely that many if not most of these
cycles involved a male factor.

A widely used, less invasive alternative to the procedures described above,
applicable at least to less severe male factor cases, is simply to combine the use
of gonadotropin therapy with IUI (Corsan & Kemmann, 1991; Dodson &
Haney, 1991). The treatment of ovulatory women with gonadotropins in this
context is often referred to as controlled ovarian hyperstimulation (COH).
Because of reduced laboratory requirements as compared with the more elabo-
rate ART techniques, combined COH/IUI treatment can be carried out in facilities not performing IVF. The use of IUI treatment for male factor infertility is
specifically addressed in Chapters 7 and 8.

Diagnostic sperm function tests and IVF

A large number of diagnostic tests have been used to determine the capability
of a given individual's semen specimen to achieve fertilization of a human
oocyte. Most commonly, this capability has been considered in the context of
the normal sequence of events leading to fertilization *in vivo* after intercourse
(Critser & Noiles, 1993). For couples considering ART, however, sperm
requirements may be different to a variable degree, depending on the individual
circumstances involved.

This section describes different assays of sperm function primarily as they
relate to IVF. Determination of sperm function prior to ART is important not
only for its prognostic value and use in modifying the procedure to improve
outcome, but also to select alternative therapies when indicated. Most of the
literature in this area has focused on the relationship between the results of a
given diagnostic sperm function study and the endpoint of the occurrence of
fertilization *in vitro*, as opposed to clinical or liveborn pregnancy rates. This is
appropriate because a substantial majority of studies have shown that once
fertilization occurs in male factor cases, pregnancy outcomes are at least as
good as those in cases without a male factor (Meacham & Lipshultz, 1990;
Hammitt, 1993). Far fewer studies have been done relating tests of sperm

function to GIFT, largely because the endpoint of fertilization cannot be directly assessed. Thus studies of GIFT must use occurrence of pregnancy as an endpoint, and as a consequence more patients are needed in order to reach valid conclusions.

When dealing with a possible male factor diagnosis, it may be useful to repeat any of the diagnostic tests described here, particularly when the initial result is considered abnormal (Critser & Noiles, 1993). This caveat relates largely to the fact that a single spermatogenic cycle in humans requires on average 70 days, not allowing for epididymal transit (Stevens, 1990). Thus an acute testicular insult may have a temporary effect on sperm function, with resolution after about 3 months. Even with no such apparent insult there is wide day-to-day variation in semen quality among normal subjects (Mallidis *et al.*, 1991).

Standard semen analysis

The initial diagnostic test done to assess sperm function is the standard semen analysis. This is descriptive in nature. The parameters assessed generally include semen volume, sperm concentration, the percentage of sperm showing forward progression (motility), and the percentage of sperm with normal morphology as analyzed by light microscopy (World Health Organization, 1992a). All these parameters have been investigated in relation to IVF results. Such investigations are complicated by the fact that frequently more than one of these parameters is abnormal.

Sperm concentration has never been considered an especially useful predictor for fertilization rate *in vitro*, particularly if other parameters are simultaneously taken into account (Liu & Baker, 1992b). On the other hand, early investigations did point to motility parameters as being important correlates of the occurrence of fertilization *in vitro*. For example, Mahadevan & Trounson (1984) reported that, of conventional semen analysis parameters, motility was the single best predictor of fertilization rate *in vitro*, with failure of fertilization consistently occurring with motilities of less than 20%. Along these lines, Battin and colleagues (1985) reported reduced fertilization rates when the ejaculate contained less than 10×10^6 motile spermatozoa. Even today, there remain prominent IVF centers at which the concentration of motile sperm is considered to be a better predictor of IVF results than morphology, particularly when a prepared specimen is evaluated (Avery & Elder, 1992). A recent study showed that assessment of motility in a specimen prepared for IVF can be combined with morphology analysis, prior to processing, to provide excellent IVF predictive ability (Duncan *et al.*, 1993).

A limited number of studies have sought to establish the relationship between semen analysis parameters and GIFT success. One investigation not involving morphology assessment found the total number of motile sperm, but not motility *per se*, to correlate well with the clinical pregnancy rate (Rodriguez-Rigau *et al.*, 1989). Another found that both motility and morphology independently affected the likelihood of successful GIFT (Guzick *et al.*, 1989).

Sperm morphology

Sperm morphologic features have been intensively studied in relation to ability to achieve fertilization both *in vivo* and *in vitro*. The differing results reported by investigators in this area can in part be attributed to different criteria used to distinguish between normal and abnormal morphology. The general trend in recent years has been towards using stricter criteria, resulting of course in a decline in the lower limit of the percentage of normal forms considered to be normal. For example, the most recent World Health Organization guidelines suggest teratozoospermia is present only when the percentage of normal forms is less than 30% (World Health Organization, 1992*b*), in contrast to the cut-off of 50% suggested 5 years earlier (World Health Organization, 1987).

The majority of studies, using different criteria, have found sperm morphologic parameters to be predictive for IVF performance. More recently, morphology has been identified as being more important than motility as a predictor of successful IVF (Liu & Baker, 1992*b*). However, no clear-cut consensus has been reached as to the superiority of morphology over other diagnostic tests in this regard (Fraser & DasGupta, 1993). Morphology results have been shown to be an important predictor of GIFT success as well (Guzick *et al.*, 1989; van der Merwe *et al.*, 1992). Not surprisingly, morphologic results generally correlate well with results of such functional tests as the sperm penetration assay (SPA) and the hemizona assay (HZA) (Fraser & DasGupta, 1993), and the human zona pellucida (ZP) has been shown to be highly selective for binding of sperm with normal morphology (Liu & Baker, 1992*a*).

Several studies have agreed that severe teratozoospermia is associated with poor IVF performance, including reduced as well as delayed fertilization, poor embryo quality, and reduced clinical and liveborn pregnancies rates (Kruger *et al.*, 1986, 1988*a*; Oehninger *et al.*, 1988*b*; Ron-El *et al.*, 1991). The most striking relationships between sperm morphology and IVF outcome have been found in studies using Kruger's so-called strict criteria (Kruger *et al.*, 1986; Menkveld *et al.*, 1990; Enginsu *et al.*, 1992*b*), according to which ejaculates with more than 14% normal forms are considered to be normal morphologically. Using these criteria, at least with ejaculates from men with relatively normal sperm concentrations and motility parameters, the fertilization rate with 4–14% normal forms has been shown to be similar to that with more than 14% normal forms (Oehninger *et al.*, 1988*b*). Interestingly, application of strict criteria has been shown to account for previously unexplained failed fertilization in selected cases (Oehninger *et al.*, 1988*a*).

It is important to note that the work discussed above had involved only assessment by light microscopy, which does not allow for visualization of organelles (Zamboni, 1992). Electron microscopy allows for a much more precise understanding of the relationship between sperm morphology and function in specific cases (Schill, 1991; Nulsen *et al.*, 1992; Zamboni, 1992), but is generally impractical for routine clinical use. A retrospective study using both scanning and transmission electron microscopy did show a relationship between specific sperm malformation patterns and fertilization *in vitro*, although interestingly there was no relationship between the percentage of normal forms and fertilization (Mashiach *et al.*, 1992).

Analysis for white blood cells

The standard semen analysis may indicate the presence of an increased number of white blood cells (WBC) in the ejaculate (see Chapter 16). A WBC concentration of greater than $10^6/ml$ is considered to be abnormal and is referred to as leukocytospermia (World Health Organization, 1992*b*). Leukocytospermia has been linked to both poor SPA performance (Berger *et al.*, 1982) and overall poor semen quality (Wolff *et al.*, 1990), and recent work has identified seminal leukocytes as a major source of reactive oxygen species (Aitken & West, 1990; Aitken *et al.*, 1992; Kessopoulou *et al.*, 1992). Not surprisingly, in an early report Cohen *et al.* (1985) noted that leukocytospermia was associated with decreased fertilization of human oocytes *in vitro*. Thus a search for, and correction of, the cause of leukocytospermia is indicated prior to the IVF cycle.

Computer-aided semen analysis

Computer-aided semen analysis (CASA) allows for an objective and systematic assessment of sperm motility parameters (Chapter 4). In an early study, Holt *et al.* (1985) showed a correlation between 'sperm swimming speed' or curvilinear velocity (VCL) in semen as assessed by a computerized technique and IVF results. A subsequent study found IVF results to be related to VCL following a swim-up preparation (Chan *et al.*, 1989). Another early report demonstrated a relationship between amplitude of lateral head displacement (ALH) and IVF results (Jeulin *et al.*, 1986). Liu and colleagues (1991) used logistic regression analysis to relate both CASA and other parameters to IVF results, and found that the fertilization rate *in vitro* was positively related to linearity (LIN) in semen, and negatively related to the proportion of sperm with poor average-path velocity (VAP) values following swim-up.

The ability of CASA to identify specific hyperactivated subpopulations of sperm (Robertson *et al.*, 1988; Ginsburg *et al.*, 1989; Burkman, 1990, 1991; Katz *et al.*, 1993; see Chapter 9) may ultimately prove most useful in the management of IVF patients. Hyperactivation rates have been shown to correlate with sperm morphology and HZA results (Coddington *et al.*, 1991) and with IVF success (Davis *et al.*, 1991).

Sperm penetration assay

The SPA (Chapter 6), using zona-free hamster oocytes, was originally designed to assess the fertilizing ability of human spermatozoa when human oocytes were not available (Yanagimachi *et al.*, 1976). It specifically measures the ability of spermatozoa *in vitro* to undergo capacitation, the acrosome reaction, membrane fusion and sperm chromatin decondensation (Aitken, 1990; Liu & Baker, 1992*b*).

There have been conflicting reports regarding the ability of the SPA to predict successful human IVF (Liu & Baker, 1992*b*) due in part to methodological differences (Bronson & Rogers, 1988). Nonetheless, most studies have shown that a normal SPA result is predictive of successful IVF, while an abnormal result appears to be of less predictive value, especially in the setting of abnormal semen parameters (Margalioth *et al.*, 1986; Coetzee *et al.*, 1989).

A number of sperm preparation methods which modify the SPA have been developed that may yield a positive SPA result for a specimen for which a conventional SPA is negative; many of these same preparation methods can also be applied therapeutically to improve IVF results, including techniques involving Percoll gradients (Berger *et al.*, 1985; McClure *et al.*, 1989; Quinn, 1993), TES and Tris (TEST)-yolk buffer incubation (Katayama *et al.*, 1989; Soffer *et al.*, 1992; Veeck, 1992), follicular fluid (Yee & Cummings, 1988; Blumenfeld & Nahhas, 1989; Ghetler *et al.*, 1990; Muller, 1992), use of a hyperosmolar medium (Aitken *et al.*, 1983; Muller, 1992), use of a calcium ionophore (Aitken *et al.*, 1984; Muller, 1992), low-temperature incubation (Sanchez & Schill, 1991; Carrell *et al.*, 1992) and others (Carrell *et al.*, 1992).

Sperm–zona pellucida binding tests

Since the human zona is known to be selective for binding of sperm with normal morphology (Liu & Baker, 1992*a*), tests assessing sperm binding should have substantial prognostic valve (Liu & Baker, 1992*b*). The hemizona assay (HZA) uses the matched halves of a microbisected zona to compare the binding capacities of a proven fertile semen specimen and a test specimen (Burkman *et al.*, 1988; Franken *et al.*, 1989, 1993; Oehninger *et al.*, 1989). In addition to its predictive value for IVF success, the HZA may be useful when used with other tests to delineate the specific gamete defect present in cases of recurrent failed fertilization (Oehninger *et al.*, 1991).

Another such test uses human oocytes which failed to fertilize *in vitro* (Liu *et al.*, 1988, 1989; Liu & Baker, 1992*b*). Equal numbers of progressively motile test and control sperm, labeled with different fluorochromes, are mixed and incubated with several salt-stored ZP. The ratio of test to control sperm bound is then determined. In particular, the results may be useful in predicting fertilizing ability *in vitro* when poor sperm morphology is present (Liu *et al.*, 1989).

Tests of acrosomal status and function

The acrosome is a flattened, membrane-bound organelle which lies as a cap surrounding the anterior aspect of the sperm nucleus. Its three components include an outer acrosomal membrane, the acrosome proper and an inner acrosomal membrane (Zaneveld *et al.*, 1991). Breakdown of the acrosome (the acrosome reaction) as a final step in capacitation (Storey, 1991; Zaneveld *et al.*, 1991) can be induced by the ZP, and is necessary for penetration of the ZP, entrance into the perivitelline space and fusion with the oolemma. The acrosome reaction involves release of several enzymes such as acrosin and hyaluronidase, and exposure of the inner acrosomal membrane. Acrosin, a serine protease, plays an important role in ZP penetration. Hyaluronidase is important since hyaluronic acid is the main component of the intercellular matrix of the cumulus cells (Tesarik, 1992).

The acrosome reaction can occur spontaneously; several agents which stimulate the acrosome reaction have also been identified (Storey, 1991; Liu & Baker, 1992*b*). Although acrosome-reacted human sperm may bind to the ZP (Morales *et al.*, 1989; Liu & Baker, 1990, 1992*b*) the sperm that actually fertilizes the oocyte must acrosome react following binding to the ZP (Tesarik *et al.*, 1988; Tesarik, 1989, 1992).

Several distinct abnormalities of acrosome morphology associated with impaired fertilizing capacity *in vivo* and *in vitro* have been described (Aitken *et al.*, 1990; Schill, 1991; Mashiach *et al.*, 1992; Zamboni, 1992). Furthermore, in semen specimens with poor morphology, the proportion of sperm with normal intact acrosomes following swim-up was correlated with fertilization *in vitro* (Liu & Baker, 1988), again demonstrating the importance of acrosomal status in assessing the functional capacity of spermatozoa.

Abnormal kinetic patterns of the acrosome reaction have been associated with markedly reduced fertilization rates *in vitro* (Takahashi *et al.*, 1992). These included both a quickly reacting kinetic pattern, by which an excessive number of sperm were acrosome-reacted after a short time period, as well as a non-reacting pattern, involving reduced numbers of acrosome-reacted sperm at all intervals studied. The proportion of spermatozoa acrosome reacting in response to a stimulus such as calcium ionophore may yield useful information related to IVF success (Muller, 1992; Pampiglione *et al.*, 1993).

Specific acrosomal activity has also been studied in relation to IVF results. Despite conflicting reports (Kruger *et al.*, 1988*b*), acrosin activity (Tummon *et al.*, 1991; De Jonge *et al.*, 1993) and hyaluronidase activity (Hirayama *et al.*, 1989) correlated with successful IVF.

Hypo-osmotic swelling test

The hypo-osmotic swelling (HOS) test, which evaluates the functional integrity of the human sperm membranes, was shown initially to correlate with SPA results (Jeyendran *et al.*, 1984, 1992). Although there have been conflicting reports (Enginsu *et al.*, 1992*a*; Hauser *et al.*, 1992; Jeyendran *et al.*, 1992; Liu & Baker, 1992*b*), it appears that an abnormal HOS test result has substantial predictive value, whereas a normal result is not predictive of IVF success (Zaneveld *et al.*, 1990; Jeyendran *et al.*, 1992).

Other diagnostic sperm function tests

Several other assays of sperm function have been investigated, including tests for sperm nuclear maturity (Liu & Baker, 1992*b*) and the sperm–mucus penetration tests (Berberoglugil *et al.*, 1993). Another test which has been evaluated in relation to IVF results involves measurement in sperm of the isoforms of creatine phosphokinase (CK), a mitochondrial enzyme involved in the production of adenosine triphosphate (Tombes & Shapiro, 1985; Cummins & Yovich, 1993), and an apparent marker of dysfunctional spermatozoa. A recent study found a significant relationship between IVF results and the ratio of CK-MM (muscle type isoform) to total CK, with substantially reduced fertilization when this ratio was below 10% (Huszar *et al.*, 1992).

Selection of pre-treatment diagnostic sperm function tests

The extent of the diagnostic sperm function tests routinely done prior to proceeding with IVF or another ART procedure varies widely between centers. A semen analysis is universally done. Many centers routinely perform antisperm antibody testing (both male and female) and at least a conventional SPA. Testing performed prior to IVF should yield information regarding the presence of sperm dysfunction which could affect IVF success, as well as suggesting the optimal specific sperm processing technique(s) (Muller, 1992).

It is important that at least two semen analyses be done, including examination of a specimen prepared as though for IVF (Avery & Elder, 1992; Muller, 1992). If preliminary testing suggests a problem, additional diagnostic studies should be performed so as to optimize ART outcome. Formal diagnostic algorithms have been devised for when preliminary testing suggests an abnormality (Muller 1992). If all testing suggests the possibility of no or poor fertilization, assisted fertilization with micromanipulation or insemination with donor semen should be offered.

Semen processing and *in vitro* modulation of motility as related to IVF

Improved IVF sperm processing techniques could benefit couples with a male factor (Quinn, 1993). The first clinically successful human IVF cycles utilized simple sperm washing centrifugation procedures to separate human spermatozoa from seminal plasma (Edwards *et al.*, 1980; Lopata *et al.*, 1980; Purdy, 1982; Wortham *et al.*, 1983). These have been replaced by more refined methods.

Swim-up techniques

Early methods used to obtain sperm specimens for IVF were the 'swim-up' techniques (Yates & de Kretser, 1987; see Chapter 8) in which fresh medium is layered over a sperm pellet obtained by centrifugation. Motile sperm swim into the overlying medium, leaving non-motile or non-progressive sperm behind. Spermatozoa obtained by swim-up have been shown to have better motility and morphology as compared with sperm from the fresh ejaculate (McDowell *et al.*, 1985). However, centrifugation of unselected sperm populations may have adverse effects on sperm function, due to generation of increased levels of reactive oxygen species (ROS) which may cause membrane lipid oxidation (Aitken & Clarkson, 1988; Mortimer, 1991). While such deleterious effects may not be important for normal semen specimens, they may be highly problematic in male factor cases, possibly leading to a lack of fertilization (Mortimer, 1991; Quinn, 1993). Spermatozoa of males with abnormal semen parameters have a substantially higher capacity to produce ROS compared with normal controls (Aitken *et al.*, 1989, 1992). Because of this concern, separation procedures involving centrifugation of unselected sperm should be avoided in male factor cases (Mortimer, 1991), not only because of generation of ROS, but also because of substantial damage from other mechanisms (Alvarez *et al.*, 1993).

Swim-up can also be performed on unprocessed semen (Lopata *et al.*, 1976; Cohen *et al.*, 1985) without an initial centrifugation step, although it is not useful when severe oligozoospermia or asthenozoospermia is present (Berger *et al.*, 1985; Aitken & Clarkson, 1988).

Gradient separation procedures

Gradients of Percoll, a suspension of polyvinylpyrollidone-coated silica particles, can be used to fractionate spermatozoa according to progressive motility (Gorus & Pipeleers 1981). Both continuous and discontinuous Percoll gradients have been described for use in IVF (Berger *et al.*, 1985; Hyne *et al.*, 1986; Mortimer, 1990; de la Calle, 1991; Avery & Elder, 1992; Quinn, 1993). The selective nature of these gradients is such that the usual damage from ROS caused by centrifugation of unselected populations does not affect the recovered sperm (Aitken & Clarkson, 1988).

The 'mini-Percoll' method (Ord *et al.*, 1990) results in improved sperm recovery from poor semen specimens, compared with more conventional Percoll techniques. It has also been useful with epididymal sperm in cases of congenital absence of the vas deferens (Ord *et al.*, 1992).

Percoll gradient techniques increase the overall yield of motile sperm compared with swim-up techniques, although the percentage of sperm with good forward progression may actually be decreased (Englert *et al.*, 1992; Ng *et al.*, 1992; Sakkas *et al.*, 1993). A combined mini-Percoll/swim-up method may provide the best results (Ng *et al.*, 1992; Baker *et al.*, 1993).

Several other gradient separation procedures, such as albumin and Nycodenz, have been developed (Mortimer, 1990), with promising results from the use of discontinuous Nycodenz gradients (Gellert-Mortimer *et al.*, 1988; Serafini *et al.*, 1990). Unfortunately, cryopreserved specimens prepared with Nycodenz did not perform as well in the SPA as Percoll-prepared specimens (Ford *et al.*, 1992).

Incubation in TES and Tris-yolk buffer

Low-temperature storage of sperm in TEST-yolk buffer (Veeck, 1992) has been shown to enhance SPA performance (Bolanos *et al.*, 1983), HZA results (Lanzendorf *et al.*, 1992) and IVF results (Katayama *et al.*, 1989; Paulson *et al.*, 1992). However, such techniques may not provide better results than those involving discontinuous Percoll gradients, particularly in male factor cases (Quinn, 1993).

Motility stimulants

Several substances have been used to enhance sperm motility and overall function (Cummins & Yovich, 1993). Pentoxifylline, a trisubstituted xanthine derivative which acts as a cyclic nucleotide phosphodiesterase inhibitor (Yovich *et al.*, 1988*b*, 1990; Yovich, 1992), improves motility secondary to increased intracellular cyclic adenosine monophosphate (cAMP) concentrations, and may enhance sperm function through a reduction in adverse effects of ROS (Gavella *et al.*, 1991; Gavella & Lipovac, 1992). Pentoxifylline has been shown to enhance multiple CASA parameters as well as the percentage of hyperactivated sperm in both normal and asthenozoospermic specimens, with little if any effect on the percent motility (Tesarik *et al.*, 1992). Pentoxifylline may also be useful in some patients with acrosome reaction abnormalities (Tesarik & Mendoza, 1993).

Caffeine, another phosphodiesterase inhibitor known to stimulate sperm motility, does not improve IVF results (Imoedemhe *et al.*, 1992*b*). In contrast, the same authors reported improved IVF results using the adenosine analog 2-deoxyadenosine in cases of asthenozoospermia (Imoedemhe *et al*, 1992*a*).

Human follicular fluid also enhances sperm motility (Mbizvo *et al.*, 1990; Mendoza & Tesarik, 1990), which may also improve IVF results in male factor patients (Ghetler *et al.*, 1990; Giorgetti *et al.*, 1992; Muller, 1992). The combination of follicular fluid and pentoxifylline has been shown to improve SPA results as compared with either agent alone (Lambert *et al.*, 1992).

Insemination using high concentrations of motile sperm

In the absence of an identified male factor, the final concentration of motile sperm for oocyte insemination ranges between 30 000 and 250 000/ml, although decreased polyploidy and increased fertilization rate may occur with the lower concentration (Wolf *et al.*, 1984; YoungLai & Daya, 1991). In the presence of an abnormal semen analysis, fertilization is more likely to occur when higher

concentrations of motile sperm are used (Hammitt, 1993). Concentrations up
to 5×10^6/ml have been used with success (Hammitt *et al.*, 1991; Hammitt,
1993). 'Microinsemination' techniques, which involve concentrating the prepared sperm specimen in a small volume for oocyte insemination, have been
described. These have successfully employed glass microcapillary tubes (van der
Ven *et al.*, 1989) or embryo cryopreservation straws following removal of the
cumulus by incubation with hyaluronidase (Hammitt *et al.*, 1991).

Antisperm antibodies in semen: processing considerations

Infertility secondary to antisperm antibodies in semen can be successfully
treated by IVF. The number of antibody-free sperm obtained can be maximized by collecting the semen specimen directly into medium, followed by
immediate processing (Elder *et al.*, 1990; Avery & Elder, 1992) (see Chapters
5,8). Increasing the number of sperm used for oocyte insemination may
provide sufficient numbers of antibody-free sperm (Hamilton *et al.*, 1989).
Proteolytic enzymes such as chymotrysin to remove bound antibody may also
be beneficial (Pattinson *et al.*, 1990; Tucker *et al.*, 1990).

Viscous semen specimens: processing considerations

Viscous specimens may also benefit from collection directly into medium
(Avery & Elder, 1992) or the use of proteolytic enzymes during processing
(Cohen & Aafjes, 1982; Tucker *et al.*, 1990). If the male partner is well hydrated
on the day of collection viscosity may not be problematic.

Selection of sperm processing method

There is wide variation among centers as to the methodology for preparation of
both normal and abnormal semen specimens for IVF. These differences and an
overall lack of proper controls in generating data make it difficult to determine
which technique is suitable for a given couple with a male factor. For less severe
male factor cases, many of the techniques reviewed here may be appropriate.
For more severe cases, use of one of the assisted fertilization techniques should
be considered. However, the mini-Percoll method (Ord *et al.*, 1993) and microinsemination using high motile sperm concentrations (Hammitt, 1993) have
also been successfully applied to severe male factor cases that might otherwise
have been treated with an assisted fertilization technique. Decisions about
which technique to use for a couple should largely be based on the ART laboratory's capabilities and experience.

Preliminary testing prior to the procedure is crucial in order to allow implementation of the optimal technique. Examination of a specimen prepared as though for IVF may reveal a previously unsuspected problem, leading to exploration of other processing techniques for the particular male involved. Modified SPA results may particularly suggest the optimal semen processing technique (Muller, 1992).

Management of couples with failed fertilization

Failure of fertilization 12–18 hours after oocyte insemination may reflect abnormal sperm function, but also raises the possibility of a specific oocyte defect such as oocyte dysmaturity. Reinseminated oocytes rarely produce viable pregnancies (Winston *et al.*, 1993), even after use of an increased concentration of motile sperm (Pampiglione *et al.*, 1990) or donor semen (Trounson & Webb, 1984). Nonetheless, reinsemination appears to be reasonable if there is a lack of fertilization, if the oocytes were initially immature and if the survival of spermatozoa at the time of assessment of fertilization is noted to be poor.

Prior to another attempt at IVF, additional testing may be indicated, perhaps using the female partner's follicular fluid specimens and ZP (Muller, 1992). If the failure is due to a male factor, such additional testing may suggest the use of a different sperm preparation method, an assisted fertilization technique, or even donor semen. However, even without such interventions, the prognosis for couples following a single cycle with no fertilization may be good. One study reported fertilization in 36 of 44 second IVF cycles with no changes in sperm processing in couples with a male factor diagnosis following an earlier attempt with no fertilization (Ben-Shlomo *et al.*, 1992). Similar results have been reported for couples with 'unexplained' infertility (Molloy *et al.*, 1991; Lipitz *et al.*, 1993).

Selection of ART procedure

As in selection of diagnostic sperm function tests and IVF sperm processing techniques, there are large differences among centers about which ART therapy is most appropriate for specific male factor cases. For example, a severe male factor might be handled by microinsemination using high concentrations of motile sperm followed by ZIFT, or by referral elsewhere for assisted fertilization and standard uterine transfer.

The absence of at least one functional tube precludes the use of combined COH/IUI therapy or tubal transfer procedures. In cases of less severe male factor, and relatively normal tubal anatomy, after a trial of IUI alone, combined COH/IUI treatment may be chosen. Clinical pregnancy rates of 15% per cycle have been reported for combined COH/IUI treatment in these patients (Dodson & Haney, 1991; Ho *et al.*, 1992).

When the degree of sperm dysfunction is more severe, or following failed COH/IUI, the choices with normal tubal anatomy include standard IVF, ZIFT or TET, and GIFT with transfer of an increased number of spermatozoa. Overall, delivery rates per retrieval for IVF, ZIFT/TET and GIFT were 15.2%, 19.3% and 26.6%, respectively (Society for Assisted Reprodutive Technology, 1993). In the presence of a male factor IVF and GIFT rates were 13% and 26.9% respectively. Interpretation of these results is complicated by the selection bids that the male factor IVF and ZIFT/TET cases probably involved substantially worse semen parameters than the male factor GIFT cases, since GIFT success rates declined dramatically with increasingly poor sperm function (Guzick *et al.*, 1989; Rodriguez-Rigau *et al.*, 1989; van der Merwe *et al.*, 1992).

For male factor cases of a greater degree of severity in the presence of normal tubal anatomy, the most appropriate therapeutic options appear to be standard IVF, ZIFT or TET. Several retrospective reports (Balmaceda *et al.*, 1988; J.L. Yovich *et al.*, 1988*a*; Hammitt *et al.*, 1990) have suggested that ZIFT or TET is preferred over standard IVF because of higher success rates. However, prospective randomized (Tanbo *et al.*, 1990; Tournaye *et al.*, 1992) and non-randomized (Toth *et al.*, 1992) studies comparing ZIFT or TET with standard IVF found no appreciable difference in outcome. Since ZIFT and TET are significantly more invasive and expensive than standard IVF, their routine use can at present be justified only at centers where clear benefits have been demonstrated.

References

Aitken, R.J. (1990). Evaluation of human sperm function. *Br. Med. Bull.*, **46**, 654–74.

Aitken, R.J. & Clarkson, J.S. (1988). Significance of reactive oxygen species and antioxidants in defining the efficacy of sperm preparation techniques. *J. Androl.*, **9**, 367–76.

Aitken, R.J. & West, K.M. (1990). Analysis of the relationship between reactive oxygen species production and leucocyte infiltration in fractions of human semen separated on Percoll gradients. *Int. J. Androl.*, **13**, 433–51.

Aitken, R.J., Wang, Y.F., Liu, J., Best, F. & Richardson, D.W. (1983). The influence of medium composition, osmolarity and albumin content on the acrosome reaction and fertilizing capacity of human spermatozoa: development of an improved zona-free hamster egg penetration assay. *Int. J. Androl.*, **6**, 180–93.

Aitken, R.J., Ross, A., Hargreave, T., Richardson, D. & Best, F. (1984). Analysis of human sperm function following exposure to the ionophore A23187: comparison of normospermic and oligospermic men. *J. Androl.*, **5**, 321–9.

Aitken, R.J., Clarkson, J.S., Hargreave, T.B., Irvine, D.S. & Wu, F.C.W. (1989). Analysis of the relationship between defective sperm function and the generation of reactive oxygen species in cases of oligozoospermia. *J. Androl.*, **10**, 214–20.

Aitken, R.J., Kerr, L., Bolton, V. & Hargreave, T. (1990). Analysis of sperm function in globozoospermia: implications for the mechanism of sperm–zona interaction. *Fertil. Steril.*, **54**, 701–7.

Aitken, R.J., Buckingham, D., West, K., Wu, F.C., Zikopoulos, K. & Richardson, D.W. (1992). Differential contribution of leucocytes and spermatozoa to the generation of reactive oxygen species in the ejaculates of oligozoospermia patients and fertile donors. *J. Reprod. Fertil.*, **94**, 451–62.

Alvarez, J.G., Lasso, J.L., Blasco, L., Nuñez, R.C., Heyner, S., Caballero, P.P. & Storey, B.T. (1993). Centrifugation of human spermatozoa induces sublethal damage: separation of human spermatozoa by a dextran swim-up procedure without centrifugation extends their motile lifetime. *Hum. Reprod.*, **8**, 1087–92.

Avery, S.M. & Elder, K.T. (1992). Routine gamete handling: semen assessment and preparation. In *A Textbook of In Vitro Fertilization and Assisted Reproduction*, ed. P.R. Brinsden & P.A. Rainsbury, pp. 171–85. Park Ridge, NJ: Parthenon Publishing Group.

Baker, H.W.G., Ng, F.L.H. & Liu, D.Y. (1993). Preparation and analysis of semen for IVF/GIFT. In *Handbook of In Vitro Fertilization*, ed. A. Trounson & D.K. Gardner, pp. 33–56. Boca Raton, FL: CRC Press.

Balmaceda, J.P., Gastaldi, C., Remohi, J., Borrero, C., Ord, T. & Asch, R.H. (1988). Tubal embryo transfer as a treatment for infertility due to male factor. *Fertil. Steril.*, **50**, 476–9.

Battin, D., Vargyas, J.M., Sato, F., Brown, J. & Marrs, R.P. (1985). The correlation between *in vitro* fertilization of human oocytes and semen profile. *Fertil. Steril.*, **44**, 835–8.

Ben-Shlomo, I., Bider, D., Dor, J., Levran, D., Mashiach, S. & Ben-Rafael, Z. (1992). Failure to fertilize *in vitro* in couples with male factor infertility: what next? *Fertil. Steril.*, **58**, 187–9.

Bennett, C.J. (1990). Assisted reproductive technologies for the anejaculatory male. *Semin. Reprod. Endocrinol.*, **8**, 265–71.

Berberoglugil, P., Englert, Y., Van den Bergh, M., Rodesch, C., Bertrand, E. & Biramane, J. (1993). Abnormal sperm–mucus penetration test predicts low *in vitro* fertilization ability of apparently normal semen. *Fertil. Steril.*, **59**, 1228–32.

Berger, R.E., Karp, L.E., Williamson, R.A., Koehler, J., Moore, D.E. & Holmes, K.K. (1982). The relationship of pyospermia and seminal fluid bacteriology to sperm function as reflected in the sperm penetration assay. *Fertil. Steril.*, **37**, 557–64.

Berger, T., Marrs, R.P. & Moyer, D.L. (1985). Comparison of techniques for selection of motile spermatozoa. *Fertil. Steril.*, **43**, 268–73.

Blumenfeld, Z. & Nahhas, F. (1989). Pretreatment of sperm with human follicular fluid for borderline male infertility. *Fertil. Steril.*, **51**, 863–8.

Bolanos, J.R., Overstreet, J.W. & Katz, D.F. (1983). Human sperm penetration of zona-free hamster eggs after storage of the semen for 48 hours at 2°C to 5°C. *Fertil. Steril.*, **39**, 536–41.

Brinsden, P.R. & Asch, R.H. (1992). Gamete intrafallopian transfer. In *A Textbook of In Vitro Fertilization and Assisted Reproduction*, ed. P.R. Brinsden & P.A. Rainsbury, pp. 227–36. Park Ridge, NJ: Parthenon Publishing Group.

Bronson, R.A. & Rogers, B.J. (1988). Pitfalls of the zona-free hamster egg penetration test: protein source as a major variable. *Fertil. Steril.*, **50**, 851–4.

Brown, D.J. & Lavy, G. (1992). Assisted reproduction and the male factor: an update. *Assist. Reprod. Rev.*, **2**, 170–2.

Burkman, L.J. (1990). Hyperactivated motility of human spermatozoa during *in vitro* capacitation and implications for fertility. In *Controls of Sperm Motility: Biological and Clinical Aspects*, ed. C. Gagnon, pp. 303–29. Boca Raton, FL: CRC Press.

Burkman, L.J. (1991). Discrimination between nonhyperactivated and classical hyperactivated motility parameters in human spermatozoa using computerized analysis. *Fertil. Steril.*, **55**, 363–71.

Burkman, L.J., Coddington, C.C., Franken, D.R., Krugen, T.F., Rosenwaks, Z. & Hogen, G.D. (1988). The hemizona assay (HZA): development of a diagnostic test for the binding of human spermatozoa to the human hemizona pellucida to predict fertilization potential. *Fertil. Steril.*, **49**, 688–97.

Bustillo, M., Munabi, A.K. & Schulman, J.D. (1988). Pregnancy after nonsurgical ultrasound-guided gamete intrafallopian transfer [letter]. *N. Eng. J. Med.*, **319**, 313.

Carrell, D.T., Bradshaw, W.S., Jones, K.P., Middleton, R.G., Peterson, C.M. & Urry, R.L. (1992). An evaluation of various treatments to increase sperm penetration capacity for potential use in an *in vitro* fertilization program. *Fertil. Steril.*, **57**, 134–8.

Cefalu, E., Cittadini, E., Balmaceda, J.P., Guastella, G., Ord, T., Rojas, F.J. & Asch, R.H. (1988). Successful gamete intrafallopian transfer following failed artificial insemination by donor: evidence for a defect in gamete transport? *Fertil. Steril.*, **50**, 279–82.

Chan, P.J., Prough, S.G., Henig, I. & Tredway, D.R. (1992). Predictive value of sperm hyperactivation measurements based on the dilution effect method in clinical *in vitro* fertilization. *Int. J. Fertil.*, **37**, 373–7.

Chan, S.Y.W., Wang, C., Chan, S.T.H., Ho, P.C., So, W.W.K., Chan, Y.F. & Ma, H.K. (1989). Predictive value of sperm morphology and movement characteristics in the outcome of *in vitro* fertilization of human oocytes. *J. In Vitro Fertil. Embryo Transf.*, **6**, 142–8.

Coddington, C.C., Franken, D.R., Burkman, L.J., Oosthuizen, W.T., Kruger, T. & Hodgen, G.D. (1991). Functional aspects of human sperm binding to the zona pellucida using the hemizona assay. *J. Androl.*, **12**, 1–8.

Coetzee, K., Kruger, T.F., Menkveld, R., Swanson, R.J., Lombard, C.J. & Acosta, A.A. (1989). Usefulness of sperm penetration assay in fertility predictions. *Arch. Androl.*, **23**, 207–12.

Cohen, J. & Aafjes, J.H. (1982). Proteolytic enzymes stimulate human spermatozoal motility and *in vitro* hamster egg penetration. *Life Sci.*, **30**, 899–904.

Cohen, J., Edwards, R., Fehilly, C., Fishel, S., Hewitt, J., Purdy, J., Rowland, G., Steptoe, P. & Webster, J. (1985). *In vitro* fertilization: a treatment for male infertility. *Fertil. Steril.*, **43**, 422–32.

Corsan, G.H. & Kemmann, E. (1991). The role of superovulation with menotropins in ovulatory infertility: a review. *Fertil. Steril.*, **55**, 468–77.

Critser, J.K. & Noiles, E.E. (1993). Bioassays of sperm function. *Sermin. Reprod. Endocrinol.*, **11**, 16.

Cummins, J.M. & Yovich, J.M. (1993). Sperm motility enhancement *in vitro. Semin. Reprod. Endocrinol.*, **11**, 56–71.

Davis, R.O., Overstreet, J.W., Asch, R.H., Ord, T. & Silber, S.J. (1991). Movement characteristics of human epididymal sperm used for fertilization of human oocytes *in vitro. Fertil. Steril.*, **56**, 1128–35.

De Jonge, C.J., Tarchala, S.M., Rawlins, R.G., Binor, Z. & Radwanska, E. (1993). Acrosin activity in human spermatozoa in relation to semen quality and *in-vitro* fertilization. *Hum. Reprod.*, **8**, 253–7.

de la Calle, J.F.V. (1991). Human spermatozoa selection in improved discontinuous Percoll gradients. *Fertil. Steril.*, **56**, 737–42.

Devroey, P., Staessen, C., Camus, M., De Grauwe, E., Wisanto, A. & Van Steirteghem, A.C. (1989). Zygote intrafallopian transfer as a successful treatment for unexplained infertility. *Fertil. Steril.*, **52**, 246–9.

Dodson, W.C. & Haney, A.F. (1991). Controlled ovarian hyperstimulation and intrauterine insemination for treatment of infertility. *Fertil. Steril.*, **55**, 457–67.

Duncan, W.W., Glew, M.J., Wang, X.-J., Flaherty, S.P. & Matthews, C.D. (1993). Prediction of *in vitro* fertilization rates from semen variables. *Fertil. Steril.*, **59**, 1233–8.

Edwards, R.G., Steptoe, P.C. & Purdy, J.M. (1980). Establishing full-term human pregnancies using cleaving embryos grown *in vitro. Br. J. Obstet. Gynaecol.*, **87**, 737–56.

Elder, K.T., Wick, K.L. & Edwards, R.G. (1990). Seminal plasma anti-sperm antibodies and IVF: the effect of semen sample collection into 50% serum. *Hum. Reprod.*, **5**, 179–84.

Enginsu, M.E., Dumoulin, J.C.M., Pieters, M.H.E.C., Bergers, M., Evers, J.L.H. & Geraedts, J.P.M. (1992*a*). Comparison between the hypoosmotic swelling test and morphology evaluation using strict criteria in predicting *in vitro* fertilization (IVF). *J. Assist. Reprod. Genet.*, **9**, 259–64.

Enginsu, M.E., Pieters, M.H.E.C., Dumoulin, J.C.M., Evers, J.L.H. & Geraedts, J.P.M. (1992*b*). Male factor as determinant of *in-vitro* fertilization outcome. *Hum. Reprod.*, **7**, 1136–40.

Englert, Y., Van den Bergh, M., Rodesch, C., Bertrand, E., Biramane, J. & Legreve, A. (1992). Comparative auto-controlled study between swim-up and Percoll preparation of fresh semen samples for *in-vitro* fertilization. *Hum. Reprod.*, **7**, 399–402.

Ford, W.C.L., McLaughlin, E.A., Prior, S.M., Rees, J.M., Wardle, P.G. & Hull, M.G.R. (1992). The yield, motility and performance in the hamster egg test of human spermatozoa prepared from cryopreserved semen by four different methods. *Hum. Reprod.*, **7**, 654–9.

Franken, D.R., Oehninger, S., Burkman, L.J., Coddington, C.C., Kruger, T.F., Rosenwaks, Z., Acosta, A.A. & Hodgen, G.D. (1989). The hemizona assay (HZA): a predictor of human sperm fertilizing potential in in vitro (IVF) treatment. *J. In Vitro Fertil. Embryo Transf.*, **6**, 44–50.

Franken, D.R., Acosta, A.A., Kruger, T.F., Lombard, C.J., Oehninger, S. & Hodgen, G.D. (1993). The hemizona assay: its role in identifying male factor infertility in assisted reproduction. *Fertil. Steril.*, **59**, 1075–80.

Fraser, L.R. & DasGupta, S. (1993). Sperm morphology: Does it have predictive value for *in vitro* fertilization? *Semin. Reprod. Endocrinol.*, **11**, 17–26.

Gavella, M. & Lipovac, V. (1992). Pentoxifylline-mediated reduction of superoxide anion production by human spermatozoa. *Andrologia*, **24**, 37–9.

Gavella, M., Lipovac, V. & Marotti, T. (1991). Effect of pentoxifylline on superoxide anion production by human sperm. *Int. J. Androl.*, **14**, 320–7.

Gellert-Mortimer, S.T., Clarke, G.N., Baker, H.W., Hyne, R.V. & Johnston, W.I. (1988). Evaluation of Nycodenz and Percoll density gradients for the selection of motile human spermatozoa. *Fertil. Steril.*, **49**, 335–41.

Ghetler, Y., Ben-Nun, I., Kaneti, H., Jaffe, R., Gruber, A. & Fejgin, M. (1990). Effect of sperm preincubation with follicular fluid on the fertilization rate in human *in vitro* fertilization. *Fertil. Steril.*, **54**, 944–6.

Ginsburg, K.A., Sacco, A.G., Moghissi, K.S. & Sorovetz, S. (1989). Variation of movement characteristics with washing and capacitation of spermatozoa. I. Univariate statistical analysis and detection of sperm hyperactivation. *Fertil. Steril.*, **51**, 869–73.

Giorgetti, C., Hans, E., Spach, J.L., Auquier, P. & Roulier, R. (1992). *In-vitro* fertilization in cases with severe sperm defect: use of a swim-across technique and medium supplemented with follicular fluid. *Hum. Reprod.*, **7**, 1121–5.

Gorus, F.K. & Pipeleers, D.G. (1981). A rapid method for the fractionation of human spermatozoa according to their progressive motility. *Fertil. Steril.*, **35**, 662–5.

Guzick, D.S., Balmaceda, J.P., Ord, T. & Asch, R.H. (1989). The importance of egg and sperm factors in predicting the likelihood of pregnancy from gamete intrafallopian transfer. *Fertil. Steril.*, **52**, 795–800.

Hamilton, F., Gutley-Yeo, A.L. & Meldrum, D.R. (1989). Normal fertilization in men with high antibody sperm binding by the addition of sufficient unbound sperm in vitro. *J. In Vitro Fertil. Embryo Transf.*, **6**, 342–4.

Hammitt, D.G. (1993). Treatment of male-factor infertility by *in vitro* insemination with high concentrations of motile sperm. *Semin. Reprod. Endocrinol.*, **11**, 72–82.

Hammitt, D.G., Syrop, C.H., Hahn, S.J., Walker, D.L., Butkowski, C.R. & Donovan, J.F. (1990). Comparison of concurrent pregnancy rates for *in-vitro* fertilization: embryo transfer, pronuclear stage embryo transfer and gamete intra-fallopian transfer. *Hum. Reprod.*, **5**, 947–54.

Hammitt, D.G., Walker, D.L., Syrop, C.H., Miller, T.M. & Bennett, M.R. (1991). Treatment of severe male-factor infertility with high concentrations of motile sperm by microinsemination in embryo cryopreservation straws. *J. In Vitro Fertil. Embryo Transf.*, **8**, 101–10.

Hauser, R., Yavetz, H., Paz, G.F., Homonnai, Z.T., Amit, A., Lessing, J.B., Peyser, M. R. & Yogev, L. (1992). The predictive fertilization value of the hypoosmotic swelling test (HOST) for fresh and cryopreserved sperm. *J. Assist. Reprod. Genet.*, **9**, 265–70.

Hirayama, T., Hasegawa, T. & Hiroi, M. (1989). The measurement of hyaluronidase activity in human spermatozoa by substrate slide assay and its clinical application. *Fertil. Steril.*, **51**, 330–4.

Ho, P.-C., So, W.-K., Chan, Y.-F. & Yeung, W.S.-B. (1992). Intrauterine insemination after ovarian stimulation as a treatment for subfertility because of subnormal semen: a prospective randomized controlled trial. *Fertil. Steril.*, **58**, 995–9.

Holt, W.V., Moore, H.D. & Hillier, S.G. (1985). Computer-assisted measurement of sperm swimming speed in human semen: correlation of results with *in vitro* fertilization assays. *Fertil. Steril.*, **44**, 112–19.

Huszar, G., Vigue, L. & Morshedi, M. (1992). Sperm creatine phosphokinase M-isoform ratios and fertilizing potential of men: a blinded study of 84 couples treated with *in vitro* fertilization. *Fertil. Steril.*, **57**, 882–8.

Hyne, R.V., Stojanoff, A., Clarke, G.N., Lopata, A. & Johnston, W.I. (1986). Pregnancy from *in vitro* fertilization of human eggs after separation of motile spermatozoa by density gradient centrifugation. *Fertil. Steril.*, **45**, 93–6.

Imoedemhe, D.A.G., Sigue, A.B., Pacpaco, E.A. & Olazo, A.B. (1992*a*). Successful use of the sperm motility enhancer 2-deoxyadenosine in previously failed human *in vitro* fertilization. *J. Assist. Reprod. Genet.*, **9**, 53–6.

Imoedemhe, D.A.G., Sigue, A.B., Pacpaco, E.A. & Olazo, A.B. (1992*b*). The effect of caffeine on the ability of spermatozoa to fertilize mature human oocytes. *J. Assist. Reprod. Genet.*, **9**, 155–60.

Jansen, R.P.S. & Anderson, J.C. (1987). Catheterisation of the fallopian tubes from the vagina. *Lancet*, **ii**, 309–10.

Jeulin, C., Feneux, D., Serres, C., Jouannet, P., Guillet-Rosso, F., Belaisch-Allart, J., Frydman, R. & Testart, J. (1986). Sperm factors related to failure of human *in-vitro* fertilization. *J. Reprod. Fertil.*, **76**, 735–44.

Jeyendran, R.S., Van der Ven, H.H., Perez-Pelaez, M., Crabo, B.G. & Zaneveld, L.J. (1984). Development of an assay to assess the functional integrity of the human sperm membrane and its relationship to other semen characteristics. *J. Reprod. Fertil.*, **70**, 219–28.

Jeyendran, R.S., Van der Ven, H.H. & Zaneveld, L.J.D. (1992). The hypoosmotic swelling test: an update. *Arch. Androl.*, **29**, 105–16.

Katayama, K.P., Stehlik, E., Roesler, M., Jeyendran, R.S., Holmgren, W.J. & Zaneveld, L.J.D. (1989). Treatment of human spermatozoa with an egg yolk medium can enhance the outcome of *in vitro* fertilization. *Fertil. Steril.*, **52**, 1077–9.

Katz, D.F., Davis, R.O., Drobnis, E.Z. & Overstreet, J.W. (1993). Sperm motility measurement and hyperactivation. *Semin. Reprod. Endocrinol.*, **11**, 27–39.

Kessopoulou, E., Tomlinson, M.J., Barratt, C.L.R., Bolton, A.E. & Cooke, I.D. (1992). Origin of reactive oxygen species in human semen: spermatozoa or leucocytes? *J. Reprod. Fertil.*, **94**, 463–70.

Kruger, T.F., Menkveld, R., Stander, F.S.H., Lombard, C.J., Van der Merwe, J.P., van Zyl, J.A. & Smith, K. (1986). Sperm morphologic features as a prognostic factor in *in vitro* fertilization. *Fertil. Steril.*, **46**, 1118–23.

Kruger, T.F., Acosta, A.A., Simmons, K.F., Swanson, R.J., Matta, J.F. & Oehninger, S. (1988*a*). Predictive value of abnormal sperm morphology in *in vitro* fertilization. *Fertil. Steril.*, **49**, 112–17.

Kruger, T.F., Haque, D., Acosta, A.A., Pleban, P., Swanson, R.J., Simmons, K.F., Matta, J.F., Morshedi, M. & Oehninger, S. (1988*b*). Correlation between sperm morphology, acrosin, and fertilization in an IVF program. *Arch. Androl.*, **20**, 237–41.

Lambert, H., Steinleitner, A., Eisermann, J., Serpa, N. & Cantor, B. (1992). Enhanced gamete interaction in the sperm penetration assay after coincubation with pentoxifylline and human follicular fluid. *Fertil. Steril.*, **58**, 1205–8.

Lanzendorf, S.E., Holmgren, W.J. & Jeyendran, R.S. (1992). The effect of egg yolk medium on human sperm binding in the hemizona assay. *Fertil. Steril.*, **58**, 547–50.

Lipitz, S., Rabinovici, J., Ben-Shlomo, I., Bider, D., Ben-Rafael, Z., Mashiach, S. & Dor, J. (1993). Complete failure of fertilization in couples with unexplained infertility: implications for subsequent *in vitro* cycles. *Fertil. Steril.*, **59**, 348–52.

Liu, D.Y. & Baker, H.W.G. (1988). The proportion of human sperm with poor morphology but normal intact acrosomes detected with *Pisum sativum* agglutinin correlates with fertilization *in vitro. Fertil. Steril.*, **50**, 288–93.

Liu, D.Y. & Baker, H.W.G. (1990). Inducing the human acrosome reaction with a calcium ionophore A23187 decreases sperm-zona pellucida binding with oocytes that failed to fertilize *in vitro. J. Reprod. Fertil.*, **89**, 127–34.

Liu, D.Y. & Baker, H.W.G. (1992*a*). Morphology of spermatozoa bound to the zona pellucida of human oocytes that failed to fertilize *in vitro. J. Reprod. Fertil.*, **94**, 71–84.

Liu, D.Y. & Baker, H.W.G. (1992*b*). Tests of human sperm function and fertilization *in vitro. Fertil. Steril.*, **58**, 465–83.

Liu, D.Y., Lopata, A., Johnston, W.I. & Baker, H.W. (1988). A human sperm–zona pellucida binding test using oocytes that failed to fertilize *in vitro. Fertil. Steril.*, **50**, 782–8.

Liu, D.Y., Clarke, G.N., Lopata, A., Johnston, W.I. & Baker, H.W. (1989). A sperm–zona pellucida binding test and *in vitro* fertilization. *Fertil. Steril.*, **52**, 281–7.

Liu, D.Y., Clarke, G.N. & Baker, H.W.G. (1991). Relationship between sperm motility assessed with the Hamilton-Thorn Motility Analyzer and fertilization rates *in vitro. J. Androl.*, **12**, 231–9.

Lopata, A., Patullo, M.J., Chang, A. & James, B. (1976). A method for collecting motile spermatozoa from human semen. *Fertil. Steril.*, **27**, 677–84.

Lopata, A., Johnston, I.W.H., Hoult, I.J. & Speirs, A.I. (1980). Pregnancy following intrauterine implantation of an embryo obtained by *in vitro* fertilization of a preovulatory egg. *Fertil. Steril.*, **23**, 117–20.

Mahadevan, M.M. & Trounson, A.O. (1984). The influence of seminal characteristics on the success rates of human *in vitro* fertilization. *Fertil. Steril.*, **42**, 400–5.

Mahadevan, M.M., Trounson, A.O. & Leeton, J.F. (1983). The relationship of tubal blockage, infertility of unknown cause, suspected male infertility, and endometriosis to success of *in vitro* fertilization and embryo transfer. *Fertil. Steril.*, **40**, 755–62.

Mallidis, C., Howard, E.J. & Baker, H.W.G. (1991). Variation of semen quality in normal men. *Int. J. Androl.*, **14**, 99–107.

Margalioth, E.J., Navot, D., Laufer, N., Lewin, A., Rabinowitz, R. & Schenker, J.G. (1986). Correlation between the zona-free hamster egg sperm penetration assay and human *in vitro* fertilization. *Fertil. Steril.*, **45**, 665–70.

Mashiach, R., Fisch, B., Eltes, F., Tadir, Y., Ovadia, J. & Bartoov, B. (1992). The relationship between sperm ultrastructural features and fertilizing capacity *in vitro. Fertil. Steril.*, **57**, 1052–7.

Matson, P.L., Blackledge, D.G., Richardson, P.A., Turner, S.R., Yovich, J.M. & Yovich, J.L. (1987). The role of gamete intrafallopian transfer (GIFT) in the treatment of oligospermic infertility. *Fertil. Steril.*, **48**, 608–12.

Mbizvo, M.T., Burkman, L.J. & Alexander, N.J. (1990). Human follicular fluid stimulates hyperactivated motility in human sperm. *Fertil. Steril.*, **54**, 708–12.

McClure, R.D., Nunes, L. & Tom, R. (1989). Semen manipulation: improved sperm recovery and function with a two-layered Percoll gradient. *Fertil. Steril.*, **51**, 874–7.

McDowell, J.S., Veeck, L.L. & Jones, H.W., Jr (1985). Analysis of human spermatozoa before and after processing for *in vitro* fertilization. *J. In Vitro Fertil. Embryo Transf.*, **2**, 23–6.

Meacham, R.B. & Lipshultz, L.I. (1990). The impact of *in vitro* fertilization on male infertility. *Semin. Reprod. Endocrinol.*, **8**, 281–9.

Mendoza, C. & Tesarik, J. (1990). Effect of follicular fluid on sperm movement characteristics. *Fertil. Steril.*, **54**, 1135–9.

Menkveld, R., Stander, F.S., Kotze, T.J., Kruger, T.F. & van Zyl, J.A. (1990). The evaluation of morphological characteristics of human spermatozoa according to stricter criteria. *Hum. Reprod.*, **5**, 586–92.

Molloy, D., Harrison, K., Breen, T. & Hennessey, J. (1991). The predictive value of idiopathic failure to fertilize on the first *in vitro* fertilization attempt. *Fertil. Steril.*, **56**, 285–9.

Morales, P., Cross, N.L., Overstreet, J.W. & Hanson, F.W. (1989). Acrosome intact and acrosome-reacted human sperm can initiate binding to the zona pellucida. *Dev. Biol.*, **133**, 385–92.

Mortimer, D. (1990). Semen analysis and sperm washing techniques. In *Controls of Sperm Motility: Biological and Clinical Aspects*, ed. C. Gagnon, pp. 263–84. Boca Raton, FL: CRC Press.

Mortimer, D. (1991). Sperm preparation techniques and iatrogenic failure of *in-vitro* fertilization. *Hum. Reprod.*, **6**, 173–6.

Muller, C.H. (1992). The andrology laboratory in an Assisted Reproductive Technologies program: quality assurance and laboratory methodology. *J. Androl.*, **13**, 349–60.

Ng, F.L.H., Liu, D.Y. & Baker, H.W.G. (1992). Comparison of Percoll, mini-Percoll and swim-up methods for sperm preparation from abnormal semen samples. *Hum. Reprod*, **7**, 261–6.

Nulsen, J.C., Metzger, D.A. & Steinhoff, M.M. (1992). Sperm electron microscopy for the evaluation of *in vitro* fertilization failures. *J. Assist. Reprod. Genet.*, **9**, 491–7.

Oehninger, S., Acosta, A.A., Kruger, T., Veeck, L.L., Flood, J. & Jones, H.W., Jr (1988a). Failure of fertilization in *in vitro* fertilization: the 'occult' male factor. *J. In Vitro Fertil. Embryo Transf.*, **5**, 181–7.

Oehninger, S., Acosta, A.A., Morshedi, M., Veeck, L., Swanson, R.J., Simmons, K. & Rosenwaks, Z. (1988b). Corrective measures and pregnancy outcome in *in vitro* fertilization in patients with severe sperm morphologic abnormalities. *Fertil. Steril.*, **50**, 283–7.

Oehninger, S., Coddington, C.C., Scott, R., Franken, D.A., Burkman, L.J., Acosta, A.A. & Hodgen, G.D. (1989). Hemizona assay: assessment of sperm dysfunction and prediction of *in vitro* fertilization outcome. *Fertil. Steril.*, **51**, 665–70.

Oehninger, S., Acosta, A.A., Veeck, L.L., Brzyski, R., Kruger, T.F., Muasher, S.J. & D. H.G. (1991). Recurrent failure of *in vitro* fertilization: role of the hemizona assay in the sequential diagnosis of specific sperm–oocyte defects. *Am. J. Obstet. Gynecol.*, **164**, 1210–15.

Ord, T., Patrizio, P., Marello, E., Balmaceda, J.P. & Asch, R.H. (1990). Mini-Percoll: a new method of semen preparation for IVF in severe male factor infertility. *Hum. Reprod.*, **5**, 987–9.

Ord, T., Marello, E., Patrizio, P., Balmaceda, J.P., Silber, S.J. & Asch, R.H. (1992). The role of the laboratory in the handling of epididymal sperm for assisted reproductive technologies. *Fertil. Steril.*, **57**, 1103–6.

Ord, T., Patrizio, P., Balmaceda, J.P. & Asch, R.H. (1993). Can severe male factor infertility be treated without micromanipulation. *Fertil. Steril.*, **60**, 110–15.

Pampiglione, J.S., Mills, C., Campbell, S., Steer, C., Kingsland, C. & Mason, B.A.

(1990). The clinical outcome of reinsemination of human oocytes fertilized *in vitro*. *Fertil. Steril.*, **53**, 306–10.

Pampiglione, J.S., Tan, S.-L. & Campbell, S. (1993). The use of the stimulated acrosome reaction test as a test of fertilizing ability in human spermatozoa. *Fertil. Steril.*, **59**, 1280–4.

Pattinson, H.A., Mortimer, D. & Taylor, P.J. (1990). Treatment of sperm agglutination with proteolytic enzymes. II. Sperm function after enzymatic disagglutination. *Hum. Reprod.*, **5**, 174–8.

Paulson, R.J., Sauer, M.V., Francis, M.M., Macaso, T.M. & Lobo, R.A. (1992). A prospective controlled evaluation of TEST-yolk buffer in the preparation of sperm for human *in vitro* fertilization in suspected cases of male infertility. *Fertil. Steril.*, **58**, 551–5.

Purdy, J.M. (1982). Methods for fertilization and embryo culture *in vitro*. In *Human Conception In Vitro*, ed. R.G. Edwards & J.M. Purdy, pp. 135–48. New York: Academic Press.

Quinn, P. (1993). Sperm processing in assisted reproductive technology: male factor. *Semin. Reprod. Endocrinol.*, **11**, 49–55.

Rainsbury, P.A. (1992). The treatment of male factor infertility due to sexual dysfunction. In *A Textbook of In Vitro Fertilization and Assisted Reproduction*, ed. P.R. Brinsden & P.A. Rainsbury, pp. 345–59. Park Ridge, NJ: Parthenon Publishing Group.

Robertson, L., Wolf, D.P. & Tash, J.S. (1988). Temporal changes in motility parameters related to acrosomal status: identification and characterization of populations of hyperactivated human sperm. *Biol. Reprod.*, **39**, 797–805.

Robinson, J.N., Lockwood, G.M., Dokras, A., Egan, D.M., Ross, C. & Barlow, D.H. (1993). A controlled study to assess the use of *in vitro* fertilization with donor semen after failed therapeutic donor insemination. *Fertil. Steril.*, **59**, 353–8.

Rodriguez-Rigau, L.J., Ayala, C., Grunert, G.M., Woodward, R.M., Lotze, E.C., Feste, J.R., Gibbons, W., Smith, K.D. & Steinberger, E.(1989). Relationship between the results of sperm analysis and GIFT. *J. Androl.*, **10**, 139–44.

Ron-El, R., Nachum, H., Herman, A., Golan, A., Caspi, E. & Soffer, Y. (1991). Delayed fertilization and poor embryonic development associated with impaired semen quality. *Fertil. Steril.*, **55**, 338–44.

Sakkas, D., Gianaroli, L., Diotallevi, L., Wagner, I., Ferraretti, A.P. & Campana, A. (1993). IVF treatment of moderate male factor infertility: a comparison of mini-Percoll, partial zona dissection and sub-zonal sperm insertion techniques. *Hum. Reprod.*, **8**, 587–91.

Sanchez, R. & Schill, W.B. (1991). Influence of incubation time/temperature on acrosome reaction/sperm penetration assay. *Arch. Androl.*, **27**, 35–42.

Schill, W.-B. (1991). Some disturbances of acrosomal development and function in human spermatozoa. *Hum. Reprod.*, **6**, 969–78.

Scholtes, M.C.W., Roozenburg, B.J., Alberda, A.T. & Zeilmaker, G.H. (1990). Transcervical intrafallopian transfer of zygotes. *Fertil. Steril.*, **54**, 283–6.

Serafini, P., Blank, W., Tran, C., Mansourian, M., Tan, T. & Batzofin, J. (1990). Enhanced penetration of zona-free hamster ova by sperm prepared by Nycodenz and Percoll gradient centrifugation. *Fertil. Steril.*, **53**, 551–5.

Silber, S.J., Balmaceda, J., Borrero, C., Ord, T. & Asch, R. (1988). Pregnancy with sperm aspiration from the proximal head of the epididymis: a new treatment for congenital absence of the vas deferens. *Fertil. Steril.*, **50**, 525–8.

Society for Assisted Reproductive Technology, The American Fertility Society (1993). Assisted reproductive technology in the United States and Canada: 1991 results from the Society for Assisted Reproductive Technology generated from The American Fertility Society Registry. *Fertil. Steril.*, **59**, 956–62.

Soffer, Y., Golan, A., Herman, A., Pansky, M., Caspi, E. & Ron-El, R. (1992). Prediction of *in vitro* fertilization outcome by sperm penetration assay with TEST-yolk buffer preincubation. *Fertil. Steril.*, **58**, 556–62.

Stevens, R.W., III (1990). Basic spermatozoon anatomy and physiology for the clinician. In *Human Spermatozoa in Assisted Reproduction*, ed. A.A. Acota, R.J. Swanson, S.B. Ackerman, T.F. Kruger, J.A. van Zyl & R. Menkveld, pp. 1–23. Baltimore: Williams & Wilkins.

Storey, B.T. (1991). Sperm capacitation and the acrosome reaction. *Ann. N.Y. Acad. Sci.*, **637**, 459–73.

Takahashi, K., Wetzels, A.M., Goverde, H.J., Bastaans, B.A., Janssen, H.J. & Rolland, R. (1992). The kinetics of the acrosome reaction of human spermatozoa and its correlation with *in vitro* fertilization. *Fertil. Steril.*, **57**, 889–94.

Tanbo, T., Dale, P.O. & Abyholm, T. (1990). Assisted fertilization in infertile women with patent fallopian tubes: a comparison of *in-vitro* fertilization, gamete intra-fallopian transfer and tubal embryo stage transfer. *Hum. Reprod.*, **5**, 266–70.

Tesarik, J. (1989). Appropriate timing of the acrosome reaction is a major requirement for the fertilizing spermatozoon. *Hum. Reprod.*, **4**, 957–61.

Tesarik, J. (1992). Control of the fertilization process by the egg coat: how does it work in humans? *J. Assist. Reprod. Genet.*, **9**, 313–17.

Tesarik, J. & Mendoza, C. (1993). Sperm treatment with pentoxifylline improves the fertilizing ability in patients with acrosome reaction insufficiency. *Fertil. Steril.*, **60**, 141–8.

Tesarik, J., Drahorad, J. & Peknicova, J. (1988). Subcellular immunochemical localization of acrosin in human spermatozoa during the acrosome reaction and zona pellucida penetration. *Fertil. Steril.*, **50**, 133–41.

Tesarik, J., Thébault, A. & Testart, J. (1992). Effect of pentoxifylline on sperm movement characteristics in normozoospermic and asthenozoospermic specimens. *Hum. Reprod.*, **7**, 1257–63.

Tesarik, J., Mendoza, C. & Carreras, A. (1993). Fast acrosome reaction measure: a highly sensitive method for evaluating stimulus-induced acrosome reaction. *Fertil. Steril.*, **59**, 424–30.

Tombes, R.M. & Shapiro, B.M. (1985). Metabolite channeling: a phosphorylcreatine shuttle to mediate high energy phosphate transport between sperm mitochondrion and tail. *Cell*, **41**, 325–34.

Toth, T.L., Oehninger, S., Toner, J.P., Brzyski, R.G., Acosta, A.A. & Muasher, S.J. (1992). Embryo transfer to the uterus or the fallopian tube after *in vitro* fertilization yields similar results. *Fertil. Steril.*, **57**, 1110–13.

Tournaye, H., Devroey, P., Camus, M., Valkenburg, M., Bollen, N. & Van Steirteghem, A.C. (1992). Zygote intrafallopian transfer or *in vitro* fertilization and embryo transfer for the treatment of male-factor infertility: a prospective randomized trial. *Fertil. Steril.*, **58**, 344–50.

Trounson, A. & Webb, J. (1984). Fertilization of human oocytes following reinsemination *in vitro*. *Fertil. Steril.*, **41**, 816–19.

Tucker, M., Wright, G., Bishop, F., Wiker, S., Cohen, J., Chan, Y.M. & Sharma, R. (1990). Chymotrypsin in semen preparation for ARTA. *Mol. Androl.*, **2**, 179–86.

Tummon, I.S., Yuzpe, A.A., Daniel, S.A.J. & Deutsch, A. (1991). Total acrosin activity correlates with fertility potential after fertilization *in vitro. Fertil. Steril.,* **56**, 933–8.

van der Merwe, J.P., Kruger, T.F., Grobler, G.M., Hulme, V., Windt, M.-L., Stander, F.S.H., Coetzee, K. & Erasmus, E. (1990). Evaluation and preparation of spermatozoa for gamete intrafallopian transfer. In *Human Spermatozoa in Assisted Reproduction,* ed. A.A. Acosta, R.J. Swanson, S.B. Ackermann, T.F. Kruger, J.A. van Zyl & R. Menkveld, pp. 256–61. Baltimore: Williams & Wilkins.

van der Merwe, J.P., Kruger, T.F., Swart, Y. & Lombard, C.J. (1992). The role of oocyte maturity in the treatment of infertility because of teratozoospermia and normozoospermia with gamete intrafallopian transfer. *Fertil. Steril.,* **58**, 581–6.

van der Ven, H.H., Hoebbel, K., al-Hasani, S., Diedrich, K. & Krebs, D. (1989). Fertilization of human oocytes in capillary tubes with very small numbers of spermatozoa. *Hum. Reprod.,* **4**, 72–6.

Veeck, L. (1992). TES and Tris (TEST)-yolk buffer systems, sperm function testing, and *in vitro* fertilization. *Fertil. Steril.,* **58**, 484–6.

Wang, C., Lee, G.S., Leung, A., Surrey, E.S. & Chan, S.Y.W. (1993). Human sperm hyperactivation and acrosome reaction and their relationships to human *in vitro* fertilization. *Fertil. Steril.,* **59**, 1221–7.

Winston, N.J., Braude, P.R. & Johnson, M.H. (1993). Are failed-fertilized human oocytes useful? *Hum. Reprod.,* **8**, 503–7.

Wolf, D.P., Byrd, W., Dandekar, P. & Quigley, M.M. (1984). Sperm concentration and the fertilization of human eggs *in vitro. Biol. Reprod.,* **31**, 837–48.

Wolff, H., Politch, J.A., Martinez, A., Haimovici, F., Hill, J.A. & Anderson, D.J. (1990). Leukocytospermia is associated with poor sperm quality. *Fertil. Steril.,* **53**, 528–36.

World Health Organization (1987). Normal values of semen variables. In *WHO Laboratory Manual for the Examination of Human Semen and Semen–Cervical Mucus Interaction,* 2nd edn, p. 27. Cambridge: Cambridge University Press.

World Health Organization (1992*a*). Collection and examination of human semen. In *WHO Laboratory Manual for the Examination of Human Semen and Sperm–Cervical Mucus Interaction,* 3rd edn, pp. 3–27. Cambridge: Cambridge University Press.

World Health Organization (1992*b*). Normal values of semen variables. In *WHO Laboratory Manual for the Examination of Human Semen and Sperm–Cervical Mucus Interaction,* 3rd edn, pp. 43–4. Cambridge: Cambridge University Press.

World Health Organization (1992*c*). Nomenclature for some semen variables. In *WHO Laboratory Manual for the Examination of Human Semen and Sperm–Cervical Mucus Interaction,* 3rd edn, p. 45. Cambridge: Cambridge University Press.

Wortham, J.W.E., Veeck, L.L., Witmyer, J. & Jones, H.W., Jr (1983). Vital initiation of pregnancy (VIP) using human menopausal gonadotropin and human chorionic ovulation induction: phase I–1981. *Fertil. Steril.,* **39**, 785–92.

Yanagimachi, R., Yanagimachi, H. & Rogers, B.J. (1976). The use of zona-free animal ova as a test-system for the assessment of the fertilizing capacity of human spermatozoa. *Biol. Reprod.,* **15**, 471–6.

Yates, C.A. & de Kretser, D.M. (1987). Male-factor infertility and *in vitro* fertilization. *J. In Vitro Fertil. Embryo Transf.,* **4**, 141–7.

Yee, B. & Cummings, L.M. (1988). Modification of the sperm penetration assay using human follicular fluid to minimize false negative results. *Fertil. Steril.*, **50**, 123–8.

YoungLai, E.V. & Daya, S. (1991). Increased fertilization of human oocytes with low sperm density at insemination. *J. In Vitro Fertil. Embryo Transf.*, **8**, 176–7.

Yovich, J.L. (1992). Assisted reproduction for male factor infertility. In *A Textbook of In Vitro and Assisted Reproduction*, ed. P.R. Brinsden & P.A. Rainsbury, pp. 311–23. Park Ridge, NJ: Parthenon Publishing Group.

Yovich, J.L., Yovich, J.M. & Edirisinghe, W.R. (1988*a*). The relative chance of pregnancy following tubal or uterine transfer procedures. *Fertil. Steril.*, **49**, 858–64.

Yovich, J.M., Edirisinghe, W.R., Cummins, J.M. & Yovich, J.L. (1988*b*). Preliminary results using pentoxifylline in a pronuclear stage tubal transfer (PROST) program for severe male factor infertility. *Fertil. Steril.*, **50**, 179–81.

Yovich, J.M., Edirisinghe, W.R., Cummins, J.M. & Yovich, J.L. (1990). Influence of pentoxifylline in severe male factor infertility. *Fertil. Steril.*, **53**, 715–22.

Zamboni, L. (1992). Sperm structure and its relevance to infertility: an electron microscopic study. *Arch. Pathol. Lab. Med.*, **116**, 325–44.

Zaneveld, L.J.D., Jeyendran, R.S., Krajeski, P., Coetzee, K., Kruger, T.F. & Lombard, C.J. (1990). Hypo-osmotic swelling test. In *Human Spermatozoa in Assisted Reproduction*, ed. A.A. Acosta, R.J. Swanson, S.B. Ackerman, T.F. Kruger, J.A. van Zyl & R. Menkveld, pp. 223–9. Baltimore: Williams & Wilkins.

Zaneveld, L.J., De Jonge, C.J., Anderson, R.A. & Mack, S.R. (1991). Human sperm capacitation and the acrosome reaction. *Hum. Reprod.*, **6**, 1265–74.

11

Microinjection techniques for male infertility

CHARLES C. CODDINGTON and SERGIO OEHNINGER

Introduction

Male factor infertility affects 25–50% of the couples presenting for evaluation and therapy (Glass, 1991). Depending upon semen quality and the underlying pathophysiologic diagnosis, some of these patients become candidates for assisted fertilization. Our aim in this chapter is to assist the reader in helping patients make decisions as to what method should be used to treat their fertility problem. Although this guidance is based upon scientific data from the litera- ture it is important that the practitioner maintain a sensitive, thorough approach to the couple when dealing with emotional, religious, ethical and financial concerns which may arise during evaluation and treatment.

In vitro fertilization (IVF) increases sperm exposure to the female gamete. Strategies that improve sperm–oocyte exposure have included altering sperm concentration and enhancing motility. For example, in teratozoospermic samples when the incubate was increased from 50 000 motile sperm to between 500 000 and 1 million motile sperm per milliliter per oocyte, fertilization rates of 75% were reported (Oehninger *et al.*, 1988a). Using a simple wash and swim- up technique, the morphology and motion parameters of the sperm exposed to the oocytes can be significantly improved (Oehninger *et al.*, 1990). Even though the fertilization and implantation success reported was excellent, there were increased numbers of spontaneous miscarriages and low term pregnancy rates (Oehninger *et al.*, 1988a).

In addition to the above, oocyte micromanipulation can assist male-factor couples. In cases of low sperm count consideration may be given to oocyte micromanipulation for assisted fertilization. Table 11.1 indicates criteria which may be helpful in selecting patients for micromanipulation (World Health Organization, 1987; Kruger *et al.*, 1988; Acosta, 1992; Coddington *et al.*, 1993a). The severe male factor patient is more likely to need these techniques when presenting with a sperm concentration $<5 \times 10^6$ /ml, progressive motility

Table 11.1   *Norfolk Program definition of male factor[a]*

Factor	Male factor	Severe
Sperm concentration	$<20 \times 10^6$/ml	$<5 \times 10^6$/ml
Sperm motility (progressive)	$<50\%$	$<10\%$
Sperm morphology	$<14\%$ (strict)	$<4\%$ (strict)
Total sperm recovered in 'swim-up'	$<10 \times 10^6$	$<1.5 \times 10^6$
Hamster penetration assay		$<10\%$
Hemizona assay index	<35	<15

Notes:
Modified from Acosta (1992) and Coddington *et al.* (1993*a*)
These factors are guidelines and should be confirmed in one's local laboratory.
[a] One or more factors may be present

$<10\%$, low normal morphology ($<4\%$ using the strict criteria of Kruger *et al.* (1988) or $<20\%$ using the WHO (1987) criteria), $<1.5 \times 10^6$ motile sperm after swim-up, and a hemizona assay (HZA) index <15 (Acosta, 1992; Oehninger *et al.*, 1992*a*; Coddington *et al.*, 1993*a*, 1994). The patient's history may also lead to use of assisted reproductive techniques including micromanipulation.

History

Certain aspects of the patient's history should expedite referral to an assisted reproductive center. Patients who have had spinal cord injury or cancer surgery in the retroperitoneal space may need assistance because of lack of ability to deliver sperm to the vagina. If other ovulation stimulation and insemination techniques are not successful, IVF and/or micromanipulation may be beneficial. Congenital absence of the vas and other obstructive lesions need to be treated in conjunction with a urologist, utilizing epididymal aspiration and micromanipulation (Silber *et al.*, 1988). With these aspiration procedures, small numbers of sperm may be obtained, increasing the potential use of micromanipulation. Cases of idiopathic oligozoospermia, with motile concentrations below 10×10^6 /ml are also candidates for assisted reproductive technologies.

Evaluation

Several semen samples must be analyzed before determining prognosis. If there are mutable factors, those need to be treated before a repeat test is performed. Men whose semen has significant agglutination should be evaluated for sperm antibodies (World Health Organization, 1987; Acosta, 1992). Factors such as altered pH or viscosity of seminal fluid may be treated simply by ejaculation into culture medium. If infection is suspected after culture and sensitivity, one should treat with an appropriate antibiotic. Medical therapies such as clomiphene citrate, tamoxifen or FSH may have been tried prior to referral to increase sperm numbers, although these seldom provide clinically significant improvement (Schill, 1979; Acosta *et al.*, 1991; Acosta, 1992). When standard IVF is not successful, micromanipulation techniques are then indicated.

Sperm morphology when assessed by strict criteria appears to be significant in IVF success rates. In a study of infertile couples evaluated prior to IVF, morphology was the best predictor of the ability of the sperm to bind to the zona pellucida ($r=0.52$, $p<0.0001$) (Oehninger *et al.*, 1992a). The hemizona index was the best predictor of the fertilization rate ($r=0.61$, $p=0.0001$) (Oehninger *et al.*, 1992a,b). Furthermore, the predictive value for successful fertilization was 95% if the hemizona index was >40–42 (Oehninger *et al.*, 1992a,b; Coddington *et al.*, 1994). When validated by other standard semen parameters, these bio-assays of sperm function will be used by clinicians to give prognostic advice to patients.

Treatment

Micromanipulation techniques have varied as technology has progressed in this area. The primary goal of micromanipulation is to overcome a functional defect of the sperm to fertilize, i.e., to bind and penetrate, the oocyte; in fact it has been reported that there is only a 25% chance of fertilization by standard IVF procedures when there was a previous failure to fertilize (Cohen *et al.*, 1992). This subfertility may be related to defects in sperm–zona binding ability, as well as zona penetration, egg fusion, decondensation and further events. Different methods to optimize gamete interaction have been described, including subzonal insemination (SUZI), partial zona dissection (PZD), zona drilling (ZD) and intracytoplasmic sperm injection (ICSI). For more detailed description of the techniques and protocols the reader is referred elsewhere (Lanzendorf *et al.*, 1988a,b; Malter & Cohen, 1989a; Cohen *et al.*, 1991; Ng *et al.*, 1991; Iritani, 1991). The following summarize the major benefits and problems of each method:

1. SUZI (Figs. 11.1, 11.2; Veeck, 1991)
Comments:

- Can be used in cases of severe oligozoospermia
- Circumvents zona binding and penetration by sperm

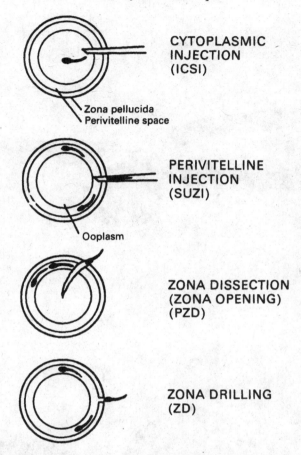

Fig. 11.1. An artist's representation of the micromanipulation techniques of SUZI, PZD, ZD and ICSI. (Modified from Iritani, 1991)

- Very poorly motile or immotile sperm can be used
- Capacitated and possibly acrosome-reacted sperm are required
- Biological selection is probably achieved with process of membrane fusion

Disadvantage

- Polyspermia may occur when multiple sperm are injected

2. PZD and ZD (Figs. 11.1, 11.3, 11.4; Veeck, 1991)
Comments:

- Only one potential sperm selection barrier, the vitelline membrane, is present
- Motile sperm must be capacitated
- ZD can be used for oligozoospermia with decreased motility

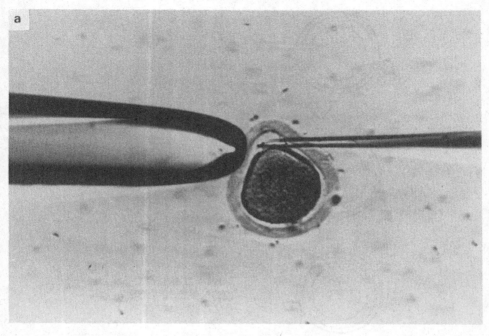

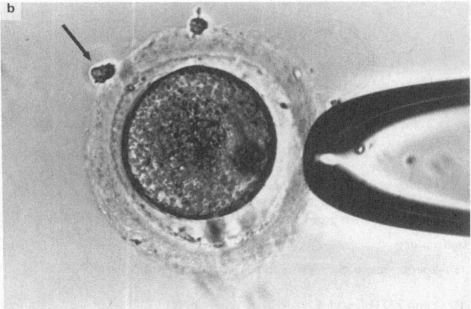

Fig. 11.2. Subzonal insertion (SUZI). (a) A sperm being inserted can be seen (*a*) at the tip of the micropipette and (b) in the arrow. (Picture of the actual case provided by Dr L.L. Veeck, Director of Embryology, The Jones Institute for Reproduction. Reprinted with permission.)

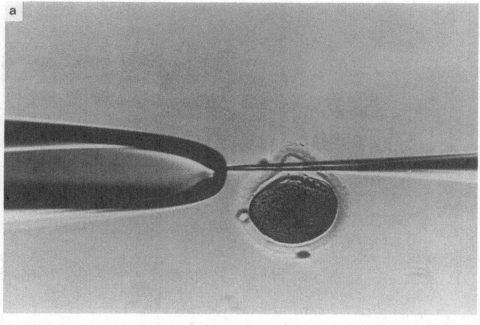

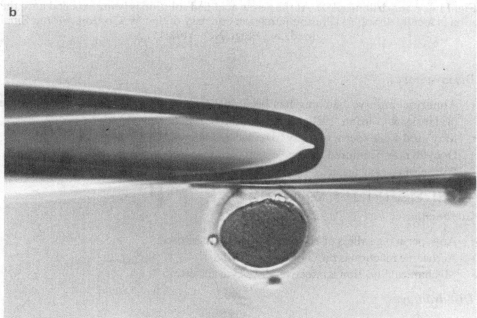

Fig. 11.3. Partial zona dissection (PZD). (a) A slit is made in the zona pellucida of a mature oocyte noted at the tip of the fine micropipette. (Picture of actual case provided by Dr L.L. Veeck, Director of Embryology, The Jones Institute for Reproduction.) (b) The microtip is rubbed gently to remove the zona pellucida.

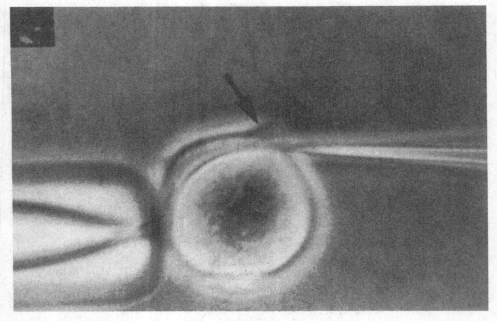

Fig. 11.4. Zona drilling (ZD). At the arrow acidified solution is being expelled until the zona is locally dissolved (Photomicrograph courtesy of Jon W. Gordon, Mount Sinai Medical Center, New York.)

Disadvantages:

- Abnormal embryo hatching has been noted after embryo transfer in the mouse (Talansky & Gordon, 1988; Malter & Cohen, 1989*b*)
- May need some sperm motility to be successful
- Oocytes may be injured to some extent
- Polyspermia may occur

3. ICSI (Figs. 11.1, 11.5; Veeck, 1991)
Comments:

- Any sperm regardless of shape or motility can be used
- Acrosome reaction is probably not needed
- Mechanical injection is effective for oocyte activation

Disadvantages:

- Damage to oocyte or ooplasm (10% of oocytes)

ICSI was first attempted in the early 1900s in animal models (Lillie, 1914), but was not successful. Since that time, improvements in assisted reproductive technologies have led to greater understanding of fertilization events as well as

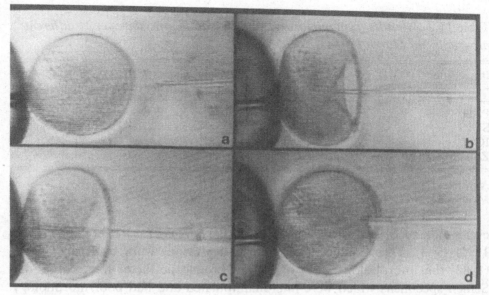

Fig. 11.5. Intracytoplasmic sperm injection (ICSI). The microneedle is placed at least halfway into the ooplasm before the ooplasm is gently aspirated and expelled to allow sperm placement. (Photomicrograph courtesy of Susan Lanzendorf, Research Division, The Jones Institute for Reproductive Medicine.)

technical improvements which optimize success. ICSI utilizes a micropipette to inject sperm directly into the ooplasm of the oocyte (Lanzendorf *et al.*, 1988*a,b*). It has been successfully used for individuals who have not conceived by other methods (IVF, SUZI, PZD) (Palermo *et al.*, 1992).

Palermo *et al.* (1992) reported the results of ICSI in 47 patients; 38 of the oocytes remained intact and 31 became fertilized. Fifteen embryos were replaced and four pregnancies occurred after eight treatment cycles, resulting in one normal set of twins, two singleton pregnancies and one preclinical abortion. Clearly, the success of these procedures is highly variable. Ng *et al.* (1991) published their results of a single sperm injection into the ooplasm of 38 oocytes in three patients. Four normal pronuclear zygotes were obtained and replaced in two patients with no resulting pregnancy.

PZD and SUZI have been compared in several studies. Cohen *et al.* (1991) reported the use of PZD and SUZI in males who had semen parameters unsuitable for IVF, in whom <50 000 motile sperm were recovered by swim-up techniques. Initial concentration was $<5 \times 10^6$ sperm/ml, motility <10% and morphology <2% by strict criteria. Sibling oocytes were used for PZD and SUZI. The fertilization results suggested SUZI to be more effective than PZD: 37/125 (30%) oocytes micromanipulated with SUZI fertilized, compared with 11/86 (13%) with PZD ($p<0.01$). However, there was no difference noted in

Table 11.2   *Results from microsurgical fertilization procedures in 21 different programs (to March 1991)*

Procedure	Cycles	Eggs fertilized (%)	Cycles with transfer (%)	Clinically pregnant (%)
PZD	715	22	57	10
SUZI	703	21	58	8
ICSI	22	36	73	0
Zona opening	93	22	57	0

Notes:
Modified from Cohen (1992).

cycles with successful fertilization: 68% SUZI versus 41% PZD (Cohen *et al.*, 1991, 1993). These studies also confirmed previous work by Kruger *et al.* (1988) that morphology is an important prognostic factor for fertilization. Semen specimens which were micromanipulated and had poor morphology (0–5% normal forms) had lower fertilization and implantation rates (48% vs 20%) (Cohen *et al.*, 1991). Fishel *et al.* (1992) studied SUZI for patients who had failed standard IVF at their institution. For 225 oocyte retrievals, fertilization occurred in 39% of patients and 16% of oocytes, with establishment of 12 clinical pregnancies. There was significant improvement in the fertilization rate utilizing SUZI in these patients (Fishel *et al.*, 1992). These studies confirm the utility of these micromanipulation procedures.

Comparison of semen parameters and the use of PZD and SUZI have also been used to determine lower limits for sperm parameters and to recommend a method of micromanipulation. In 250 patient cycles, several relationships between fertilization and implantation were seen. For couples with 0 normal forms, there was a 15% fertilization rate (16 cycles and 123 oocytes micromanipulated) and 22% of the cycles had at least one replacement embryo (Cohen *et al.*, 1993). Furthermore, whether one, two or three semen abnormalities (oligozoospermia, asthenozoospermia, teratozoospermia) were noted, did not appear to influence the outcome of the microsurgical procedure. The percentage of oocytes which fertilized in each group ranged from 17% to 22%, and embryo replacements were reported in 15–22% of cycles (Cohen *et al.*, 1993). On the basis of these findings, these techniques may be useful in patients regardless of the exact seminal defect encountered.

Cohen (1992) reported the results of a worldwide microsurgical fertilization inquiry from 21 different programs. Important outcome variables from this report are presented in Table 11.2. By 1992, over 60 babies had been born worldwide from these techniques (Cohen, 1992). The reported fertilization rates ranged from 20% to 30%. Not surprisingly, the numbers of patients who had embryos replaced are reduced when compared with standard IVF. Nevertheless, miscarriage and implantation rates appear unaffected and the babies born are healthy and karyotypically normal (Cohen, 1992) in this small initial cohort. More data are needed to determine the true efficiency of these procedures in terms of implantation and pregnancy outcome when utilizing severely abnormal sperm for micromanipulation.

At the Jones Institute of Reproductive Medicine initial (1988) ICSI procedures did not result in any viable pregnancies (Veeck *et al.*, 1989), while an overall fertilization rate of 25% with term delivery of healthy babies has been achieved with PZD and SUZI (unpublished data).

Since initial pregnancies reported by Palermo *et al.* (1992) using ICSI Van Steirteghem *et al.* (1993*a*, *b*) have published remarkable results on this technique. Patients with severe oligo-astheno-teratozoospermia, or with previous fertilization failure, can be treated by ICSI with an overall fertilization rate to 60%, and a pregnancy rate between 20 and 30% per attempt. ICSI can be used not only with ejaculated sperm (irrespective of the abnormality found), but also with epididymal and testicular sperm obtained by aspiration of biopsy. Patients with azoospermia (obstructive and non-obstructive) can be offered a combined urologic/ICSI approach with good chances of success. During 1994, of 102 ICSI cycles performed, the diploid fertilization rate was 60.9%, the transfer rate was 95%, and the delivery rate was 26.8% per cycle. None of the sperm parameters of the original or processed semen analysis correlated with ICSI outcome. Remarkably, female age had a significant impact on pregnancy rate (<34 years, 48.9%; 35–39 years, 22.9%, ≥40 years, 5.9% clinical pregnancy rate per transfer) (Oehninger *et al.*, 1995).

Severe male factor disorders leading to complete fertilization failure occur in up to 8% of IVF cycles (Oehninger *et al.*, 1988*b*). Couples with recurrent IVF failure have been studied to establish a pathophysiologic diagnosis for specific functional defects of sperm–oocyte interactions, and to develop a serial diagnostic scheme for managing these clinical problems (Oehninger *et al.*, 1991). The results of predictive fertilization bioassays (HZA and sperm penetration assay (SPA)), IVF treatment, fertile donor cross-match tests with either sperm or oocytes, and oocyte micromanipulation techniques for assisted fertilization are shown in Table 11.3. All patients had recurrent failed fertilization in multiple IVF attempts. The sequential analysis depicted allowed the establishment of probable specific diagnosis of sperm–oocyte defects in each case. Results have indicated that specific defects could be demonstrated at the level of sperm–zona binding, zona penetration and sperm–oocyte fusion (Oehninger *et al.*, 1991, 1992*c*).

Failure of fertilization due to defective sperm–zona pellucida interaction may be a relatively common problem, underscoring the potential of the HZA as an

Table 11.3   *Example of sequential analysis for the diagnosis of sperm oocyte defects*

Couple no.	HZ index (%)	SPA: control vs test (%)	Conventional IV results[a]	Oocyte micromanipulation results[b]	Cross-match test in IVF[c]		
					Donor sperm[a]	Donor oocyte[a]	Probable sperm defect
1	30	40–20	0/7	0/3 (PZD)	2/2	0/3	—
2	27	31–21	0/13	2/6 (PZD)	–	–	—
3	20	–	0/12	2/5 (SZI)	–	–	—
4	75	28–27	0/11	2/7 (ICSI); 0/2 (PZD)	2/3	0/1	—
5	65	100–0	0/18	6/10 (ICSI); 0/2 (PZD)	3/3	0/2	—
6	0	32–0	0/4	–	–	–	—
7	100	25–20	0/7	–	–	1/1	—
8	12	–	0/20	0/3 (SZI)	7/15	–	—

Adapted from Oehninger *et al.* (1991).
HZ, hemizona.
[a] Expressed as oocytes fertilized/oocytes inseminated.
[b] Expressed as oocytes fertilized/oocytes micromanipulated.
[c] When micromanipulation failed.

important diagnostic predictive test (Burkman *et al.*, 1988). However, post-zona binding defects may also occur. Patients with fertilization disorders should therefore be assessed utilizing other bioassays which assess complementary sperm functions. The order of progression of the predictive bioassays is important, and tests should assess steps in sperm–oocyte interaction in the same order that they occur *in vivo*. For example, it is important to evaluate sperm–oocyte interaction when tight binding to the zona pellucida or its penetration is defective. Accordingly, the HZA should be applied first. If results show adequate tight binding or penetration under HZA conditions, further tests of the acrosome reaction, oolemma fusion, decondensation and pronuclear formation should be done in sequence. The results will help clinicians in the management of these difficult cases, and assist in the selection of optimum therapies such as micro-insemination methods, medical therapies if validated, or oocyte micromanipulation for assisted fertilization.

Comparison of the different micromanipulation techniques is difficult due to multiple variables such as patient selection (male factors with severe alteration of the semen profile, patients with normal semen parameters and previous IVF failure, and male factor patients with previous failed IVF); presence or absence of IVF-inseminated sibling oocytes at the time of performing micro-

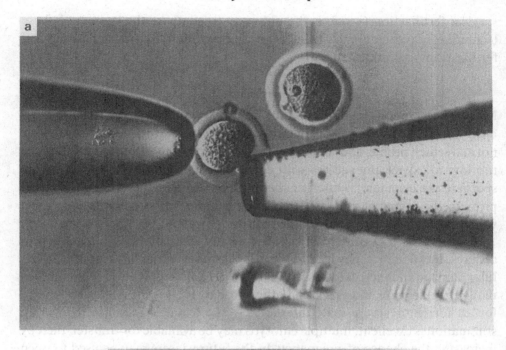

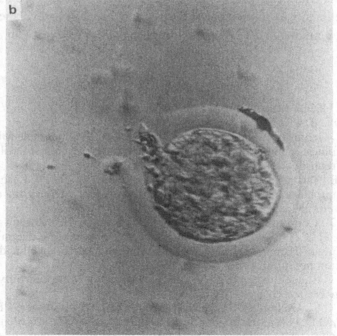

Fig. 11.6. (a) YAG laser energy was used to micromanipulate the oocyte and (b) sperm had access to the ooplasm through the opening.

surgical fertilization (which is the only way to compare the success of these techniques); and combined transfer of embryos derived from microsurgical fertilizations and 'standard' IVF.

Conclusion

Micromanipulation techniques should be available to those patients with previously failed fertilization who demonstrate either severe sperm disorders or normal semen profile, and to those whose sperm concentration and motility are too low to expect any success with conventional IVF ($<5 \times 10^6$ total motile sperm in the ejaculate). Different sperm preparation methods should be tried prior to the attempt, such as Percoll versus swim-up, in order to determine which method will enrich the motile fraction.

SUZI, PZD, ZD and ICSI are technically difficult, time-intensive procedures. Inexperience may lead to handling the oocytes harshly resulting in cellular damage and increased susceptibility to pH and temperature. The embryos require greater care and precise handling. Today, ICSI is the method of choice for all forms of severe male infertility. If the female's response to ovarian stimulation is excellent, multiple embryos may be available for transfer, thereby increasing the chance of pregnancy. In the future, lasers may be used to open the zona pellucida to allow sperm access and hence improve sperm–oocyte interaction (Blanchet *et al.*, 1992; Coddington *et al.*, 1993*b*; Laufer *et al.*, 1993) (Fig. 11.6).

References

Acosta, A.A. (1992). Male factor in assisted reproduction. *Infert. Reprod. Med. Clin. North Am.*, **3**, 487–503.

Acosta, A.A., Oehninger, S., Ertunc, H. & Philput, C. (1991). Possible role of pure human follicle-stimulating hormone in the treatment of male infertility by assisted reproduction: preliminary report. *Fertil. Steril.*, **55**, 1150–6.

Blanchet, G.B., Russell, J.B., Fincher, C.R. & Portmann, M. (1992). Laser micromanipulation in the mouse embryo: a novel approach to zona drilling. *Fertil. Steril.*, **57**, 1337–41.

Burkman, L.T., Coddington, C.C., Franken, D.R., Kruger, T.F., Rosenwaks, Z. & Hodgen, G.D. (1988). The hemizona assay: development of a diagnostic test for the binding of human spermatozoa to the human hemizona pellucida to predict fertilization potential. *Fertil. Steril.*, **49**, 688–97.

Coddington, C.C., Oehninger, S. & Acosta, A.A. (1993*a*). Male infertility update. *Contemp. Obstet. Gynecol.*, **38**, 29–37.

Coddington, C.C., Oehninger, S., Olive, D.L., Franken, D.R., Kruger, T.F. & Hodgen, G.D. (1994). Hemizona Index (HZI) demonstrates excellent predictability when evaluating sperm fertilizing capacity in *in vitro* fertilization patients. *J. Androl.*, **4**, 250–4.

Coddington, C.C., Veeck, L.L., Swanson, R., Simonetti, S. & Bocca, S. (1993*b*). YAG laser used in micromanipulation to transect the zona pellucida of hamster oocytes. *J. Assist. Reprod. Genet.*, **9**, 557–63.

Cohen, J. (1992). A review of clinical microsurgical fertilization. In *Micromanipulation of Human Gametes and Embryos*, ed. J. Cohen, H. Malter, B. Talansky & J. Grifo, pp. 163–90. New York: Raven Press.

Cohen, J., Alikani, M., Malter, H., Alder, A., Talansky, B. & Rosenwaks, Z. (1991). Partial zona dissection or subzonal insertion: microsurgical fertilization alternatives based on evaluation of sperm and embryo morphology. *Fertil. Steril.*, **56**, 696–706.

Cohen, J., Talansky, B., Alder, A., Alikani, M. & Rosenwaks, Z. (1992). Controversies and opinions in clinical microsurgical fertilization. *J. Assist. Reprod. Genet.*, **9**, 94–7.

Cohen, J., Adler, A., Alikani, M., Ferrara, T., Kissin, E., Reing, A., Suzman, M., Talansky, B. & Rosenwaks, Z. (1993). Assisted fertilization and abnormal sperm function. *Semin. Reprod. Endocrinol.*, **11**, 83–94.

Fishel, S., Timson, J., Lisi, F. & Rinaldi, L. (1992). Evaluation of 225 patients undergoing subzonal insemination for the procurement of fertilization *in vitro. Fertil. Steril.*, **57**, 840–9.

Glass, R.H. (1991). Infertility. In *Reproductive Endocrinology*, 3rd edn, ed. S.S.C. Yen & R.B. Jaffe, p. 689. Philadelphia: W.B. Saunders.

Iritani, A. (1991). Micromanipulation of gametes for *in vitro* assisted fertilization. *Mol. Reprod. Dev.*, **28**, 199–207.

Kruger, T.F., Acosta, A.A., Simmons, K.F., Swanson, R.J., Matta, J.R. & Oehninger, S. (1988). Predictive value of abnormal sperm morphology in *in vitro* fertilization. *Fertil Steril.*, **49**, 112–17.

Lanzendorf, S., Mahony, M., Veeck, L.L., Slusser, J., Hodgen, G. & Rosenwaks, Z. (1988*a*). A preclinical evaluation of pronuclear formation by microinjection of human spermatozoa into human oocytes. *Fertil. Steril.*, **49**, 835–47.

Lanzendorf, S., Mahony, M., Ackerman, S., Acosta, A. & Hodgen, G. (1988*b*). Fertilizing potential of acrosome-defective sperm following microsurgical injection into eggs. *Gamete Res.*, **19**, 329–37.

Laufer, N., Palanker, D., Shufaro, Y., Safran, A., Simon, A. & Lewis, A. (1993). The efficacy and safety of zona pellucida drilling by a 193-mm excimer laser. *Fertil. Steril.*, **59**, 889–95.

Lillie, F.R. (1914). Studies of fertilization. IV. The mechanisms of fertilization in *Arabia. J. Exp. Zool.*, **16**, 523.

Malter, H. & Cohen, J. (1989*a*). Partial zona dissection of the human oocyte: a non-traumatic method using micromanipulation to assist zona pellucida penetration. *Fertil. Steril.*, **51**, 139–48.

Malter, H.E. & Cohen, J. (1989*b*). Blastocyst formation and hatching *in vitro* following zona drilling of mouse and human embryos. *Gamete Res.*, **24**, 67–80.

Ng, S., Bongso, A. & Rotnam, S. (1991). Microinjection of human oocytes: a technique for severe oligoastheno-teratozoospermia. *Fertil. Steril.*, **56**, 1117–23.

Oehninger, S., Acosta, A., Morshedi, M., Veeck, L., Swanson, R., Simmons, K. & Rosenwaks, Z. (1988*a*). Corrective measures and pregnancy outcome in *in vitro* fertilization in patients with severe sperm morphology abnormalities. *Fertil. Steril.*, **50**, 238–87.

Oehninger, S., Acosta, A., Kruger, T., Veeck, L., Flood, J. & Jones, H.W. (1988*b*). Failure of fertilization in IVF: the 'occult' male factor. *J. In Vitro Fert. Embryo Transf.*, **5**, 181–7.

Oehninger, S., Acosta, R., Morshedi, M., Philput, C., Swanson, R.J. & Acosta, A.A. (1990). Relationship between morphology and motion characteristics of human spermatozoa in semen and swim-up fractions. *J. Androl.*, **11**, 446–52.

Oehninger, S., Acosta, A., Veeck, L., Brzyski, R., Kruger, T., Muasher, S. & Hodgen,

G. (1991). Recurrent failure of IVF: role of the hemizona assay in the sequential diagnosis of specific sperm–oocyte defects. *Am. J. Obstet. Gynecol.*, **164**, 1210–15.

Oehninger, S., Toner, J., Muasher, S., Coddington, C.C., Acosta, A. & Hodgen, G.D. (1992a). Prediction of fertilization *in vitro* with human gametes: is there a litmus test? *Am. J. Obstet. Gynecol.*, **167**, 1760–7.

Oehninger, S., Acosta, A.A., Toner, J.P., Swanson, R.J., Coddington, C.C., Kruger, T.F., Franken, D.R. & Hodgen, G.D. (1992b). Sperm–zona pellucida binding: predicting fertilizing potential of human gametes by hemizona assay. *ARTA*, **3**, 1–14.

Oehninger, S., Franken, D., Alexander, N. & Hodgen, G. (1992c). Hemizona assay and its impact on the identification and treatment of human sperm dysfunctions. *Andrologia*, **24**, 307–21.

Oehninger, S., Veeck, L. Lanzendorf, S., Maloney, M., Toner, J., Muasher S. (1995). Intracytoplasmic sperm injection: achievement of high pregnancy rates in couples with severe male factor infertility is dependent primarily upon female and not male factors. *Fertil. Steril.*, **64**, 977–81.

Palermo, G., Joris, H., Devroey, P. & Van Steirtegham, A.C. (1992). Pregnancies after intracytoplasmic injection of a single spermatozoon into an oocyte. *Lancet*, **340**, 17–18.

Schill, W.B. (1979). Recent progress in pharmacological therapy of male subfertility: a review. *Andrologia*, **11**, 77–80.

Silber, S., Balmaceda, J., Borrero, C., Ord, T. & Asch, R. (1988). Pregnancy with sperm aspiration from the proximal head of the epididymis: a new treatment for congenital absence of the vas deferens. *Fertil. Steril.*, **50**, 525–8.

Tadir, Y., Wright, W.H., Vofa, O., Ord, T., Asch, R. & Berns, M.W. (1990). Force generated by human sperm correlated to velocity and determined using a laser trap. *Fertil. Steril.*, **53**, 944–7.

Talansky, B.E. & Gordon, J.W. (1988). Cleavage characteristics of mouse embryos inseminated and cultured after zona pellucida drilling. *Gamete Res.*, **21**, 227–87.

Van Steirteghem, A.C., Liu, J., Joris, H., Nagy, Z. Janssenwillem, C., Tournaye, H., *et al.* (1993a). Higher success rates by intracytoplasmic sperm injection than by subzonal insemination: report on a second series of 300 consecutive treatment cycles. *Hum. Reprod.*, **8**, 1055–60.

Van Steirteghem, A.C., Nagy, Z., Joris, H., Liu, J., Staessen, C., Soritz, J., *et al.* (1993b). High fertilization and implantation rates after intracytoplasmic sperm injection. *Hum. Reprod.*, **8**, 1061–6.

Janssenwillem, C., Tournaye, H., *et al.* (1993a). Higher success rates by intracytoplasmic sperm injection than by subzonal insemination: report on a second series of 300 consecutive treatment cycles. *Hum. Reprod.*, **8.**, 1055–60.

Veeck, L.L. (1991). *Atlas of the Human Oocyte and Early Conceptus*, pp. 305–68. Philadelphia: Williams and Wilkins.

Veeck, L., Oehninger, S., Acosta, A. & Muasher, J. (1989). Sperm microinjection in a clinical *in vitro* fertilization program. Presented at the Forty-fifth Annual Meeting of the American Fertility Society, 13–16 November 1989, San Francisco, 0–121, S51.

World Health Organization (1987). *Laboratory Manual for the Examination of Human Semen and Semen–Cervical Mucus Interaction*, 2nd edn. Cambridge: Cambridge University Press.

12

Therapeutic donor insemination: screening, indications and technique

KENNETH A. GINSBURG and VALERIE MONTGOMERY
RICE

Introduction

Despite significant advances in both the diagnosis and treatment of male infertility, for some there is still the possibility of unsuccessful medical or surgical therapy. In these situations, and others where no therapy can be offered, when it is refused, or when therapy fails to result in conception, therapeutic donor insemination (TDI) may be the only chance for pregnancy.

Demand for TDI and human semen cryobanking has been increasing worldwide. The number of patients requesting TDI increased four-fold in the United States between 1971 and 1976 (Jacobson, 1976). The process is certainly not new, with observations of the effects of low temperature on spermatozoa being reported by Spallanzani in the eighteenth century. Human semen cryobanking and resulting *in vivo* fertilization were then reported by Bunge and Sherman in their landmark articles appearing in 1953 and 1954 (Bunge & Sherman, 1953; Bunge *et al.*, 1954). Thirty years later, data compiled by the United States Congress Office of Technology Assessment (US Congress OTA, 1988) estimated that approximately 30 000 births occurred *annually* as a result of donor insemination. While several factors may account for this tremendous increase in the utilization of donor insemination services (such as increased incidence and prevalence of infertility, greater willingness to utilize TDI by clinicians and fewer adoptive infants), much can be attributed to the established safety and efficacy of cryopreserved donor semen for therapeutic insemination (Table 12.1).

Ten years ago most donor inseminations used fresh semen specimens. Because of concern regarding the transmission of sexually transmitted diseases (STDs), including acquired immune deficiency syndrome (AIDS), practice shifted in the mid-1980s to the exclusive use of cryopreserved semen. This chapter will examine the status of TDI from that perspective, reviewing the current practice of TDI in the United States and Europe including legal and

Table 12.1   *Key developments in the history of human sperm cryobanking for therapeutic donor insemination*

Year	Historical development
1866	Mantegazza first suggested use of human semen cryobanking
1909	First report in a medical journal of TDI, which occurred in the USA in 1884 without either husband's or wife's consent, using semen from a medical student. The male partner was ultimately told, but not the woman
1938	Jahnel demonstrated that human sperm will survive after cooling to −269°C and storage at −79°C
1942	The vitrification process was described by Hoagland and Pincus
1949	Polge *et al.* reported the use of glycerol as a cryoprotective agent, making possible large-scale freezing and banking of mammalian sperm, especially in animal husbandry programs
1953	The first human offspring from therapeutic donor insemination reported by Bunge and Sherman
1962	The nitrogen vapor technique for freezing and storage of sperm at −196°C is described and births from the technique reported by Sherman; normal offspring are reported in 1972 following 10 years' storage of cryopreserved semen
Late 1980s	Guidelines for TDI using cryopreserved semen are promulgated by a number of groups (including the American Fertility Society and the American Association of Tissue Banks) in response to growing concern regarding transmission of sexually transmitted diseases including AIDS. These guidelines include the use of quarantined samples and specify donor screening practices. Some states enact legislation covering these issues

ethical issues, indications, selection and screening of donors, technique of TDI, success rates, risks and side effects. This discussion is timely since the success of other assisted reproductive technologies, notably intracytoplasmic injection of sperm into human oocytes *in vitro*, forces a reappraisal of the role of TDI for those couples in whom even a few motile sperm can be recovered. Many cases previously thought amenable only to TDI can now attempt pregnancy with homologous semen. Discussions of related issues including intrauterine insemination and assisted reproduction for male factor infertility as alternatives to the TDI process, are found in Chapters 8, 10 and 11.

Notes on the current status of therapeutic donor insemination

England and France have developed national TDI programs that merit brief review. In England, many of the issues regarding the current practice of TDI are governed by the Human Fertilization and Embryology Act 1990, which took form from the Warnock Report entitled *Report of an Inquiry into Human Fertilization and Embryology* issued in 1984. This report was commissioned by the British government following the birth in 1978 of the first baby by *in vitro* fertilization (IVF). Interestingly, the background upon which the issues leading to the Warnock Report were discussed included unsuccessful attempts by the Archbishop of Canterbury in the 1950s to introduce legislation making TDI a criminal offense, another government report (the Feversham Report, 1960) which failed to give legal recognition to TDI, and a British Medical Association commission recommendation in 1973 that TDI be made a part of the National Health Service. The Human Fertilization and Embryology Act 1990 recommended regulation of IVF, surrogacy and experimentation using human embryos in Great Britain. In particular, the following points regarding donor insemination were addressed:

- Authority to control and license centers and practioners of TDI, and provide penalties for non-compliance, including suspension or revocation of licensure
- A registry of children conceived as a result of TDI, and mandated record maintenance
- Guidelines for semen storage
- Development of a code of practice concerning the selection of donors, number of times a donor is allowed to provide samples, payment for semen samples, etc., including mechanisms for periodic review and revision
- Mandated regulatory issues including consent, counselling of donors and recipients, selection criteria, legal definitions of maternity and paternity, and disclosure of information to children conceived by TDI once they reach the age of majority in England

The French national program organized in 1973, by the Centre d'Etude et de Conservation du Sperme Humain (CECOS), has standardized the practice of TDI, much as the Fertilization and Embryology Act 1990 has attempted to do in England. In the CECOS program, all banks operate with the same procedures for donor recruitment, sample cryopreservation and recipient selection, and results are collated, analyzed and reported annually. Donors are not paid for specimens. Investigative protocols are administered across centers, with sufficient numbers of patients to provide timely answers to research questions.

In the United States, a shift in the practice of donor insemination occurred during the mid to late 1980s. Prior to that time many practitioners used fresh semen when available, and cryopreserved semen only when fresh specimens could not be obtained. Beginning in the early 1980s the dimensions of the AIDS epidemic and the spread of other STDs had sensitized the medical and lay community to the dangers *possibly* inherent in the use of fresh semen for

Table 12.2   *Summary of findings from the United States Congress Office of Technology Assessment Report on Donor Insemination, 1988*

• Eighteen percent of physicians surveyed do not present other options to donor insemination such as adoption, and 15% of physicians do not discuss risks of TDI such as infection, multiple births, birth defects, pregnancy complications or psychological complications

• Over 90% of physicians and banks surveyed require a personal medical, fertility and family history along with a physical examination, while only about half require any type of psychological evaluation. Seventy-four percent require laboratory screening of the recipient, including infertility tests and tests for infectious diseases. Eighty percent of screened recipients are ultimately accepted

• Potential recipients of TDI are rejected because of marital status, psychological contraindications, sexual orientation, socioeconomic status (e.g., welfare dependency), history of child abuse, drug abuse, alcohol abuse

• When donor semen is used for artificial insemination, the source is evenly divided between commercial sperm banks and physician-selected and -evaluated donors. Interestingly, in cases of physician-selected donors, only 66% evaluate each ejaculate for sperm motility, morphology or other parameters, while 22% do not screen for HIV and 52% do not screen for genetic disorders

• Seventy-two percent of physicians practicing TDI make some attempt to find a donor that matches at least some recipient specifications, such as (in order of importance) race, eye color, complexion, height, ethnic or national origin. Educational level, IQ, religion, hobbies, income and age are uncommonly used as criteria for matching samples with recipients

• Fifty-four percent of physicians performing TDI maintain records that would allow identification of the sperm donor although a significant majority would not provide this information to recipients or offspring under any circumstances.

TDI. Few cases documenting the actual transmission of disease vectors by semen had been reported. However, it seemed likely that frozen semen, quarantined for a period sufficient to allow the donor to be rescreened for certain diseases, would be safer. Several professional societies, including the American Fertility Society and the American Association of Tissue Banks, suggested that only cryopreserved (and quarantined) semen be used for donor insemination. Indeed several jurisdictions enacted legislation prohibiting the use of fresh semen for this purpose.

By 1988 only cryopreserved semen was recommended for TDI, although clearly not all practitioners had adopted these recommendations. Practice perspectives at that time can be extracted from a survey of 1473 physicians practicing TDI published by the Office of Technology Assessment (US Congress OTA, 1988). A summary of the key points from the OTA Report is found in Table 12.2. Important conclusions include (1) the fact that whether for fresh or frozen use, donor screening practices are quite consistent among sperm banks that sell frozen semen but vary widely among individual practitioners who process their own semen samples; (2) the majority of physicians and banks surveyed favor national standards for donor insemination, whether voluntary or mandatory; and (3) 85% of the respondant physicians do not belong to a fertility society, and thus might be missed if information and guidelines are disseminated only through these established channels.

According to the survey, the financial impact of donor insemination services in the United States is significant: 172 000 women underwent TDI in 1986–7, with the average cost of $953.00 per woman amounting to $164 million expenditure during that year for donor insemination services. Only 51% of these patients had health insurance, and slightly less than half of those found that the fees associated with TDI were covered by their insurance plans. Thus patients are paying about three-fourths of the costs for donor insemination, approximately $130 million, out of their pockets. It is thus appropriate to require that such a common and expensive service as TDI be made as safe, efficacious and cost-effective as possible.

In the United States, as the public and medical practitioners consider a national health program, donor insemination programs in England and France may indeed be the prototype for a domestic national TDI program. Drawing upon the French and English experience, parts of these programs to incorporate into a national one might include establishment of consistent guidelines and policies for donor screening and sample procurement, minimum practice standards for centers and practitioners of TDI, and development of standardized policies regarding legal and regulatory issues such as payment for samples, consent, disclosure and anonymity.

Ethical and legal issues in the donor insemination process

Ethical issues

Ethical debate centers on the development and revision of rules by which members of a society function and interact. At times these ethical principles are codified by a society into laws, which then *govern* what is right and wrong. With regard to reproduction, some rules have been formalized and enacted into law, such as statutes regarding incest or procreation by minors, while others remain informal but socially enforced, as in the selection of suitable partners for children by their parents and the arranged marriages that result. The ethical rules regarding reproduction vary between societies, as well as within a society over time. Given this, it is not surprising that there is no agreement among different societies and cultures as to what are morally, ethically and legally acceptable deviations from the norm in reproduction. Therapeutic donor insemination initiates intense ethical debate.

Ethical issues concerning donor insemination include anonymity of the donor and recipient, secrecy, autonomy regarding reproductive choice, changes in family relationships that impact upon personal identity, the sanctity of human life, the right to bear children, professional judgment and the rights of children yet to be born. There is no right or wrong view in any of these issues. To cite but one example of how these ethical issues can threaten the use of TDI, psychologists and sociologists relate that a person's sense of identity depends to a great extent on the relationships associated with parenting and family. When donor sperm is used to impregnate a woman, these relationships are perceived by some to have been undermined or destroyed. The resulting identity crisis can be difficult not only for the family accepting TDI, but also for the donor relinquishing that parental relationship. Further, while most relatives share a common biological inheritance, the spousal relationship is unique in that it is formed not through common ancestry but rather when their genes are combined through the conception of their offspring. According to this view, because the male partner's genes do not contribute to the offspring, the spousal and family relationships can be eroded with TDI. Even when the child is not informed of his or her roots, the parents know that their child conceived through TDI is different from a child who is biologically linked to them or who links them to each other (Snowden, 1993). An opposing view would argue, of course, that the identity of both partners is strengthened by raising the child they would otherwise not have had.

Because these issues can stress the spousal relationship and even lead to psychopathology, some insemination services request that a couple contemplating TDI undergo a psychological evaluation. Often the counselor, or another member of the TDI team, is called upon to help one or both partners overcome the feeling that the child must be their 'flesh and blood' in order to establish a healthy parent–child relationship. In these situations the psychological relationship between partners and child must be stressed, rather than the biologic relationship.

Unresolved ethical questions regarding TDI include medical confidentiality and secrecy of the TDI treatment, the acceptability and medical justification of treating the woman and exposing her to the risks of TDI, however small, when the male has the fertility problem, the acceptability of single woman insemination, whether it is proper to sell semen when other organs are donated freely, the purpose of record maintenance and disclosure, and the function of donor anonymity (who is protected, what information is released to the recipient and, under what circumstances, what information is given to the donor about children conceived). These ethical controversies have become legal ones in some jurisdictions.

Legal issues

No court has ever stated that TDI is illegal. Six states (California, Oklahoma, Virginia, Washington, Alaska and Oregon) have statutes that limit the practice of TDI to physicians, while 28 states have enacted laws specifying that a child conceived by means of artificial insemination with the consent of the husband is the legal offspring of the couple (Alabama, Alaska, Arkansas, California, Colorado, Connecticut, Florida, Georgia, Idaho, Illinois, Kansas, Louisiana, Maryland, Michigan, Minnesota, Montana, Nevada, New Jersey, New York, North Carolina, Oklahoma, Oregon, Tennessee, Texas, Virginia, Washington, Wisconsin and Wyoming), a precedent supported by case law involving litigation. Fifteen of these states also specifically provide that a man who furnishes sperm for artificial insemination of someone other than his wife is not the child's legal father. In fact, the courts have never held an anonymous donor responsible for supporting the child. Legally, TDI is not considered adultery unless actual sexual intercourse has taken place.

Of central importance is the anonymity between child and donor, which must be guaranteed to prevent legal problems and disputes regarding inheritance rights, support and custody. In jurisdictions where there is a statutory right of every child to know his or her biologic father, such as Germany, this ethical issue of anonymity can be violated by the legal consideration of the right to paternal identity. Violation of anonymity would also occur if proceedings were initiated to adopt a TDI-conceived child, as has been advocated by some. Many of these concerns for donor anonymity could be resolved by legislation clearly defining TDI, parental rights and the legal role of the participants. A second problem can occur in jurisdictions where birth certificates are documents defining paternity, rather than a document defining a spousal relationship in which paternity is implied but not specifically stated. In this situation, the physician who enters the husband as the father of a child knowing that the pregnancy resulted from TDI could be found guilty of falsifying records. This has occurred in England, where a physician was convicted and jailed for three years for such an offense. An obvious solution to this problem would be that the physician who performs the successful TDI should not attend the birth nor sign the birth certificate.

Another area in which the legal issues are unsettled is the limitation on monetary reimbursement for semen donation imposed by some jurisdictions.

This practice could severely limit semen donation under the present system, since nearly 90% of semen samples for TDI are obtained from paid donors. To circumvent this restriction, any written agreement between a sperm bank or physician and donor should indicate that payment to the donor is for expenses incurred in providing the sample rather than direct payment for the semen.

Nineteen states have statutes prohibiting TDI of single women. On the basis of prevailing case law, there is little doubt that these statutes would be ruled unconstitutional upon challenge and review. However, many of the issues regarding the status of the child conceived through TDI to a single woman remain unresolved.

The physician practicing TDI is advised to keep abreast of the legal developments in his or her jurisdiction to comply with changing statutes. Since many of the legal issues regarding TDI are poorly defined, written informed consent from both partners and the donor is advised. These forms should state at a minimum that conception cannot be guaranteed and that the patient and her husband relinquish the right to discover the identity of the donor. With regard to informing the child of his or her biologic origin, the predominant view is that a child conceived by TDI should not be so informed.

Indications for donor insemination

Using semen from the male partner of an infertile couple, insemination is offered in situations where semen quality is poor, cervical or immunologic factors are identified, coital factors prevent successful intercourse, and in special circumstances where semen must be cryopreserved during periods of absence or prior to surgery, radiation or chemotherapy. Homologous artificial insemination is also offered as empiric treatment for unexplained infertility. Donor insemination, on the other hand, is appropriate when intractable male fertility factors are present, as indicated in Table 12.3. In these situations, when the male partner is sterile or infertile, TDI may provide the only opportunity for the couple to experience a pregnancy.

TDI can be used for genetic indications. When a couple has a child with an autosomal recessive trait, a heterozygous carrier state in both parents is evident. In this situation, TDI provides a change in the gene pool which lessens the risk of recurrence in subsequent pregnancies. Exposure of the male to environmental agents with mutagenic potential is a valid indication for donor insemination as well. Finally, immunologic incompatibility between the male and female partner, such as Rh incompatibility or antisperm antibodies which prevent successful sperm transport or sperm–egg interaction, could be treated with TDI.

Table 12.3 *Indications for therapeutic donor insemination*

• Azoospermia (Klinefelter's syndrome, hypergonadotropic hypogonadism, intractable azoospermia, prior vasectomy)

• Failed medical or surgical therapy for oligozoospermia, teratozoospermia, asthenozoospermia or seminal fluid abnormality

• Known inheritable disease in the male such as Tay–Sachs disease, Huntington's chorea, sickle cell disease or juvenile diabetes with a high risk of transmission

• Incompatability between male and female partners (e.g., Rh factor incompatibility with a sensitized female), immunologic infertility reflected by immobilization or agglutination of the husband's sperm in the wife's mucus or failed gamete interaction during *in vitro* fertilization

• Non-correctable ejaculatory disorders such as retrograde ejaculation from trauma, surgery or medication

• Exposure to environmental agents with mutagenic potential

Idiopathic infertility or failed conventional therapy

Single females

Despite the disadvantages of sperm cryopreservation with regard to fertilization potential, cryopreservation of semen affords several distinct advantages over the use of fresh semen in a donor insemination program. There are more frozen donor samples available than fresh donor specimens. This larger donor pool with cryopreserved TDI minimizes the risk of inbreeding, consanguinity or spreading harmful recessive genes that the donor may be carrying. Also the matching of donors to recipients is potentially closer when the available (cryopreserved) donor pool is larger. Couples often request that a second pregnancy be initiated with the same donor that established the first pregnancy, a possibility with cryopreserved semen which is much less likely when fresh semen is used. Frequently, an ejaculate is frozen into several aliquots and used to inseminate more than one individual, potentially decreasing the cost per insemination. Beyond these advantages, the most compelling advantage of frozen over fresh semen is the ability to quarantine frozen semen to guard against transmission of disease.

Selection and screening of donors

In evaluating a potential donor for inclusion in a TDI program, the goal is not only to assure his general health and absence of genetic or sexually transmissible disease, but also to obtain a reasonable expectation of fertility. Most centers prefer younger donors who are below the age of 40 years. Many exclude the donor if his semen does not result in a pregnancy within a predetermined number of insemination cycles in several recipients. Prior to the early 1970s, most semen banks were located within universities, after which private semen banking facilities began to appear as TDI became more accepted and widespread. Because of the location of semen banks, most donors are medical students, residents or other university graduate students. These men are a select group with presumably above-average intelligence and health. The homogeneous, non-random characteristics of this donor pool may also explain the low rates of congenital anomalies and first-trimester spontaneous abortion seen in TDI-conceived pregnancies.

Tests and protocols are available which can, with reasonable assurance, ensure the health status of a potential sperm donor. More problematic is the inability to reliably evaluate and predict a donor's fertility potential. While desirable, proven fertility is not necessarily a requirement for inclusion in most donor programs. Several semen samples should have a sufficient volume, motile concentration and normal morphology such that acceptable numbers of motile sperm can be provided in each vial of cryopreserved and thawed semen. Using American Fertility Society guidelines, at least 50 million motile sperm per milliliter with 60% progressive motility, normal morphology and at least 50% of initial motility after cryostorage should be obtained (American Fertility Society, 1993). Test freezing is performed early in the evaluation of a potential donor, since many will be found to have suboptimal semen characteristics after cryopreservation despite normal characteristics in the fresh sample (Chauhan *et al.*, 1988). This early screening obviates the need for expensive and perhaps unnecessary laboratory testing when the donor would otherwise be excluded because of poor semen cryosurvival.

Because of the considerable time and effort spent in recruiting and screening donors, and in preparing and storing donor semen, only the most fertile specimens are cryopreserved. Various tests are available to aid in this selection process. In addition to routine semen analysis, the number of leukocytes present in the ejaculate should be assessed. Leukocytes release reactive oxygen species (ROS) capable of peroxidating lipid membranes and potentially impairing membrane fusion events associated with fertilization, such as the acrosome reaction or development of the equatorial segment (Barratt *et al.*, 1990). While not routinely performed, a functional test of spermatozoa useful in the evaluation of semen for TDI is the zona-free hamster egg sperm penetration assay, which together with videomicrographic sperm movement analysis has been shown to predict the fertilizing potential of samples in a TDI program with 80% accuracy – considerably better than with semen analysis alone (Irvine & Aitken, 1986; Marshburn *et al.*, 1992). Other tests of male fertility, such as the evaluation of cervical mucus penetration, biochemical assessment of semen, hypoosmotic swelling or acrosome reaction evaluation have not yet proven helpful in predicting pregnancies from a donor population, and hence are not recommended.

Few states require that donors be screened for either an infectious disease or a genetic abnormality, and in few cases does the law specify that specific tests must be done. Rather, information supplied by the donor can be relied upon to determine these aspects of his medical history. Genetic and general health screening of potential donors can be accomplished by questionnaire, helping to exclude current or past health problems, drug exposure, environmental exposure and family medical history that may be associated with a higher risk of transmissible disease. Many sperm banks (US Congress OTA, 1988) screen for genetic diseases of ethnic origin such as sickle cell disease, thalassemia or Tay-Sachs disease. Karyotypic analysis is not a requirement, and few centers perform routine chromosome analysis since the frequency of balanced trans-locations in the general population is estimated to be less than 2/1000, the majority of which would not lead to viable balanced offspring. Complete physical examination allows exclusion of donors with documented or suspected congenital abnormalities, and routine laboratory examination (complete blood count, automated chemistry panel, urinanalysis) can be performed. In addition to detection of current illness, the questionaire and physical examination should find those individuals whose lifestyle places them at a higher risk for future acquisition of STDs including AIDS (e.g., homosexuals, bisexuals, intravenous drug users or men whose partners are members of these groups).

Laboratory screening for STDs is most important in the evaluation of potential donors and continued surveillance of established donors. Considerable evidence has accumulated confirming the potential transmission of a number of organisms by semen (reviewed by Greenblatt *et al.*, 1986). In addition to the woman receiving TDI, there are also possible risks to the fetus and neonate for STDs acquired via TDI. Although accurate data may be difficult to obtain because of reporting bias, subclinical and hence unrecognized infection, long latent period from exposure to infection, potential lack of an immune response despite infection (a problem inherent in serologic tests for infectious disease) and difficulty tracing the infection to its TDI source, it must be stressed that STD transmission from semen appears to be very uncommon. Despite the fact that regulations and laws regarding semen cryopreservation, quarantine and testing are based on low-frequency transmission data, the severity of illnesses such as hepatitis and AIDS demand that strict protocols for STD identification and semen quarantine be followed.

The most recent version of the American Fertility Society Guidelines for Gamete Donation: 1993 (American Fertility Society, 1993) provides a protocol for donor selection and screening. Recognizing that there is no absolute method to completely ensure that infectious agents will not be transmitted by TDI, serologic tests for syphilis, hepatitis B surface antigen and core antibody, hepatitis C, HTLV-III antibodies and cytomegalovirus (CMV) should be obtained initially along with semen and/or urethral cultures for *Neisseria gonorrhoeae*, *Chlamydia trachomatis* and *Mycoplasma hominis*. The semen is then frozen and stored for a minimum of 6 months. On the basis of epidemiologic and infectious disease data suggesting that the time from AIDS infection to seroconversion is 12–15 weeks, a 95% confidence interval from infection to seroconversion was 5.8 months (Horsburgh *et al.*, 1989). Other professional societies and government bodies that require 6 month quarantine followed by reevaluation of the donor before release of the semen, include the Centers for Disease Control and the Food and Drug Administration (Center for Disease Control, 1988) and the American Association of Tissue Banks (American Association of Tissue Banks, 1989). No test is currently available to directly detect the viruses in question in the semen, and, therefore, evidence of infection must be obtained from serologic data of a systemic immune response. The continuing surveillance of donors should include periodic monitoring of health status. Changes in sexual partners or health status require rescreening followed by quarantine with possible interruption of semen donation for an appropriate interval. Permanent confidential records of this testing should be maintained, along with records of conceptions attributable to the donor. The latter is to limit the number of pregnancies for which a given donor is responsible, to reduce the risk of consanguinity. Several states, including New York, Michigan, Illinois and Indiana, have enacted specific legislation specifying donor screening and quarantine periods for cryopreserved semen.

The effectiveness of these regulations in preventing transmission of STDs via TDI is difficult to establish due to the low transmission rates in semen, reporting bias, long incubation periods from seroconversion to clinical illness (Alexander, 1990), and other factors. The impact of this shift to cryopreserved and quarantined semen has, however, had other effects. These include increased charges for donor semen samples because of higher costs associated with the additional tests performed more frequently on each donor. Another issue relates to the use of donors who are CMV-positive. The AFS Guidelines (American Fertility Society, 1993) recommend that these donors be used only with recipients who are CMV-positive. However, acknowledging that virus transmission via frozen semen has not been demonstrated, this view may be questioned since multiple strains of CMV exist and a patient with demonstrable antibody to one strain may still be at risk for infection with a different serotype. Because regulations may change (e.g., recent requirement for hepatitis C testing of donors), many banks are now attempting to maintain a relationship with donors for continued surveillance after termination of donation, in addition to long-term storage of serum samples for future testing as better methods to detect diseases become available or when new clinical entities are recognized. What to do with samples obtained prior to the institution of suggested screening protocols and quarantine and, if these samples are not used, how to recover the costs associated with their procurement and storage are unsettled issues.

Technique of donor insemination

Donors are selected to match the physical characteristics of the male partner, including race, complexion, height and body habitus, eye and hair color and hair texture. Most semen banks and TDI services do not select donors on the basis of intellect, profession, income, hobbies, religion or other such criteria, although these might be considered by the recipient couple. When indicated, consideration must be given to any special medical circumstances, such as a recipient who is Rh-negative or who tests negative for CMV antibody. If it is impossible to meet the couple's requirements, the situation should be discussed and an alternative agreed upon. Because the medicolegal and regulatory issues regarding TDI are at present not settled, it is wise to maintain permanent confidential records of donors (including their genetic and infectious disease testing) and recipients indefinitely. Appropriate informed consent should also be obtained from both partners. Specific consent forms for the single woman recipient should be used.

Three variables appear to be important determinants in the success of TDI: timing of insemination, number of inseminations relative to ovulation, and site of insemination (intracervical versus intrauterine). Since the oocyte is fertilizable for only a short time following ovulation and with intrauterine insemination the cervical sperm reservoir is not established, timing of TDI is a critical variable in its success. In addition, now that only cryopreserved semen is recommended for TDI, the fertilizing life span of cryopreserved and thawed sperm becomes an issue as well. Comparison of fresh with frozen/thawed sperm has shown in the past a significant reduction in motility (Critser *et al.*, 1988), acrosome integrity (Critser *et al.*, 1987*a,b*), intracellular function (Sawada *et al.*, 1967; Ackerman, 1968, 1970, 1971) and longevity in the female reproductive tract (Keel & Black, 1980) of the latter compared with the former. The nature of the latent or overt cryoinjury leading to this decrease in fertility potential is not understood. Judging by fecundity rates, the longevity and functional capacity of frozen sperm appear to have improved, and are dependent on the preparation of the sample, the cryoprotectant and cryopreservation technique, as well as the type of insemination (see below).

Consideration of TDI timing is important not only with regard to decreased fecundity, but also because of the increased costs associated with cryopreservation, quarantine and extensive donor testing. More cycles are required for conception using cryopreserved compared with fresh donor semen. As the cost of each insemination increases along with the number of inseminations required to obtain a pregnancy, manipulations that even minimally increase the efficiency per insemination become important. Various methods are available to predict ovulation in the female partner so as to time insemination accurately (see Chapter 18). Several studies have analyzed and compared ovulation detection methods, with the conclusion that there is no demonstrable benefit to the use of expensive serial ultrasonography for TDI timing in the usual setting. Basal body temperature charting with or without urinary LH detection in the normally ovulating woman are adequate for timing of insemination and are economically advantageous (Mortimer & Templeton, 1982; Oden *et al.*, 1991). Patients who do not ovulate regularly achieve more accurate results with the urinary LH surge detection kit. Even with documented prior ovulatory cycles, some women may require the use of ovulation stimulation to assist in regulating their cycle, since the incidence of ovulatory disturbances manifesting after beginning TDI is significant. Glezerman (1981) found anovulation in 22% of 270 women after beginning donor inseminations. Disturbed luteal function was also seen in these women, emphasizing the need for continuous ovulatory monitoring during TDI. When TDI is utilized in gonadotropin-stimulated cycles, timing of insemination is based on ultrasonographic changes, serum estradiol levels and hCG administration. In these cycles insemination is performed within 24–36 hours after administration of the ovulatory dose of hCG (Hurst *et al.*, 1992).

In addition to timing of the insemination, the number of inseminations per cycle is an important determinant of success. Most physicians inseminate patients twice each cycle, and a minority use only one insemination. Several studies have prospectively examined the benefit of one versus two inseminations. Using urinary LH surge detection, fecundity appears to be higher when two inseminations are performed beginning on the day of the LH surge (Centola & Mattox, 1990; Oden *et al.*, 1991). Prospective studies comparing pregnancy rates following a single insemination on the day after an LH surge with those following two consecutive inseminations starting on the day of an LH surge demonstrate a benefit of two inseminations (Table 12.4). Centola &

Table 12.4 *Pregnancy rates following single versus two inseminations with cryopreserved semen*

Reference	Pregnancy rate with single insemination (%)	Pregnancy rate with two inseminations (%)
Byrd *et al.*, 1990 (*n*=238 cycles)	7.0	11.6
Centola & Mattox, 1990 (*n*=213 cycles)	15.2	39.6
Silverberg *et al.*, 1992 (*n*=9 cycles)[a]	0.0	33.0

Notes:
[a] In controlled ovarian hyperstimulation cycles with menopausal gonadotropins.

Mattox also observed a decrease in the number of cycles per patient to achieve pregnancy in those receiving two inseminations compared with a single insemination. It thus appears that the optimal time for intracervical insemination extends from the time of the serum LH peak to 10 hours after the peak. In contrast, the optimal time for intrauterine insemination occurs between 11 and 20 hours after the LH peak (Byrd *et al.*, 1990).

Donor insemination can be performed using either an intravaginal, intracervical or intrauterine technique. Intravaginal insemination can be performed at the center or by the couple at home, since exposure of the cervix is not required. This type of insemination is infrequently employed, however, because placement of the ejaculate is not optimal. Techniques for intracervical insemination (ICI) range from bathing the cervix with the sperm preparation via a cervical cap to inserting the sperm preparation high into the endocervical canal (Byrd *et al.*, 1990; Urry *et al.*, 1988; Patton *et al.*, 1992). Pericervical and intracervical inseminations are usually performed concomitantly. Following placement of the specimen into the cervix, a device is placed on or against the cervix to retain the fluid in proximity with the cervical os. Although no scientific data exist to support the practice, most patients are told to remain in a supine position with their hips elevated for at least 15 minutes following ICI or intravaginal insemination.

While intrauterine insemination (IUI) was initially introduced as a treatment option for cervical factor infertility, many centers now utilize it as the preferred technique for TDI with cryopreserved semen. Comparisons of the cycle fecundity of ICI with IUI using cryopreserved sperm are shown in Table 12.5. These studies suggest that higher fecundity rates are achieved with IUI of the thawed sperm. The basis for the enhanced sperm function as reflected in the higher fecundity remains unclear, but may involve avoidance of the cervical mucus, effects of the actual washing or other processing for IUI, or placement of

Table 12.5   *Relative cycle fecundity for intrauterine and intracervical cryopreserved donor insemination cycles*

Reference	Intracervical cycle fecundity [a]	Intrauterine cycle fecundity [a]
Patton *et al.*, 1992	4/79 (5%)	19/82 (23%)
Byrd *et al.*, 1990	9/229 (4%)	23/238 (10%)
Kossoy *et al.*, 1989	14/110 (13%)	
Chauhan *et al.*, 1989	37/207 (17.8%)	
Silverberg *et al.*, 1992		3/9 (33%)

Notes:
[a] Pregnancies per treatment cycle (%).

sperm into the uterine cavity. The higher fecundity achieved with IUI versus ICI is seen with the use of fresh donor sperm as well as insemination with the male partner's sperm (Urry *et al.*, 1988).

Most institutions now wash or otherwise separate the sperm from the seminal plasma and cryoprotectant in which it was frozen prior to IUI. It is a requirement of IUI that the sperm preparation be concentrated into a smaller volume (0.2–0.3 ml) to avoid distention of the uterine cavity, resultant cramping and possible expulsion of the inseminate. To perform the insemination itself, the vaginal and cervical area is initially wiped free of mucus, then the insemination catheter is gently inserted through the cervical os into the upper fundal area of the uterine cavity. The sperm suspension is slowly injected. Several catheters have been developed especially for IUI, although none has been shown to have a more beneficial effect on outcome over any other device (Irianni *et al.*, 1990). The patient is instructed to remain supine for 15 minutes after insemination. Some centers place a pack into the vagina or a cap over the cervix to maintain the fluid against the cervix. Forceps, tenaculum and/or cervical dilators are sometimes required to negotiate the cervical canal successfully. IUI may result in a loss of the reservoir effect of the cervix as well as the filtering and capacitation functions of cervical secretions, and these changes may be detrimental in some circumstances. Potential problems of IUI include the risk of infection and painful uterine contractions due to residual prostaglandins or uterine distention.

Mixing the donor sperm suspension with the partner's semen has potential psychological advantages to the couple. However, there is the potential risk of immobilization or agglutination of the donor sperm by the partner's semen if there are seminal antisperm antibodies. Despite this objection, some centers recommend the process with the rationale that the partner becomes more

Table 12.6 *Representative pregnancy rates using cryopreserved sperm for donor artificial insemination*

Reference	No. of patients	Pregnancy rate (%)
Behrman & Sawada, 1966	28	43
Steinberger & Smith, 1973	59	61
Friedman, 1977	174	67
Matthews *et al.*, 1979	133	54
Emperaire *et al.*, 1982	131	64

involved in the TDI process and can better identify himself as the father. Sexual intercourse after insemination can achieve these same benefits.

Success rates of insemination with cryopreserved donor sperm

Donor insemination using fresh semen compares favorably with pregnancy rates in fertile couples. After 12 cycles, cumulative pregnancy rates near 90% are seen in both groups. The cumulative results from a number of studies appearing in the literature from 1959 through 1982, show that 70% of women inseminated with fresh donor semen will conceive. The method of insemination (pericervical, vaginal, intracervical, use of a cap) did not determine success. Of those that do conceive, roughly 50% do so within the first three treatment cycles and nearly 80–90% within the first six cycles (Yeh & Seibel, 1987). Only 10% of those women who do not conceive in the first six treatment cycles would be expected to conceive subsequently (Dixon & Buttram, 1976).

More important is the question of efficacy of cryopreserved semen. Pregnancy rates using cryopreserved semen were initially reported to be lower than with fresh semen. A representative sample of studies from the literature (Table 12.6) in 525 patients shows a mean TDI pregnancy rate of 54%. This agrees with the estimate by Brotherton (1990) that 55% of recipients will eventually achieve pregnancy using cryopreserved semen. Tyler (1973) reviewed inseminations in 196 women, in whom 22 pregnancies were achieved after one to three inseminations, 29 required four to six inseminations, 24 required seven to ten inseminations, and 17 required eleven or more inseminations. Fifty-five percent of all pregnancies occurred within the first 6 months of therapy, which was lower than insemination with fresh donor semen. The cumulative expectation for pregnancy is about 10–20% lower with frozen semen, and the monthly fecundity of frozen semen appears to be one-half to three-fourths that of insemination with fresh semen. Conception will occur 2–3 months later with frozen than with fresh semen.

The optimal number of cryopreserved sperm necessary to achieve pregnancy with donor IUI or ICI varies between studies. Brown *et al.* (1988) demonstrated that increasing the number of motile sperm used for ICI from 29 million to 67 million doubled the gross fecundity from 5% to 10.4%. Patton *et al.* (1992) used a similar number of motile sperm per insemination for IUI (43.7 million) or ICI (49.2 million), finding more pregnancies in the IUI group. There was no difference in the number of motile cells inseminated in women who conceived compared with those who did not. Data suggest that the optimal pregnancy rates are achieved using a minimum of 15 million motile sperm per IUI insemination (Byrd *et al.*, 1990). Not surprisingly, motility characteristics of cryopreserved sperm after thawing and washing affect pregnancy expectations. Marshburn *et al.* (1992) found that pregnancy following IUI with cryopreserved sperm correlated with average curvilinear and straight line sperm velocity and the total number of motile sperm in the thawed specimen as determined by computer-assisted videomicrographic analysis.

The sex ratio of infants conceived after donor insemination with cryopreserved semen approaches that of the corresponding natural population. Data from the United States and five European countries demonstrate a sex ratio of 49.7% males to 50.3% females – a slight decrease in male births compared with results obtained with fresh donor semen (Mortimer & Richardson, 1982). For both fresh and cryopreserved semen used in DTI, the incidence of spontaneous abortion and congenital anomalies approximates that in the general population. Chong (1985) has reported spontaneous abortion rates of 23% with fresh semen and less than 10% with frozen semen. These rates, as low as or lower than in the naturally reproducing population, may be due to abnormal sperm failing to survive the freeze–thaw cycle and to the 'beneficial' effects of donor selection (see above). Also, because of this donor selection and preconceptual care afforded the recipient, children conceived by TDI may be expected to be physically and mentally superior to naturally conceived cohorts. Indeed Iizuka (1991) found that the intelligence quotients (IQs) of 54 children born following TDI was in a higher range than those of control children at 2½ years of age or older. In no case was the physical or mental development of children conceived through TDI inferior to that of the control group. Studies such as these are poorly controlled, and resulting conclusions must be viewed with caution. These caveats aside, however, it seems clear that cryopreserved TDI pregnancies have no higher risk of abortion, birth defects or other untoward outcomes than TDI with fresh sperm or naturally conceived pregnancies.

In summary, the success of TDI depends on three factors: the recipient woman's fertility potential, the quality and fertilizing ability of the sperm sample, and the timing and frequency of insemination relative to ovulation.

Female factors which appear to influence the success of TDI include age of the recipient (Dixon & Buttram, 1976; Glezerman, 1981; Yeh & Seibel, 1987), duration of infertility, development of subtle ovulatory disturbances, prior pelvic surgery and the presence of endometriosis. Indeed Aiman (1982) has concluded that such considerations as number of inseminations per cycle, sperm concentration and motility, timing of insemination, etc., were not important determinants of conception in 103 women inseminated for six cycles. This emphasizes the status of the female in determining TDI success, and further underscores the difficulty in comparing studies in the literature in which recipient screening and evaluation may have differed.

Risks and side effects of therapeutic donor insemination

The most important risk associated with TDI using donor insemination, beyond that actually attendant in the pregnancy itself, is the risk of STDs. Review of the literature concerning cases when fresh donor semen was used indicates that this risk is exceedingly low. Now, with the virtual exclusive use of cryopreserved and quarantined donor semen, that risk appears to be even lower. TDI recipients must understand, however, that some risk, even when of an exceedingly small magnitude, is inherent in the procedure. Their signed informed consent should reflect this understanding.

IUI and ICI are not without potential complications. Introduction of microorganisms into the upper genital tract and peritoneal cavity remains the major concern of IUI in particular. Stone *et al.* (1986) retrieved peritoneal fluid which contained microorganisms from five of nine patients undergoing IUI and only one of ten undergoing ICI. Following hydrotubation the number of positive peritoneal cases increased in both groups. These findings remain to be substantiated at other centers. Because of the careful screening of donors, infections resulting from IUI and cases of pelvic inflammatory disease after IUI are very rare. Other risks of insemination, including uterine discomfort or genital tract bleeeding, do not appear to be significant.

Conclusions

It is apparent that many factors influence the success of cryopreserved donor TDI, including the status of the female, the quality of the ejaculate or washed specimen, whether or not it was cryopreserved, and when, where or how it is placed into the female reproductive tract. Unfortunately, other than the reassurring data regarding pregnancy rates with cryopreserved semen noted above, little is known about the cryoinjury which accompanies sperm freezing and thawing, and its effect, if any, upon pregnancy outcome. The impression has always been that conception rates are lower with cryopreserved semen due to cryoinjury, despite the body of evidence now emerging which indicates that in couples where the inseminations are properly timed using contemporary methods to predict and detect ovulation, few differences are found between success rates with frozen and fresh semen (Steinberger & Smith, 1973; Iddenden *et al.*, 1985). Basic research into the mechanisms and effects of cryo-injury using contemporary cell and molecular biological techniques, along with additional large clinical investigations using cryopreserved semen, will further establish the efficacy of cryopreserved semen now that fresh semen has been abandoned for therapeutic insemination. In turn, development of national standards fcr sperm banks and donor insemination practice will do much to ensure a safe and effective therapy for the thousands of patients who will avail themselves of this treatment in the future.

References

Ackerman, D.R. (1968). Damage to human spermatozoa during storage at warming temperatures. *Int. J. Fertil.*, **13**, 220–5.

Ackerman, D.R. (1970). Hyaluronidase in human semen and sperm suspensions subjected to temperature shock to freezing. *J. Reprod. Fertil.*, **23**, 521–3.

Ackerman, D.R. (1971). Variation due to freezing in the citric acid content of human semen. *Fertil. Steril.*, **22**, 58–60.

Aiman, J. (1982). Factors affecting the success of donor insemination. *Fertil. Steril.*, **37**, 94–9.

Alexander, N.J. (1990). Sexual transmission of human immunodeficiency virus: virus entry into the male and female genital tract. World Health Organization, programme in acquired immune deficiency syndrome. *Fertil. Steril.*, **54**, 1–18.

American Association of Tissue Banks (1989). *Standards for Tissue Banking.* Arlington, Virginia: AATB.

American Fertility Society (1993). Guidelines for gamete donation: 1993. *Fertil Steril.*, **59**, 1S–9S.

Barratt, C.L.R., Bolton, A.E. & Cooke, I.D. (1990). Functional significance of white blood cells in the male and female reproductive tract. *Hum. Reprod.*, **5**, 639–48.

Behrman, S.J. & Sawada, Y. (1966). Heterologous and homologous inseminations with human semen frozen and stored in a liquid-nitrogen refrigerator. *Fertil. Steril.*, **17**, 457–66.

Brotherton, J. (1990). Cryopreservation of human semen. *Arch. Androl.*, **25**, 181–95.

Brown, C.A., Boone, W.R. & Shapiro, S.S. (1988). Improved cryopreserved semen fecundability in an alternating fresh-frozen artificial insemination program. *Fertil. Steril.*, **50**, 825–7.

Bunge, R.G., Keettel, W.C. & Sherman, J.K. (1954). Clinical use of frozen semen. *Fertil. Steril.*, **5**, 520.

Bunge, R.G. & Sherman, J.K. (1953). Fertilizing capacity of frozen human spermatozoa. *Nature*, **172**, 767.

Byrd, W., Bradshaw, K., Carr, B., Edman, C., Odom, J. & Ackerman, G. (1990). A prospective randomized study of pregnancy rates following intracervical and intrauterine insemination using frozen donor sperm. *Fertil Steril.*, **53**, 521–7.

Center for Disease Control (1988). Semen banking, organ and tissue transplantation and HIV antibody testing. *MMWR Morb. Mortal. Wkly Rep.*, **37**, 1.

Centola, G.M. & Mattox, J.H. (1990). Pregnancy rates after double versus single insemination with frozen donor semen. *Fertil. Steril.*, **54**, 1089–92.

Chauhan, M., Barratt, C.L.R., Cooke, S. & Cooke, I.D. (1988). A rationalized and objective protocol for the recruitment and screening of semen donors for an AID programme. *Hum. Reprod.*, **3**, 773–6.

Chauhan, M., Barratt, C.L., Cooke, S.M. & Cooke, I.D. (1989). Differences in the fertility of donor insemination recipients: a study to provide prognostic guidelines as to its success and outcome. *Fertil. Steril.*, **51**, 815–19.

Chong, A.P. (1985). Artificial insemination and sperm banking: clinical and laboratory considerations. *Semin. Reprod. Endocrinol.*, **3**, 193–200.

Critser, J.K., Arneson, B.W., Aaker, D.V., Huse-Benda, A.R. & Ball, G.D. (1987a). Cryopreservation of human spermatozoa. II. Postthaw chronology of motility and of zona-free hamster ova penetration. *Fertil. Steril.*, **47**, 980–4.

Critser, J.K., Huse-Benda, A.R., Aaker, D.V., Arneson, B.W. & Ball, G.D. (1987b). Cryopreservation of human spermatozoa. I. Effects of holding procedure and seeding on motility, fertilizability and acrosome reaction. *Fertil. Steril.*, **47**, 656–63.

Critser, J.K., Huse-Benda, A.R., Aaker, D.V., Arneson, B.W. & Ball, G.D. (1988). Cryopreservation of human spermatozoa. III. The effect of cryoprotectant on motility. *Fertil. Steril.*, **50**, 314–20.

Dixon, R.E. & Buttram, V.C. (1976). Artificial insemination using donor semen: a review of 171 cases. *Fertil. Steril.*, **27**, 130–4.

Emperaire, J.C., Gauzere-Soumireu, E. & Audebert, A.J. (1982). Female fertility and donor insemination. *Fertil. Steril.*, **37**, 90–3.

Friedman, S. (1977). Artificial donor insemination with frozen human semen. *Fertil. Steril.*, **28**, 1230–3.

Glezerman, M. (1981). Two hundred and seventy cases of artificial donor insemination: management and results. *Fertil. Steril.*, **35**, 180–7.

Glezerman, M. & Potashnik, G. (1988). Artificial insemination using fresh donor semen. *Andrologia*, **20**, 384–8.

Greenblatt, R.M., Handsfield, H.H., Sayers, M.H. & Homes, K.K. (1986). Screening therapeutic donors for sexually transmitted diseases: overview and recommendations. *Fertil. Steril.*, **46**, 351–64.

Horsburgh, C.R.J., Ou, C.Y., Jason, J., Holmberg, S.D., Longini, I.M., Schable, C., Mayer, K.H., Lifson, A.R., Schochetman, G. & Ward, J.W. (1989). Duration of human immunodeficiency virus infection before detection of antibody. *Lancet*, **ii**, 637–49.

Hurst, B.S., Tjaden, B.L., Kimball, A., Schlaff, W.D., Damewood, M.D. & Rock, J.A. (1992). Superovulation with or without intrauterine insemination for the treatment of infertility. *J. Reprod. Med.*, **37**, 237–41.

Iddenden, D.A., Sallam, H.N. & Collins, W.P. (1985). A prospective randomized study comparing fresh semen and cryopreserved semen for artificial insemination by donor. *Int. J. Fertil.*, **30**, 50–6.

Iizuka, R. (1991). Artificial insemination: progress and clinical application. *Ann. N.Y. Acad. Sci.*, **626**, 399–413.

Irianni, F.M., Acosta, A.A., Oehninger, S. & Acosta, M.R. (1990). Therapeutic intrauterine insemination (TII): controversial treatment for infertility. *Arch. Androl.*, **25**, 147–67.

Irvine, D.S. & Aitken, R.J. (1986). Predictive values of *in-vitro* sperm function tests in the context of an AID service. *Hum. Reprod.*, **1**, 539–45.

Jacobson, E. (1976). Up 400%: artificial insemination. *Sexual Med. Today*, [Dec 6].

Keel, B.A. & Black, J.B. (1980). Reduced motility longevity in thawed human spermatozoa. *Arch. Androl.*, **4**, 213–15.

Kossosy, L.R., Hill, G.A., Parker, R.A. & Rogers, B.J. (1989). Luteinizing hormone and ovulation timing in a therapeutic donor insemination program using frozen semen. *Am. J. Obstet. Gynecol.*, **160**, 1169–72.

Marshburn, P.B., McIntire, D., Carr, B.R. & Byrd, W. (1992). Spermatozoal characteristics from fresh and frozen donor semen and their correlation with fertility outcome after intrauterine insemination. *Fertil. Steril.*, **58**, 179–86.

Matthews, C.D., Broom, T.J., Crawshaw, K.M. & Hopkins, R.E. (1979). The influence of insemination timing and semen characteristics on the efficiency of a donor insemination program. *Fertil. Steril.*, **31**, 45–7.

Mortimer, D. & Richardson, D.W. (1982). Sex ratio of birth resulting from artificial insemination. *Br. J. Obstet. Gynecol.*, **89**, 132–5.

Mortimer, D. & Templeton, A.A. (1981). Sperm transport in the human female reproductive tract in relation to semen analysis characteristics and time of ovulation. *J. Reprod. Fertil.*, **64**, 401–8.

Odem, R.R., Durso, N.M., Long, C.A., Pineda, J.A., Strickler, R.C. & Gast, M.J. (1991). Therapeutic donor insemination: a prospective randomized study of scheduling methods. *Fertil. Steril.*, **55**, 976–82.

Patton, P.E., Burry, K.A., Thurmond, A., Novy, M.J. & Wolf, D.P. (1992). Intrauterine insemination outperforms intracervical insemination in a randomized, controlled study with frozen donor semen. *Fertil. Steril.*, **57**, 559–64.

Sawada, Y., Ackerman, D.R. & Behrman, S.J. (1967). Motility and respiration of human spermatozoa after cooling to various low temperatures. *Fertil. Steril.*, **18**, 775–81.

Silverberg, K.M., Johnson, J.V., Olive, D.L., Burns, W.N. & Schenken, R.S. (1992). A prospective, randomized trial comparing two different intrauterine insemination regimens in controlled ovarian hyperstimulation cycles. *Fertil. Steril.*, **57**, 357–61.

Snowden, R. (1993). Ethical and legal aspect of donor insemination. In *Donor Insemination*, ed. C.L.R. Barratt & I.D. Cooke, pp. 193–203. Cambridge: Cambridge University Press.

Steinberger, E. & Smith, K.D. (1973). Artificial insemination with fresh or frozen semen: a comparative study. *JAMA*, **223**, 778–83.

Stone, S.C., de la Maza, L.M. & Peterson, E.M. (1986). Recovery of microorganisms from the pelvic cavity after intracervical or intrauterine artificial insemination. *Fertil. Steril.*, **46**, 61.

Tyler, E.T. (1973). Clinical use of frozen semen banks. *Fertil. Steril.*, **24**, 413–16.

Urry, R.L., Middleton, R.G., Jones, K., Poulson, M., Worley, R. & Keye, W. (1988). Artificial insemination: a comparison of pregnancy rates with intrauterine versus cervical insemination and wash sperm versus serum swim-up sperm preparations. *Fertil. Steril.*, **49**, 1036.

US Congress OTA (1988). *Artificial Insemination: Practice in the United States*: Summary of a 1987 survey: background paper. OTA-BP-BA-48. Washington, DC: US Government Printing Office.

Yeh, J. & Seibel, M.M. (1987). Artificial insemination with donor sperm: a review of 108 patients. *Obstet. Gynecol.*, **70**, 180–7.

13

Endocrine assessment and hormone treatment of the infertile male

REBECCA Z. SOKOL

Introduction

Male factor infertility is a heterogeneous disorder. The majority of subfertile men do not have an identifiable cause of their infertility (Sokol, 1987, 1992). For example, 74% of 1041 patients seen in Melbourne, Australia, for evaluation of their infertility were diagnosed with idiopathic infertility, even though they presented with azoospermia, oligozoospermia, asthenozoospermia or normo-zoospermia (Baker *et al.*, 1985). The investigators reported that as semen quality improved there was less of a chance of identifying a cause for the disturbed testicular function (Baker & Burger, 1986). Most treatment regimens for idiopathic male infertility have been unsuccessful. However, a small percentage of men will present with a clearly definable disorder that may lend itself to a therapeutic intervention. The selection of the treatment regimen depends on both the underlying endocrine abnormality and the patient's semen analysis. This chapter will review the endocrine factors leading to disordered sperm function, the evaluation needed to diagnose those conditions, and the available treatment options.

Physiology of the hypothalamic–pituitary–testicular axis

The hypothalamic–pituitary–testicular axis is a closely integrated series of closed loop feedback systems involving the higher centers in the central nervous system, the hypothalamus, the pituitary and the testicular endocrine and germinal compartments.

The hypothalamus produces gonadotropin releasing hormone (GnRH), which is transported to the pituitary gland by a short portal system connecting the two areas. Extrahypothalamic neurotransmitters, norepinephrine and dopamine, regulate GnRH synthesis and its pulsatile release into the hypophyseal portal veins. Norepinephrine facilitates GnRH secretion, while dopamine appears to have both stimulatory and inhibitory effects (Steinberger, 1979; di Zerega & Sherins, 1981).

The neural mechanism responsible for generating the hypothalamic drive to the pituitary gonadotropes is referred to as the GnRH pulse generator, which is thought to serve as a major site for the integration of neural, hormonal, and perhaps metabolic signals that control gonadotropin secretion and gonadal function (Barraclough, 1982; Plant, 1986). The intermittent discharge of GnRH into the hypophyseal portal circulation results in ultradian fluctuations in the concentration of this releasing factor into portal blood (Plant, 1986). This pulsatile GnRH signal, generated by the brain, is an obligatory component for hypophysiotropic stimulation of pituitary gonadotropes. If the neuro-humoral link between the brain and pituitary gland is interrupted, pituitary function is abolished and gonadal function arrested (Plant, 1986).

Binding of GnRH to GnRH receptors on the gonadotropes of the pituitary gland stimulates, via calcium, the synthesis and release of the gonadotropic hormones LH and FSH (Conn *et al.* 1987). Both are composed of alpha and beta subunits. Within a species, a single gene codes for the alpha subunit of all glycoprotein pituitary hormones (i.e., LH, FSH, TSH), whereas different genes code for the beta subunits (Papavasiliou *et al.*, 1986*a*). Concentrations and production rates of beta subunits thus determine amounts of bioactive hormone (Papavasiliou *et al.*, 1986*b*).

Abnormalities in the biologic actions of LH have been reported in various disease states. This is manifested as *immunologically* measurable LH but *biologically* less active LH (as measured in an LH bioassay *in vitro*). Such discrepancy in the biologic/immunologic LH ratio has been demonstrated during normal sexual maturation, in renal failure, and after GnRH agonist treatment, suggesting that disruption and/or changes in the signals between hypothalamus and pituitary may induce an abnormally acting LH (Acbers & Smith, 1985; Yuan *et al.*, 1988).

LH and FSH are secreted by the pituitary gland into the general circulation, by which they are carried to the testes. There they stimulate gonadal steroid secretion and are important in the maturation and maintenance of spermatogenesis (Steinberger, 1979; Sokol & Swerdloff, 1984).

Testosterone is the major steroid hormone produced by the testis. Ninety-eight percent of testosterone circulates bound to carrier proteins including sex hormone binding globulin (SHBG) and albumin (Partridge, 1981). It is the 2% of testosterone which circulates in the unbound or 'free' state in the plasma that is able to enter cells where it exerts its metabolic effects. Changes in the amount of available SHBG alter tissue entry of testosterone (Dunn *et al.*, 1981) and hence its biologic effect.

Twenty-five percent of circulating estradiol is secreted by the testes. The majority of circulating estradiol is derived from the peripheral conversion of testosterone and androstenedione (Longcope *et al.*, 1984). Estrogens play a role in regulation of GnRH and LH secretion (Santen, 1975; Winters & Troen, 1975). Dihydrotestosterone (DHT), the most potent androgen, is derived from the *in situ* peripheral conversion of testosterone (Ito & Horton, 1971). DHT is necessary for external virilization during embryogenesis, puberty and adulthood (Griffin & Wilson, 1985).

In addition to their steroid production, the testes also produce a nonsteroid substance, inhibin (McCullagh, 1932). Inhibin, secreted by the sertoli cells, is thought to act at the pituitary level where it selectively inhibits the secretion of FSH (Ying, 1988). It may also exert local regulatory effects on spermatogenesis (Demoulin *et al.*, 1981) in a paracrine or autocrine fashion.

Prolactin, a polypeptide hormone synthesized and secreted from the pituitary gland, may be required in physiologic amounts for the maintenance of testosterone biosynthesis (Magrini *et al.*, 1976; Klemcke *et al.*, 1984). Elevated levels of prolactin *suppress* testosterone synthesis in men, by interfering with the catecholaminergic regulation of GnRH, and by inhibiting its release from the hypothalamus (Ben-Jonathan, 1986), resulting in reduced LH secretion and hence lower testosterone levels. The hypothalamic regulation of prolactin secretion is predominantly inhibitory through dopamine (Ben-Jonathan, 1986). Psychotropic drugs such as thorazine, antihypertensives such as reserpine, and abused drugs such as amphetamines, interfere with dopamine release, resulting in the elevation of prolactin.

Control and coordination of testicular function occurs via both positive and negative feedback signals exerted by the hormones secreted at each level of the hypothalamic–pituitary–testicular axis. These signals include testicular steroid inhibition of hypothalamic GnRH secretion and pituitary (LH) responsiveness to GnRH, and inhibition of pituitary FSH production and release by inhibin and, possibly, circulating estrogens. Any disruption of the delicate interaction between the components of this axis may lead to hypogonadism and/or infertility.

Clinical evaluation

The evaluation of the hypothalamic–pituitary–testicular axis is initiated with the history and the physical examination, especially since a number of genetic congenital and secondary disorders are associated with hypogonadism. For example, Klinefelter's syndrome, the most common disorder causing male hypogonadism, occurs in approximately 0.20% of adults (Winter, 1987). Other disorders resulting in hypogonadism are listed in Table 13.1.

Table 13.1   Classification of hypogonadism

HYPOGONADOTROPIC HYPOGONADISM
Hypothalamic disease
Gonadotropin deficiency
  Congenital
    Kallmann's syndrome
    Prader–Labhart–Willi syndrome
    Laurence–Moon–Biedl syndrome
  Acquired
    Trauma
    Tumor
    Malnutrition
    Chronic disease
      Liver failure
      Uremia
      Emotional disorders
      Collagen vascular diseases
    Infiltrative disease
      Sarcoidosis
      Tuberculosis
      Fungal
      Histiocytosis
Secondary to hyperprolactinemia
Drug and toxin induced
  Reproductive Hormones and their antagonists
  Cimetidine
  Spironolactone
  Tranquilizers and opioids
  Metoclopramide
  Lead
  Cocaine (possibly)
  Alcohol (possibly)

Pituitary disease
Tumor
Diseases
  Hemachromatosis
  Autoimmune hypophysitis

HYPERGONADOTROPIC HYPOGONADISM
Gonadal defects
Genetic
  Klinefelter's syndrome
  XYY syndrome
  Down's syndrome
  Myotonic dystrophy
  Other autosomal and chromosomal translocations

(*cont.*)

Table 13.1   *cont.*

Orchitis
  Mumps
  Misc. viruses
  Autoimmune

Drug and toxin induced
Alcohol
Marijuana
Heavy metals
Gossypol (cotton-seed oil)
Insecticides, herbicides and fungicides
Ketoconazole
Ionizing radiation

Enzymatic defects in androgen synthesis

Anatomic castration

Paraplegia

Hormone resistance

History

A detailed account of the patient's developmental history is essential: age of testicular descent, age of puberty, congenital abnormalities of the urinary tract or central nervous system, history of gynecomastia and fertility history. Any changes in libido and/or potency should be noted. Other pertinent aspects of the history to elicit include surgery of the central nervous system and genito-urinary system (i.e. orchiopexy, pelvic or retroperitoneal surgery, herniorrhaphy, vasectomy); infectious disease, including sexually transmitted diseases, mumps, tuberculosis and epididymitis; use of drugs and medications; past and present occupations; and proximity of the patient's residence to areas of chemical exposure.

Physical examination

The physician can frequently ascertain whether hypogonadism presented prior to or following puberty on the basis of specific physical findings. Inadequate Leydig cell function or androgen action during embryogenesis may manifest itself by the presence of hypospadias, cryptorchidism or microphallus (Griffin & Wilson, 1985). If Leydig cell failure occurs prior to puberty, sexual maturation will not occur, and the individual will develop the features termed eunuchoidism (Griffin & Wilson, 1985). The cardinal feature of eunuchoidism is the failure of androgen-induced closure of the epiphyses of the long bones, their continued growth resulting in an arm span more than 5 cm greater than the height, and a lower body segment (pubis to heel) more than 5 cm longer than the upper body segment (crown to pubis). Other findings associated with prepubertal onset of hypogonadism include sparse body, pubic and facial hair, poor development of skeletal muscles, absence of male pattern baldness, infantile genitalia with small firm testes (less than 15 cc) and, occasionally, a small phallus, failure of voice to deepen, and possibly gynecomastia.

Leydig cell failure which commences after puberty presents with more subtle physical findings. The most important physical finding is soft, smaller (than normal) testes. Other features include a female body habitus with female fat distribution, a decrease in skeletal muscle mass, gynecomastia and a decrease in facial hair (Sokol, 1992).

Laboratory assessment

Laboratory investigation of testicular function begins with basic screening tests; more specialized tests are ordered to isolate specific abnormalities in selected patients when indicated (Sokol, 1988).

Hormonal baseline assessment

Evaluation of the endocrine status of the hypothalamus, pituitary, and testes requires the measurement of serum LH, FSH and testosterone. A sample of 10 ml of whole blood collected in the morning, thus minimizing diurnal variation, is adequate (Baum *et al.*, 1988). However, due to the pulsatile nature of hormone secretion in man, single random serum levels may not accurately reflect the mean concentration of LH, FSH and testosterone over a prolonged period of time (Santen & Bardin, 1973). If an abnormal result is obtained multiple samples (three samples collected through an indwelling cannula at 20 minute intervals) should be re-evaluated. By pooling three samples an integrated measure of basal hormone secretion is obtained (Santen & Bardin, 1973).

Estradiol measurements are indicated when a patient presents with gynecomastia. Prolactin measurement is included if a patient presents with impotence and/or evidence for a central nervous system tumor, as well as in men with a history of drug abuse. The measurement of DHT is indicated when a disorder of testosterone conversion to DHT is suspected.

Stimulation tests

Dynamic tests available to determine the physiologic state of the hypothalamic–pituitary–testicular axis include stimulation test with GnRH and hCG. The GnRH test evaluates the functional capacity of the gonadotropes to release LH and FSH (Santen, 1987). The single-dose GnRH test consists of a bolus injection of 100 µg GnRH. Three measurements of plasma LH concentration precede the injection, after which plasma is collected at 30, 60 and 90 minutes for measurement of LH concentration. A doubling of LH concentration is normal (Santen, 1987).

In states of reduced endogenous GnRH secretion, the pituitary cells producing LH and FSH are not primed, which results in blunting of the response to a single bolus of GnRH. Thus a low LH response to a single-dose GnRH stimulation may not reliably distinguish between hypothalamic and pituitary disease. If an equivocal result is obtained, a multiple-dose GnRH priming test can be performed. The principle of this test is to prime the pituitary gonadotropes with repeated low-dose stimulation, which recreates the physiologic conditions in which the pituitary gland is exposed to regular pulses of GnRH. GnRH is administered either as an infusion (0.25 µg/min) over a four hour period, or as a single injection every day for 7 days. Serum is collected for LH analysis before and after 'priming' (Snyder *et al.*, 1979).

The ability of the testes to secrete testosterone is tested with the administration of hCG. hCG is used as a stimulus of testosterone secretion because of the close structural similarity between the biologically active subunits of hCG and LH, and its long half-life. Traditional test procedures use multiple injections of hCG on a daily basis (Santen, 1987). However, data suggest that such high doses interfere with Leydig cell responsiveness (Padron *et al.*, 1980). The recommended procedure is to give one intramuscular injection of 1500–4000 IU hCG, followed by plasma testosterone measurement before, and 5 days after, the injection. A doubling of the initial testosterone level is considered normal in an adult man.

Specialized tests

Free testosterone and sex hormone binding globulin (SHBG)

The measurement of free (unbound) testosterone is a more accurate marker of available and hence physiologically active testosterone than is total testosterone level when conditions of altered SHBG concentrations or binding exist (Vermeulen *et al.*, 1969). Reduced SHBG levels occur in association with obesity, acromegaly and hypothyroidism. Increased SHBG levels occur in association with early hepatic cirrhosis and hypogonadism. Estrogens stimulate and androgens inhibit the biosynthesis of SHBG (Santen, 1987), and many other natural and synthetic steroids alter the binding of SHBG (Pugeat *et al.*, 1981).

SHBG can be indirectly measured by a variety of radioreceptor assays. Unbound free testosterone can be measured by radioimmunoassay after equilibrium dialysis, or indirectly calculated from measurements of SHBG levels. The proportion of testosterone that is 'free' is inversely related to the SHBG (Handelsman & Swerdloff, 1985).

Bioassay of LH

Certain medical conditions can induce gonadotropin molecular heterogeneity, which then presents as a disparity between the measurable levels of LH and testosterone, and the clinical picture. The LH *in vitro* bioassay is designed to measure immunologically assayable LH, which is not biologically active. The *in vitro* production of testosterone by Leydig cells isolated from rodents is measured (Smith *et al.*, 1983). Plasma samples are simultaneously assayed for LH by radioimmunoassay. The ratio of biologic to immunologic activity (B/I ratio) is then determined. A 1:1 ratio indicates equal immunologic and biologic activity.

Summary of diagnostic categories

Patients with evidence of hypogonadism and/or infertility will present with a history, physical examination, semen analysis and baseline hormone testing consistent with one of three diagnostic categories: (1) hypogonadotropic hypogonadism, (2) irreversible seminiferous tubular failure and (3) idiopathic oligospermia.

Hypogonadotropic hypogonadism

Patients with hypogonadotropic hypoganadism present with low testosterone, low LH, low FSH and oligozoospermia or azoospermia, and possibly elevation of prolactin and estradiol levels. The differential diagnosis of hypogonadotropic hypogonadism includes hypothalamic or pituitary tumor, congenital LH deficiency (Kallman's syndrome), severe malnutrition, anorexia nervosa, specific genetic disorders, and infectious diseases (see Table 12.1). The GnRH stimulation test aids the differentiation between hypothalamic and pituitary disease in these patients. Occasionally, the endocrine evaluation of some patients will reveal a low testosterone concurrent with 'normal' gonadotropin levels, suggesting abnormalities in SHBG or the biologic action of LH. This can be evaluated by measuring free testosterone and the biologic activity of LH, respectively. In the former, the free testosterone will fall within the normal range, while in the latter condition the biologic activity of LH will be less than the amount of LH measured by radioimmunoassay.

Irreversible seminiferous tubular failure

Irreversible seminiferous tubular failure can ·be divided into hyper-gonadotropic hypogonadism and primary germ cell failure. Patients with hypergonadotropic hypogonadism present with low testosterone and elevated LH and FSH, and oligozoospermia or azoospermia. Estradiol may be elevated. Differential diagnosis includes gonadal defects and hormone resistance. The hCG stimulation test is rarely indicated.

Patients with primary germ cell failure present with normal testosterone and LH levels, and elevated FSH levels. The primary complaint is oligozoospermia and infertility. In the future, the measurement of serum inhibin levels may clarify this diagnosis.

Idiopathic oligozoospermia

Patients with idiopathic oligozoospermia have normal LH, FSH, testosterone and estradiol levels. Their primary complaint is infertility and oligozoospermia.

Treatment

Hypogonadotropic hypogonadism

The etiology of hypogonadotropic hypogonadism is either congenital or acquired. The former, Kallmann's syndrome, or idiopathic hypogonadotropic hypogonadism, is an abnormality of the secretion of GnRH. Acquired causes of hypogonadotropic hypogonadism include tumor, infection, infiltrative diseases, and autoimmune hypophysitis. Prolactin-secreting pituitary tumors in men are large at the time of discovery, and therapy must be directed at reduction of tumor mass. The hyperprolactinemia may be treated with dopamine agonists to normalize testicular hormone levels and spermatogenic function (Winters & Troen, 1984).

Men with hypogonadotropic hypogonadism are deficient in LH and FSH, which results in a deficiency in testosterone secretion and spermatogenesis. Spermatogenesis can be initiated, and pregnancies achieved in the partners of many of these hypogonadotropic hypogonadal men, following treatment with exogenous gonadotropins or pulsatile GnRH. Selection of the type of therapy, as well as the ultimate success of the therapy, depends on the severity. of the defect. The most frequently prescribed preparations are hCG and human menopausal gonadotropin (hMG).

hCG binds to its receptor and stimulates Leydig cell secretion of testosterone and estradiol, required for spermatogenesis. Paradoxically, however, the increase in sex steroid levels results in suppression of FSH via the feedback mechanism on the hypothalamus and pituitary gland. Nonetheless, hCG is usually the first-line drug for the treatment of nonhyperprolactinemic hypogonadotropic hypogonadism to attempt to restore spermatogenesis. Treatment with hCG alone in patients with partial gonadotropin deficiency may increase sperm counts, with resultant pregnancies. The hCG is administered at a dose of 6000–8000 IU two or three times per week for 18–24 weeks. Ultimately, the majority of patients with partial defects, as well as those with complete hypogonadotropic hypogonadism, will require the addition of hMG to their regimens (Sherins, 1984; Sherins & Howards, 1986).

In both groups of patients, hCG is administered until normal serum testosterone levels are achieved, and there is no further increase in testicular growth or improvement in sperm production. At that point, hMG, which contains both LH and FSH, is added to the regimen. The hMG is administered at a dose of 75 IU twice weekly until the patient produces ejaculates containing 5 million or more sperm per milliliter, or until pregnancy is achieved. The hMG can then be withdrawn, and spermatogenesis will usually be maintained by continued administration of hCG alone (Sherins & Howards, 1986).

Although this preceding regimen is the standard for gonadotropin replacement, other investigators have suggested an alternate regimen. Lunenfeld & Berezin (1988) recommended daily injections of one ampule hMG (containing 75 IU LH and 75 IU FSH), for at least 90 days. If an inadequate response is observed in 120 days, the hMG dose is doubled. Every 5 days, one ampule of 5000 IU hCG is also injected intramuscularly. Of the 62 patients treated with this regimen, 29 had an improvement in sperm production, and 22 fathered 39 children. Interestingly, 20 of the 29 patients had previously received hCG therapy alone for 6 months to 3 years without initiation of spermatogenesis. Following the hMG and hCG treatment course, spermatogenesis could be maintained with hCG alone in 3 of 29 patients. These data are in sharp contrast to those of Sherins (1984), who reported that 8 of 9 men who responded positively to combined therapy were able to maintain spermatogenesis for at least 1 year on hCG alone.

Prior long-term treatment of these men with testosterone does not affect the subsequent success of gonadotropin therapy (Ley & Leonard, 1985; Hamman & Berg, 1990). Side effects have been reported during treatment with hCG and hMG, including headaches, gynecomastia, breast tenderness, and the development of anti-hCG antibodies.

Men with idiopathic hypogonadotropic hypogonadism may also be treated by replacement therapy with GnRH. By definition, GnRH therapy is effective only in cases in which the pituitary gland is intact. In preliminary studies, Hoffman & Crowley (1982) administered long-term, episodic low-dose GnRH therapy by a portable subcutaneous infusion pump to patients with idiopathic hypogonadotropic hypogonadism. Gonadotropin levels increased to normal adult ranges within 1 week of treatment, and spermatogenesis was restored after 3–5 weeks of therapy.

In these initial studies, the patients were treated with 25 mg/kg of native GnRH every 2 hours by a portable infusion pump. Crowley and co-workers also explored the possibility that GnRH dose requirements may vary from patient to patient. In their follow-up study, 11 men were treated with initial doses of 10–25 mg/kg of GnRH, which were increased over several months until serum testosterone levels increased to the mid-normal adult male range (Crowley, 1988). They concluded that there may be a specific threshold dose required for each individual patient prior to initiation of gonadal steroid secretion in that patient. The data also suggested that pituitary or gonadal responsiveness may increase in men with idiopathic hypogonadotropic hypogonadism during long-term GnRH therapy. Other investigators have also reported pregnancies in the partners of men treated with GnRH by infusion pump (Donald *et al.*, 1983; Skarin *et al.*, 1982). Administration of GnRH by the nasal route has also been studied (Klingmuller & Schweikert, 1985), with the maintenance of spermatogenesis by large doses of an intranasal preparation. Although both these treatment approaches appear to be effective, the clinical experience available is limited.

Recently, Shoham and co-workers (1992) treated four patients with hypogonadotropic hypogonadism who had failed to respond adequately to conventional therapy using a combination of growth hormone (GH) and gonadotropin therapy. For 24 weeks patients received 4 IU human GH, three times per week; 150 IU FSH and 150 IU LH three times per week; and 2500 IU hCG twice a week. Following the treatment, three patients increased testosterone secretion, and two produced semen samples with sperm concentrations of 12 and 13 million/ml, respectively. The former patient's partner became pregnant. One patient showed no improvement in either serum testosterone level or sperm concentration. Based on their data and the theory that IGF-I, like GH is capable of augmenting FSH hormonal action on the Sertoli and Leydig cells, the authors suggest that combined treatment with gonadotropins and GH may offer a new approach to the treatment of these men. Definitive conclusions regarding the efficacy of this treatment regimen await the results of larger clinical trials.

Irreversible germ cell failure

Men with irreversible seminiferous failure can be subdivided into two major groups: (1) men with spermatogenic failure who present only with elevated serum FSH levels, normal LH and testosterone levels, and small testes, and (2) men who present with classic hypergonadotropic hypogonadism, identified by elevated gonadotropins, low testosterone, and severe oligozoospermia or azoospermia. There is currently no therapy available for the treatment of infertility in these two groups of men. Artificial insemination with donor semen (AID) or adoption are the recommended options if assisted reproductive technologies such as ICSI are not feasible. Those men who present with both an abnormality of spermatogenesis and hypogonadism should be treated with androgens to maintain secondary sexual characteristics (Sokol & Swerdloff, 1982).

Idiopathic oligozoospermia

There is no proven treatment for idiopathic oligozoospermia. These patients present with normal gonadotropins and normal testosterone and low sperm counts. Idiopathic oligozoospermia results from a variety of abnormalities, each causing a reduction in sperm concentration. Treating all patients with the same drug will not uniformly result in improvement of fertility. The drugs used in the treatment of idiopathic oligozoospermia include androgens, gonadotropins, antiestrogens, and prostaglandin inhibitors. Few placebo-controlled studies have been published that evaluate the efficacy of these drugs in the treatment of male infertility.

Androgen therapy

There are two forms of androgen therapy: low-dose testosterone and high-dose testosterone regimens. In the low-dose testosterone regimen, androgens are given in oral doses of either 10–50 mg/day methyltestosterone, 50–70 mg/day of mesterolone, or 5–20 mg/day fluoxymesterone for at least 3 months in an effort to supplement inadequate endogenous production of testosterone and thus stimulate spermatogenesis. These regimens have been shown to be ineffective (Giarola, 1974; Brown, 1975; Keough *et al.*, 1976; Steinberger, 1986), probably because they fail to alter intratesticular testosterone concentrations significantly.

Rebound testosterone therapy involves the administration of higher doses of testosterone, most frequently testosterone enanthate, 200–250 mg intramuscularly every 2 weeks. These doses have been shown to suppress LH and spermatogenesis (Peterson *et al.*, 1968; Franchimont *et al.*, 1975; Keough *et al.*, 1976). Following the cessation of therapy, sperm prodution usually resumes and, in some patients, sperm concentrations may rebound to a higher level. On the basis of conception rates, treatment does not appear to improve fertility (Schill, 1979; Baker, 1983).

Most recently, Gerris *et al.* (1991) treated 52 patients with idiopathic oligoasthenozoospermia and/or teratozoospermia with either 150 mg/day mesterolone or placebo for 12 months. Similar semen improvement was noted in
both the treated and control patients. The pregnancy rate in the mesterolone-
treated cases was 26%. The pregnancy rate in the placebo-controlled cases was
48%. Comhaire (1990) treated 25 men with idiopathic oligozoospermia,
asthenozoospermia, or teratozoospermia, with either 240 mg/day testosterone
undecanoate or placebo. One group received 3 months of placebo followed by
3 months of testosterone undecanoate, and another group received 6 months
of testosterone undecanoate. Changes in sperm concentration, motility, and
morphology were similar in both groups. Two pregnancies occurred: one
during the first month of placebo intake and the other during the second
month of treatment with testosterone undecanoate. Androgen therapy cannot be recommended in contemporary practice for treatment of idiopathic
oligozoospermia.

Gonadotropins

Investigators have administered gonadotropins to patients with idiopathic
oligozoospermia using regimens similar to those for patients with hypogonadotropic hypogonadism. Unfortunately, gonadotropins have not
enhanced the fertility of these men (Lunenfeld, *et al.*, 1967; Troen *et al.*, 1970;
Rosenberg, 1976; Sokol, 1982).

Recently, Acosta and co-workers (1992) have suggested that therapy with
pure human FSH may play a role in the treatment of severe male infertility by
assisted reproductive techniques. Fifty men with abnormal semen analyses
were treated with 150 IU pure FSH three times per week for at least 3 months.
One group had a history of failed fertilization in previous IVF attempts, and
one group had not undergone an IVF attempt. Although no significant
changes were observed in serum LH levels, testosterone levels or semen parameters, the fertilization rates of pre-ovulatory oocytes were significantly
improved. Unfortunately, no control arm was included in the study, and the
number of men in some of the groups was too low to reach definite conclusions
regarding significance. The efficacy of FSH treatment of infertile men as
adjunctive treatment during IVF remains to be proven.

Antiestrogens

The most popular drugs used to treat oligozoospermia are the antiestrogens,
clomiphene and tamoxifen, which act as competitive inhibitors of estrogen
action by occupying estrogen receptors. Testolactone, an aromatase inhibitor
which prevents the conversion of testosterone to estradiol (Vigersky & Glass,

1981) is also used in this setting. Androgens and estrogens modulate hypothalamic and pituitary functions to regulate gonadotropin production. Antiestrogens thus interfere with (block) the normal negative feedback signals of circulating or locally produced steroids on the hypothalamus and pituitary. As a result, secretion of GnRH stimulates increased gonadotropin secretion, which in turn increases testosterone production, and would theoretically enhance germ cell maturation. Antiestrogens may also have a direct effect on the testis by blocking the inhibitory action of estradiol on Leydig cell function. Decreasing the effective levels of estradiol by administering an estrogen inhibitor or an aromatase inhibitor was suggested as a mechanism to increase sperm production in men with oligozoospermia (Adashi, 1985).

Clomiphene has been the most commonly used drug in the treatment of male infertility. Some previous studies indicated improvement of sperm motility and infertility on clomiphene regimens, whereas others reported no improvement in fertility. In the few studies that did include controls, the investigators concluded that clomiphene could not be considered an effective agent (Foss *et al.*, 1973; Masala *et al.*, 1978; Micic & Dotlic, 1985; Wang *et al.*, 1983; Weiland *et al.*, 1972).

Weiland *et al.* (1972) administered 5 mg or 10 mg of clomiphene per day for 12 weeks, then placebo for 12 weeks. Although sperm concentrations were increased with clomiphene, the increase was erratic and there were no pregnancies. Masala *et al.* (1978) administered clomiphene, 50 mg, twice daily for 5 days to 10 oligozoospermic men and 10 control subjects. There were no statistical differences in hormonal response between the two groups. Foss *et al.* (1973) gave either clomiphene (100 mg/day) or a placebo for 10 days in each of 3 months. Although 19 pregnancies occurred, it was not clear if they were due to the clomiphene treatment.

Pregnancy rates of 36% and 22% were observed in partners of men receiving 25 mg and 50 mg of clomiphene citrate, respectively. Pregnancy occurred when initial sperm concentrations were greater than 10 million sperm per milliliter. Of the seven control patients studied, in one series, only two began the study with sperm concentrations between 10 and 15 million sperm per milliliter. The prognosis for fertility with treatment was more favorable for patients with higher initial sperm concentrations (Wang *et al.*, 1983). These results were not confirmed by Micic & Dotlic (1985), who reported no differences in pregnancy rates between men treated with placebo and those treated with clomiphene.

In a longitudinal prospective study, 21 men were treated with either clomiphene citrate, 50 mg/day, or placebo daily for 12 months. All spouses of participants in the study were carefully screened for any evidence of infertility and were included only if they were considered to be potentially fertile by two independent evaluations. There were no significant differences in sperm concentrations, sperm penetration into zona-free hamster eggs, or pregnancy rates between the treatment group and the placebo group (Sokol *et al.*, 1988). During the entire time course of the study all sperm counts increased in both the placebo and the clomiphene groups. Similar results have been observed by others (Baker *et al.*, 1981; Baker & Burger, 1986).

Investigators evaluating testolactone and tamoxifen citrate as antiestrogen therapies for men with idiopathic oligozoospermia have similarly reported variable results (Comhaire, 1976, 1982; Willis *et al.*, 1977; Vermeulen & Comhaire, 1978; Vigersky & Glass, 1981; Buvat *et al.*, 1983; AinMelk *et al.*, 1987).

Tamoxifen citrate is an antiestrogen with weaker intrinsic estrogenic activity than clomiphene and a similar mechanism of action. Vermeulen & Comhaire (1978) reported that sperm concentration or motility improved in 12 men with idiopathic oligozoospermia. Although Willis *et al.* (1977) reported no statistically significant improvement in the sperm concentration of oligozoospermic men, one of the partners conceived. Comhaire (1976) reported an increase in sperm concentration, with three pregnancies. Buvat *et al.* (1983) treated 25 normogonadotropic oligozoospermic men with tamoxifen (20 mg/day) for 4–12 months. The mean sperm concentration was significantly increased ($P<0.001$), and 10 pregnancies were reported during the treatment period. In contrast, AinMelk *et al.* (1987) reported no differences in pregnancy rates between tamoxifen-treated men and placebo-treated men.

Testolactone, an aromatase inhibitor, may also stimulate spermatogenesis. One gram orally each day for 6–12 months resulted in a significant increase in sperm concentration in eight of nine men with idiopathic oligozoospermia (Vigersky & Glass, 1981). There were no significant changes in motility or semen volume, or in the response to GnRH stimulation at the end of the treatment period. Estradiol levels decreased, testosterone levels increased, and LH, FSH, and prolactin levels did not change. In marked contrast, Clark & Sherins (1989) reported no differences between placebo and testolactone treatment groups in a controlled, crossover trial.

Miscellaneous drugs

Several investigators have suggested that spermatogenesis is improved by treatment with prostaglandin synthetase inhibitors, because testosterone secretion and spermatogenesis are inhibited in male rodents treated with prostaglandin E or E_2. The addition of prostaglandin E to semen samples results in the inhibition of motility of human spermatozoa (Abbatiello *et al.*, 1973; Bartke *et al.*, 1976). In a clinical trial, Barkay *et al.* (1984) compared the effects of various doses of indomethacin and ketoprofen with placebo in 100 patients with oligozoospermia. Serum LH, FSH, and sperm concentration and motility significantly improved in all patients treated with indomethacin, whereas sperm concentration remained unchanged in semen of patients treated with ketoprofen. A significantly greater number of pregnancies were reported in the groups treated with the drugs than in the placebo group. The highest proportion of pregnancies (35%) occurred in women whose partners were receiving 75 mg of indomethacin per day.

A variety of other pharmacologic agents have been empirically administered to men with idiopathic infertility. These include triiodothyronine, vitamins A, C, and E, zinc and bromocriptine. None of these has proved successful in the treatment of idiopathic male infertility.

Summary

The majority of infertile men present with disorders that are either non-treatable or questionably amenable to treatment. Endocrine therapy has rarely proven successful except in cases of hypogonadotropic hypogonadism, where exogenous gonadotropins or GnRH replace deficiencies. In the remaining patients their pathogenic heterogeneity probably prevents discovery of a suitable endocrine therapy.

In addition, the importance of controlled therapeutic trials of male fertility drugs, in which 'spontaneous cures' and placebo effects are included, cannot be overemphasized. Investigators in Australia and England have analyzed pregnancy rates by life-table analyses. For example, Glazner *et al.* (1987) reported a 30% conception rate in women without infertility factors after 18 months of unprotected intercourse with partners whose motile sperm densities were less than 4 million sperm per milliliter. Baker & Burger (1986) reported similar 25% pregnancy rates after 24 months in presumptively fertile women whose partners had sperm concentrations of less than 5 million sperm per milliliter.

Viewed upon this background, empiric endocrine therapy of the patient with idiopathic infertility provides little reason for optimism.

References

Abbatiello, E.R., Kaminsky, M. & Weisbroth, S. (1973). The effect of prostaglandins and prostaglandin inhibitors on spermatogenesis. *Int. J. Fertil.*, **20**, 177.

Acbers, G. & Smith, F. (1985). Effects of site-specific amino acids modification on protein interactions and biologic function. *Annu. Rev. Biochem.*, **54**, 597.

Acosta, A.A., Khalifa, E. & Oehninger, S. (1992). Pure human follicle stimulating hormone has a role in the treatment of severe male infertility by assisted reproduction: Norfolk's total experience. *Hum. Reprod.*, **7**, 1067.

Adashi, E.Y. (1985). Clomiphene citrate: mechanism(s) and site(s) of action. A hypothesis revisited. *Fertil. Steril.*, **42**, 331.

AinMelk, Y., Belisle, S., Caimel, M., *et al.* (1987). Tamoxifen citrate therapy in male infertility. *Fertil. Steril.*, **48**, 113.

Baker, H.W.G. (1983). Male infertility of undetermined etiology. In *Current Therapy in Endocrinology*, p. 366. Philadelphia: B.C. Decker.

Baker, H.W.G. & Burger, H.G. (1986). Male infertility. In *Reproductive Medicine*, ed. A. Steinberger, G. Frajese & E. Steinberger, p. 187. New York: Raven Press.

Baker, H.W.G., Burger, H.G., DeKretser, D.M., *et al.* (1981). Factors affecting variability of semen analysis results in infertile men. *Int. J. Androl.*, **4**, 609.

Baker, H.W.G., Burger, H.G. & DeKretser, D.M. (1985). Relative incidence of etiologic disorders in male infertility. In *Male Sexual Dysfunction*, ed. R.J. Santen & R.S. Swerdloff, p. 341. New York: Marcel Dekker.

Barkay, J., Harpaz-Kerpel, S., Ben-Ezra, S., Gordon, S. & Zuckerman, H. (1984). The prostaglandin inhibitor effect of anti-inflammatory drugs in the therapy of male infertility. *Fertil. Steril.*, **42**, 406.

Barraclough, C.A. (1982). The role of catecholamines in the regulation of pituitary LH and FSH secretion. *Endocr. Rev.*, **3**, 91.

Bartke, A., Kupper, D. & Dalterio, S. (1976). Prostaglandins inhibit testosterone secretion by mouse testes *in vitro*. *Steroids*, **28**, 81.

Baum, J., Langenin, R., D'Costta, M., Sanders, R.M. & Hucker, S. (1988). Serum pituitary and steroid hormone levels in the adult male: one value is as good as the mean of three. *Fertil. Steril.*, **49**, 123.

Ben-Jonathan, N. (1986). Dopamine: a prolactin-inhibiting hormone. *Endocr. Rev.*, **6**, 564.

Brown, J.S. (1975). The effect of orally administered androgens on sperm motility. *Fertil. Steril.*, **26**, 305.

Buvat, J., Ardaens, K., Lemaire, A., *et al.* (1983). Increased sperm count in 25 cases of idiopathic normogonadotropic oligospermia following treatment with tamoxifen. *Fertil. Steril.*, **39**, 700.

Clark, R.V. & Sherins, R.J. (1989). Clinical trial of testolactone for treatment of idiopathic male infertility. *J. Androl.*, **10**, 240.

Comhaire, F.H. (1976). Treatment of oligospermia with tamoxifen. *Int. J. Fertil.*, **21**, 232.

Comhaire, F.H. (1982). Tamoxifen. In *Treatment of Male Infertility*, ed. J. Bain, W.B. Schill & S. Schwarzstein, p. 45. Berlin: Springer.

Comhaire, F.H. (1990). Treatment of idiopathic testicular failure with high-dose testosterone undecanoate: a double-blind pilot study. *Fertil. Steril.*, **54**, 689.

Conn, P.M., Hucle, W.V. & McArdle, C.A. (1987). The molecular mechanism of action of gonadotropin releasing hormone (GnRH) in the pituitary. *Recent Prog. Hormone Res.*, **43**, 29.

Crottaz, R., Senn, A., Reymond, M.J., Rey, F., Germond, M. & Gomez, F. (1992). Follicle-stimulating hormone bioactivity in idiopathic normogonadotropin oligospermia: double-blind trial with gonadotropin releasing hormone. *Fertil. Steril.*, **57**, 1034.

Crowley, W.F. (1988). Hypogonadotropic hypogonadism with gonadotropin-releasing hormones. In *Current Therapy of Infertility*, vol. 3, ed. C.-R. Garcia *et al.*, p. 192. Philadelphia: B.C. Decker.

Demoulin, A., Hustin, J., Lambotte, R. & Franchimont, P. (1981). Effect of inhibin on testicular function. In *Intragonadal Regulation of Reproduction*, ed. P. Franchimont & C.P. Channing, p. 327. New York: Academic Press.

Donald, R.A., Wheeler, M., Sonksen, P.H., *et al.* (1983). Hypogonadotropic hypogonadism resistant to hCG and response to LHRH: report of a case. *Clin. Endocrinol.*, **18**, 385.

Dunn, J.F., Nisula, B.C. & Rodbard, D. (1981). Transport of steroid hormones: binding of 21 endogenous steroids to both testosterone binding globulin and corticosteroid binding globulin in human plasma. *J. Clin. Endocrinol. Metab.*, **53**, 58.

Forest, M.G. (1983). How should we perform the human chorionic gonadotropin (hCG) stimulation test? *Int. J. Androl.*, **6**, 1.

Foss, G.L., Tindall, V.R. & Birkett, J.P. (1973). The treatment of subfertile men with clomiphene citrate. *J. Reprod. Fertil.*, **32**, 167.

Franchimont, P., Chari, S. & Demoulin, A. (1975). Hypothalamus–pituitary–testis interaction. *J. Reprod. Fertil.*, **44**, 335.

Gerris, J., Comhaire, F., Hellemans, P., *et al.* (1991). Placebo-controlled trial of high-dose mesterolone treatment of idiopathic male infertility. *Fertil. Steril.*, **55**, 603.

Giarola, A. (1974). Effect of mesterolone in the spermatogenesis of infertile patients. In *Male Fertility and Sterility*, ed. F. Mancini & E. Martini, p. 479. Proceedings of the Serono Symposia. New York: Academic Press.

Glazner, C.M.A., Kelly, N.J., Weir, M.J.A., *et al.* (1987). The diagnosis of male infertility: prospective time-specific study of conception rates related to seminal analysis and post-coital sperm–mucus penetration and survival in otherwise unexplained infertility. *Hum. Reprod.*, **2**, 665.

Griffin, J.E. & Wilson, J.D. (1985). Disorders of the testes and male reproductive tract. In *Williams Textbook of Endocrinology*, ed. J.D. Wilson & D.W. Foster, p. 259. Philadelphia: W.B. Saunders.

Hamman, M. & Berg, A.A. (1990). Long-term androgen replacement therapy does not preclude gonadotropin-induced improvement of spermatogenesis. *Scand. J. Urol. Nephrol.*, **24**, 17.

Handelsman, D.J. & Swerdloff, R.S. (1985). Male gonadal dysfunction. *Clin. Endocrinol. Metab.*, **14**, 89.

Hoffman, A.R. & Crowley, W.F. (1982). Induction of puberty in men by long-term pulsatile administration of low-dose gonadotropin-releasing hormone. *N. Engl. J. Med.*, **307**, 1237.

Ito, T. & Horton, R. (1971). The source of plasma DHT in man. *J. Clin. Immunol.*, **50**, 1621–71.

Keough, E.J., Burger, H.G., deKretser, D.M., *et al.* (1976). Non-surgical management of male infertility. In *Human Semen and Fertility Regulation in Men*, ed. E.S.E. Hafez, p. 452. St Louis: C.V. Mosby.

Klemcke, H.G., Bartke, A. & Borer, K.T. (1984). Regulation of testicular prolactin and luteinizing hormone receptors in golden hamsters. *Endocrinology*, **114**, 594.

Klingmuller, D. & Schweikert, H.U. (1985). Maintenance of spermatogenesis by intranasal administration of gonadotropin-releasing hormone in patients with hypothalamic hypogonadism. *J. Clin. Endocrinol. Metab.*, **61**, 868.

Ley, S.B. & Leonard, J.M. (1985). Male hypogonadotropic hypogonadism: factors influencing response to human chorionic gonadotropin and human menopausal gonadotropin, including prior endogenous androgens. *J. Clin. Endocrinol. Metab.*, **61**, 746.

Longcope, C., Sato, K., McKay, C. & Horton, R. (1984). Aromatization by splanchnic tissue in men. *J. Clin. Endocrinol. Metab.*, **58**, 1089.

Lunenfeld, B. & Berezin, M. (1988). Hypogonadotropic hypogonadism with gonadotropins. In *Current Therapy of Infertility*, vol. 3, ed. C.-R. Garcia *et al.*, p. 187. Philadelphia: B.C. Decker.

Lunenfeld, B., Mor, A. & Mani, M. (1967). Treatment of male infertility. I. Human gonadotropins. *Fertil. Steril.*, **18**, 581.

Magrini, G., Elvina, J.R., Burckhardt, P. & Fellier, J.P. (1976). Study in the relationship between plasma prolactin levels and androgen metabolism in man. *J. Clin. Endocrinol. Metab.*, **43**, 944.

Masala, A., Delitala, G., Alagna, S., *et al.* (1978). Effect of clomiphene citrate on plasma levels of immunoreactive luteinizing hormone-releasing hormone, gonadotropin, and testosterone in normal subjects and in patients with idiopathic oligospermia. *Fertil. Steril.*, **29**, 424.

McCullagh, D.R. (1932). Dual endocrine activity of the testes. *Science*, **76**, 19.

Micic, S. & Dotlic, R. (1985). Evaluation of sperm parameters in clinical trial with clomiphene citrate of oligospermic men. *J. Urol.*, **133**, 221.

Padron, R.S., Wischusen, J., Hudson, B., Burger, H.G. & DeKretser, D.M. (1980). Prolonged biphasic response of plasma testosterone to single intramuscular injections of human chorionic gonadotropin. *J. Clin. Endocrinol. Metab.*, **50**, 1100.

Papavasiliou, S.S., Zmeili, S., Khoury, S., Landefeld, T.D., Chin, W.W. & Marshall, J.C. (1986*a*). Gonadotropin-releasing hormone differentially regulates expression of the genes for luteinizing hormone alpha and beta subunits in male rats. *Proc. Natl Acad. Sci. USA*, **83**, 4026.

Papavasiliou, S.S., Zmeili, S., Herbon, L., Duncan-Weldon, J., Marshall, J.C. & Landefeld, T.D. (1986*b*). Alpha and luteinizing hormone beta messenger ribonucleic acid (RNA) of male and female rats after castration: quantitation using an RNA dot blot hybridization assay. *Endocrinology*, **119**, 691.

Partridge, W.M. (1981). Transport of protein-bound hormones into tissues *in vivo*. *Endocr. Rev.*, **2**, 103.

Peterson, N.T., Midgely, A.R. & Jaffee, R.B. (1968). Regulation of human gonadotropins. III. Luteinizing hormone and follicle-stimulating hormone in sera from adult males. *J. Clin. Endocrinol. Metab.*, **28**, 1473.

Plant, T.M. (1986). Gonadal regulation of hypothalamic gonadotropin releasing hormone release in primates. *Endocr. Rev.*, **7**, 75.

Pugeat, M.M., Dunn, J.F. & Nisula, B.C. (1981). Transport of steroid hormones: interaction of 70 drugs with testosterone-binding globulin and corticosteroid-binding globulin in human plasma. *J. Clin. Endocrinol. Metab.*, **53**, 69.

Rosenberg, E. (1976). Medical treatment of male infertility. *Andrologia*, **8** (Suppl 1), 95.

Santen, R.J. (1975). Is aromatization of testosterone to estradiol required for inhibition of LH secretion in men? *J. Clin. Immunol.*, **156**, 1555.

Santen, R.J. (1987). The testis. In *Endocrinology and Metabolism*, ed. P. Felig, J.D. Baxter, A.E. Broadus & L.A. Frohman, p. 821. New York: McGraw-Hill.

Santen, R.J. & Bardin, C.W. (1973). Episodic luteinizing hormone secretion in man: pulse analysis, clinical interpretation, physiologic metabolism. *J. Clin. Immunol.*, **52**, 2617.

Santen, R.J. & Kuelin, H.E. (1981). Hypogonadotropic hypogonadism and delayed puberty. In *The Testis*, ed. H.G. Burger & D.M. deKretser, p. 329. New York: Raven Press.

Schill, W.B. (1979). Recent progress in pharmacological therapy of male subfertility: a review. *Andrologia*, **11**, 77.

Sherins, R.J. (1984). Evaluation and management of men with hypogonadotropic hypogonadism. In *Current Therapy of Infertility*, ed. C.-R. Garcia *et al.*, p. 10. Philadelphia: B.C. Decker.

Sherins, R.J. & Howards, S.S. II (1986). Male infertility. In *Campbell's Urology*, p. 640. Philadelphia: W.B. Saunders.

Shoham, Z., Conway, G.S., Ostergaard, H., Lah Lou N., Bouchard, P. & Jacobs, H.S. (1992). Cotreatment with growth hormone for induction of spermatogenesis in patients with hypogonadotropic hypogonadism. *Fertil. Steril.*, **57**, 1044.

Skarin, G., Nillius, S.J. & Wibell, L. (1982). Chronic pulsatile low dose GnRH therapy for induction of testosterone production and spermatogenesis in a man with secondary hypogonadotropic hypogonadism. *J. Clin. Endrocrinol. Metab.*, **55**, 723.

Smith, M.A., Perrin, M.H. & Vale, W.W. (1983). Desensitization of cultured pituitary cells to gonadotropin-releasing hormones: evidence for a post-receptor mechanism. *Mol. Cell. Endocrinol.*, **30**, 85.

Snyder, P.J., Rubenstein, R.S., Garder, D.F. & Rothman, J.C. (1979). Repetitive infusion of GnRH distinguishes hypothalamic from pituitary hypogonadism. *J. Clin. Endocrinol. Metab.*, **48**, 864.

Sokol, R.Z. (1987). Pharmacologic treatment of infertility. In *Problems in Urology*, ed. R.-V. White, p. 461. Philadelpia: J.B. Lippincott.

Sokol, R.Z. (1988). Endocrine evaluation in the assessment of male reproductive hazards. *Reprod. Toxicol.*, **2**, 217.

Sokol, R.Z. (1992). Medical endocrine therapy of male factor infertility. *Infertil. Reprod. Med. Clin. North Am.*, **3**, 389.

Sokol, R.Z. & Swerdloff, R.S. (1984). Male reproductive physiology and male infertility: diagnosis and medical management. In *Infertility: Diagnosis and Management*, ed. J. Aiman, p. 185.

Sokol, R.Z., Palacios, A., Campfield, L.A., Saul, C. & Swerdloff, R.S. (1982). Comparison of the kinetics of injectable testosterone in eugonadal and hypogonadal men. *Fertil. Steril.*, **37**, 425.

Sokol, R.Z., Steiner, B.S., Bustillo, M., *et al.* (1988). A controlled comparison of the efficacy of clomiphene citrate in male infertility. *Fertil. Steril.*, **49**, 865.

Steinberger, E. (1979). Hormonal control of spermatogenesis. In *Endrocrinology*, ed. L.J. DeGroot *et al.*, p. 1535. New York: Grune and Stratton.

Steinberger, A. (1986). Clinical assessment of treatment results in male infertility. In *Male Reproductive Dysfunction*, ed. R.J. Santen & R.S. Swerdloff, p. 370. New York: Marcel Dekker.

Swerdloff, R.S., Overstreet, J.W., Sokol, R.Z., *et al.* (1985). Infertility in the male. *Ann. Intern. Med.*, **103**, 906.

Troen, P., Yanihar, T., Nankin, H., *et al.* (1970). Assessment of gonadotropin therapy in infertile males. In *The Human Testis*, ed. E. Rosenberg & C.A. Paulsen. New York: Plenum Press.

Vermeulen, A. & Comhaire, F. (1978). Hormonal effects of an antiestrogen, tamoxifen, in normal and oligospermic men. *Fertil. Steril.*, **29**, 320.

Vermeulen, A., Verdonck, L., Vander Straeten, M. & Orie, M. (1969). Capacity of the testosterone binding globulin in human plasma and influence of specific binding by testosterone on its metabolic clearance rate. *J. Clin. Endocrinol. Metab.*, **29**, 1470–80.

Vigersky, R.A. & Glass, A.R. (1981). Effects of delta-1-testosterone on the pituitary–testicular axis in oligospermic men. *J. Clin. Endocrinol. Metab.*, **52**, 897.

Wang, C., Chan, C.W., Wong, K.K., *et al.* (1983). Comparison of the effectiveness of placebo, clomiphene citrate, mesterolone, pentoxifylline, and testosterone rebound therapy for the treatment of idiopathic oligospermia. *Fertil. Steril.*, **40**, 358.

Weiland, R.G., Ansari, A.H., Klein, D.E., *et al.* (1972). Idiopathic oligospermia: control observations and response to cis-clomiphene. *Fertil. Steril.*, **23**, 471.

Willis, K.J., London, D.R., Bevis, M.A., *et al.* (1977). Hormonal effects of tamoxifen in oligospermic men. *J. Endrocrinol.*, **73**, 171.

Winter, J.S.D. (1987). Sexual differentiation. In *Endocrinology and Metabolism*, ed. P. Felig, J.D. Baxter, A.E. Broadus & L.A. Frohman, p. 983. New York: McGraw-Hill.

Winters, S.J. & Troen, P. (1975). Evidence for a role of endogenous estrogen in the hypothalamic control of gonadotropin secretion. *J. Clin. Endocrinol. Metab.*, **61**, 842.

Winters, S.J. & Troen, P. (1984). Altered pulsatile secretion of luteinizing hormone in hypogonadal men with hyperprolactinemia. *Clin. Endocrinol.*, **21**, 257.

Ying, S.Y. (1988). Inhibins, activins and follistatins: gonadal proteins modulating the secretion of follicle-stimulating hormone. *Endocr. Rev.*, **9**, 267.

Yuan, Q.X., Swerdloff, R.S. & Bhasin, S. (1988). Differential regulation of rat luteinizing hormone alpha and beta subunits during the stimulatory and down-regulatory phases of gonadotropin releasing hormone action. *Endocrinology*, **122**, 504.

diZerega, G.S. & Sherins, R.J. (1981). Endocrine control of adult testicular function. In *The Testis*, ed. H. Berger & D. deKretser, p. 127. New York: Raven Press.

14

The urologic evaluation of the infertile male

JEAN L. FOURCROY

Introduction

Infertility is defined as the failure to achieve pregnancy after unprotected coitus for at least 1 year. Approximately 15% of couples attempting their first pregnancy are unsuccessful. Diagnosis and treatment are often costly, time consuming, intrusive and for many diagnoses there is a variable but low chance of success. According to the Office of Technology Assessment (OTA, 1988), 2.4 million married couples were defined as infertile in 1982. Voluntary delayed child-bearing may also complicate this situation. The child-bearing potential of a couple is less dependent on the age of the male than the age of the female partner; the average woman experiences a gradual deterioration of her reproductive potential between the ages of 24 and 50 years (Speroff *et al.*, 1989) which may not be apparent in the older man (Nieschlag *et al.*, 1982).

Secondary infertility is defined as the inability to conceive after 1 year of unprotected intercourse following a previously documented pregnancy. Male fertility may have been altered by reproductive toxicants, drugs, inflammatory conditions, varicocele, or unknown factors. A 'male factor' is considered important in 40–50% of infertility evaluations (Jouannet *et al.*, 1988).

The evaluation of the infertile couple must be thorough, blameless and should include a review of possible previous pregnancies of both partners. This chapter will discuss the male fertility examination from the perspective of the urologist as andrologist, with an overview of the normal and abnormal male reproductive system.

The male evaluation

The andrologist should emphasize the role of prevention long before the couple presents for evaluation. Education must begin much earlier regarding workplace toxicants and occupational hazards, use of both prescribed and

abused drugs, and the long-term role of genital tract infections. Sexually transmitted diseases (STDs) may be a significant cause of infertility, and an estimated 20% of the cases in the United States may be preventable (OTA, 1988).
Condoms and spermicidal protection should be encouraged by the clinician to
decrease the incidence of STDs and long-term sequelae of these infections for
both the male and female. The physician must also understand the effects of a
number of other chronic diseases as well as various medications used to treat
the patient.

The physician who evaluates the male partner should coordinate the care
with the female partner's evaluation. The request to evaluate the male is made
early during the couple's investigation because the woman's evaluation involves
more expensive and invasive procedures. Often, the request is made to define
the man's 'fertility' rather than the couple's potential. The initial male evaluation should include a thorough medical, surgical, sexual, developmental and
environmental assessment. The history, the physical examination and at least
one semen analysis (World Health Organization, 1987) should provide critical
information for the fertility consultation.

Physical examination

The testis

The adult testis is a spheroid approximately 4.5 cm × 2.5 cm × 3 cm. Each testis
contains 500–1000 seminiferous tubules each containing 800 million germ cells.
The tubules are surrounded by 700 million Leydig cells in the interstitium of
the testis. Between 80% and 90% of the volume of the testis consists of seminiferous tubules and intratubular cells. A decrease in tubular width will be
reflected in the decreased volume of the testis. Determination of the size, shape
and consistency of the testis is an important part of the infertility evaluation.
The use of standardized measurement by either orchiometers, calipers or ultrasound is strongly encouraged (Takihara, 1983; Kulin & Santner, 1986; Rivkees
et al., 1987).

The Leydig cells in the interstitial compartments secrete testosterone (see
excellent reviews by Saez, 1994). The Sertoli cells are necessary for
spermatogenesis, for maintaining the blood–testis barrier, and for secretion of
important proteins including transferrin, androgen binding protein (ABP), and
inhibin which acts to inhibit FSH release from the pituitary. The levels of circulating inhibin and FSH reflect the reversibility of impaired spermatogenesis. An
increase in FSH reflects a loss of germ cells. Several reproductive toxicants are
known to affect Sertoli cell development, including 5-bromodeoxyuridine,

cyclophosphamide and a plasticizer used in the production of medical devices and in food packaging (Dostal *et al.*, 1988; Schrader *et al.*, 1988, 1993). The number of Sertoli cells per tubule also decreases with age (Johnson *et al.*, 1984; Cortes *et al.*, 1987). An important cause of maturation arrest may well be a reflection of Sertoli cell dysfunction. The reader is referred to Russell & Griswold (1993) for a review of Sertoli cell physiology.

Toxicants can affect testicular function at many levels. Ethylene dibromide (EDB) exerts its effects on post-testicular stages by reducing sperm velocity and ejaculate volume (Ratcliffe *et al.*, 1987), while exposure to dibromochloro-propane (DBCP) reduces sperm concentration and damages spermatogonia (Whorton *et al.*, 1979). Finasteride is associated with diminished ejaculate volume but with no demonstrated changes in sperm count, volume, or motility (Physician's Desk Reference, 1994).

Cystic structures and their contribution to fertility potential must be identified and assessed. Rete cysts can represent an important loss of continuity from the seminiferous tubules (Fourcroy *et al.*, 1994). Epididymal or adnexal cysts may include benign adenomatoid tumors as well as cystadenomas which will be associated with von Hippel–Lindau disease. Adnexal remnants of Müllerian structures have been demonstrated in a small group of men with Persistent Müllerian Duct Syndrome (Fourcroy & Belman, 1982). Cysts adjacent to the epididymis, possibly remnants of the Müllerian duct, have been identified in the male children of women treated during gestation with high doses of diethylstilbestrol (DES) (Gill *et al.*, 1977; Whitehead & Leiter, 1981; Conley *et al.*, 1983).

The epididymis

The efferent ductules form the critical bridge between the rete testis and the epididymis. The epididymis is a highly convoluted structure, rich in vascular supply and innervation. It is thought to be important for storage, phagocytosis and maturation of spermatozoa. This single tube needs to be carefully palpated for continuity; it should not be indurated or thickened. For a full review of congenital abnormalities of the testis and epididymis see Scorer & Farrinton (1971) and Turek *et al.* (1994).

The vas deferens

The vas deferens (ductus deferens) is a thick muscular tube, 2–3 mm in diameter and about 46 cm long, that propels and transports sperm. The vas is easily felt on examination in the scrotum. If it can not be easily palpated, a scrotal ultrasound scan may be used to exclude agenesis of the vas (Schellen & van

Stratten, 1980; Christensen *et al.*, 1987). As many as 4.5% of the men who present for infertility evaluation have absence of one or both vas deferens and possible agenesis of ipsilateral renal units (Christenson *et al.*, 1987). Complete or partial obstruction of the ductal system can result in azoospermia, oligo-zoospermia and asthenozoospermia. Both the physical examination and use of imaging techniques such as ultrasound may help in the complete evaluation of the entire ductal system (Porch, 1978; Paterson & Jarow, 1990; Pryor & Hendry, 1991; Hellerstein *et al.*, 1992; Arnold, 1993).

Accessory glands

The paired seminal vesicles are convoluted alveolar sacs posterior to the bladder. They can contribute up to 80% of the total volume of the ejaculate. Fructose is the major secretory product of the seminal vesicles, and its absence from the ejaculate has long been used as an indication of congenital bilateral absence of the seminal vesicles or obstruction of the ducts (Eliasson, 1976). The seminal vesicles are not normally palpated.

The prostate gland is a complex fibromuscular and glandular organ which sits below the bladder and surrounds the posterior urethra. The development of the prostate gland is dependent on dihydrotestosterone as early as 12 weeks of gestation. This complex and poorly understood organ contributes at least 30% to the total semen volume.

The ejaculatory duct is the short 2 cm termination of the vas deferens opening into the prostatic urethra on each side of the prostatic utricle. Obstruction of the distal ejaculatory ducts due to trauma, congenital atresia or infection is an uncommon problem but is treatable by transurethral resection of the terminal ejaculatory ducts (Porch, 1978).

Additional accessory glands adding components to the seminal fluid include the urethral glands of Littre, and Cowper's or the bulbourethral glands. Both these glands add important secretory components to the ejaculate (Eliasson, 1976).

The examination of the male should include an examination of the penis and identification of the normal position of the meatus. Any signs of STDs need to be treated since infection may affect fertility. Identification of any penile curvatures and/or angulation as well as the identification of the normal site of the urethral meatus are important for the effective deposition of the ejaculate in the vagina.

Family history

Obtaining the family history allows the clinican to review with the patient any familial factors that may alter fertility or affect the fetus. It is the responsibility of the fertility team to identify any genetic problems and provide counseling as appropriate. The couple should be questioned as to autosomal dominant or X-linked disorders in first-degree relatives (American Fertility Society, 1993). If an individual has an autosomal dominant condition, the risk of transmission to the unborn child is up to 50% dependent on penetrance. The couple can then be counseled appropriately. Other genetic disorders are discussed below.

Medical history

The medical history must include a complete and organized review of the patient's history, identifying any factor that could affect the male's fertility potential. In 3–20% of infertile couples no apparent cause of infertility can be determined (OTA, 1988). Any review should include a history of acute and chronic illnesses, especially any possible urologic infections and STDs (Krieger, 1990), disabilities (Haseltine *et al.*, 1993), cancer, the use and abuse of any drugs, lifestyles of the patient and his partner, as well as occupational and avocational hazards. The evaluation should include a wide range of factors known to affect fertility in either direct or indirect ways. Visual changes, headaches or impaired visual fields may suggest central nervous system tumors; anosmia is associated with Kallmann's syndrome (Kallmann *et al.*, 1944); recurrent respiratory infections and the associated inherited immotile cilia syndromes may suggest Kartagener's syndrome (Eliasson *et al.*, 1977; Jonsson *et al.*, 1982) Young's syndrome (Jequier, 1985; Handelsman *et al.*, 1984; Hendry *et al.*, 1993) or cystic fibrosis (Kaplan *et al.*, 1968; Taussig *et al.*, 1972; Matwijiw, 1987; Rigot *et al.*, 1991; Anguiano *et al.*, 1992). Bronchiectasis (de Santi *et al.*, 1985) as well as any illness with fever over the last 6 months may also affect fertility. One should also consider autosomal recessive cystic fibrosis with absent or rudimentary vasa deferentia (Anguiano *et al.*, 1992). Possible androgen receptor deficiencies should also be considered (Wilson, 1992).

Both prenatal and early childhood diseases and time of onset of puberty should be discussed with the patient.

Cancer and survivors

More than 26 000 men in the United States between the ages of 17 and 50 years are afflicted with cancer each year and more than 70% of these men survive the malignancy and multiple therapeutic regimens (Jaffe *et al.*, 1988). Male sterility has been a major concern in the young men who survive a childhood cancer, since the testis is sensitive to chemotherapeutic alkylating agents (Chapman, 1983; Clifton & Bremner, 1983; Hahn *et al.*, 1983; Da Cunha *et al.*, 1984; Damewood & Grochow, 1986; Averett *et al.*, 1990; Morrish *et al.*, 1990) and radiation (Meistrich, 1986; Lione, 1987) in a dose-dependent manner (Sanders *et al.*, 1983; Oates & Lipshultz, 1989).

Testicular cancer is the most common cancer in this age group accounting for 1% of all male malignancies and 2–3 new cases per 100 000 males in the United States each year. Eighty per cent of these patients are oligozoospermic at the time of diagnosis (Hendry, 1981; Morrish *et al.*, 1990). The survival rate following treatment has improved dramatically in the last two decades with a current survival rate of 90% (Einhorn, 1993). Many of these men will be candidates for sperm banking. Their future fertility is dependent primarily on the radiation or chemotherapeutic regimes. Surgery such as retroperitoneal lymph node dissection may cause loss of sympathetic input resulting in retrograde ejaculation (because of lost bladder neck closure) or interference with emission and sexual function in up to 40% of the patients. However, in the experience of Indiana University at least one-third of patients treated with chemotherapy alone have been able successfully to father children without congenital anomalies, confirming previous data (see review by Einhorn *et al.*, 1993).

The other malignancies seen in men during these peak reproductive years include lymphomas and leukemia. Hodgkin's lymphoma is associated with a high incidence of irreversible infertility and gonadal dysfunction, although improved outcomes have been suggested with some therapeutic protocols (Whitehead *et al.*, 1982; Viviani *et al.*, 1985).

The impact of any disabilities or chronic diseases on fertility potential must be evaluated. Venereal infections (STDs) have long-lasting sequelae on the genital tract. Viral episodes such as mumps can result in permanent damage in the pubertal male and, if bilateral, may result in hypergonadotropic hypogonadism (Werner, 1950).

Other illnesses that should be considered include: diabetes, which may be associated with neuropathy and small vessel disease; sickle cell anemia; myotonic dystrophy, which is associated with small testes; low plasma testosterone levels and elevated plasma LH and FSH levels. Consideration should be given to premature frontal baldness, posterior subcapsular cataracts, cardiac conduction defects (Lubinsky, 1983), celiac disease with elevated plasma testosterone and LH levels consistent with testicular dysfunction (Farthing *et al.*, 1983). The andrologist is in a unique position to identify these relationships that could be associated with infertility.

Table 14.1 *Drugs and compounds suspected to affect fertility*

Agricultural chemicals
Dibromochlorpropane (DBCP)
Nematocide

Antimicrobials/antibiotics
Nitrofurantoin

Drugs currently approved for medical use
Amiodarone (an antiarrhythmic)
Unknown: cholesterol synthesis inhibitors?
Cimetidine
Cyclophosphamide
Sulfasalazine
Antiandrogens – spironolactone

Drugs of abuse and addiction
Alcohol
Heroin
Tobacco

Elements
Cadmium
Lead

Polyhalogenated biphenyls
Polybrominated biphenyls
Polychlorinated biphenyls (PCBs)

Notes:
Compiled from: Dixon (1986), OTA (1988), Dobs *et al.* (1991), Fourcroy (1993) and
Physician's Desk Reference (1994).

Drugs

Many drugs (Table 14.1) adversely affect the male reproductive system by
affecting hormone metabolism, altering spermatogenesis, spermiogenesis or
motility of the mature sperm (Handelsman & Turtle, 1983). Some drugs may
affect libido: antihypertensive drugs may be the cause of impotence and antide-
pressants and beta blockers such as propranolol have been reported to decrease
libido. Alcohol may induce neuropathy and increase estrogens (Van Thiel *et al.*,
1975, 1979). Cigarette smoking may contribute to vasoconstriction and erectile
problems. Additional drugs which may decrease available androgens include
digoxin, spironolactone, phenothiazines, tetrahydrocannabinol (marijuana),
and ketoconazole (Dobs *et al.*, 1991; see review by Dixon, 1986).

Sulfasalazine, which was first used in the 1940s for inflammatory bowel
disease causes reversible decreased sperm count and motility (Hudson *et al.*,

1982; Riley, 1987). This drug is thought to affect the sperm acrosomal membrane enzymes during late stage development (Cosentino *et al.*, 1984; O'Morain *et al.*, 1984). Antibiotics used to treat sexually transmitted diseases or urinary tract infections must also be suspect (Schlegel *et al.*, 1991; Fourcroy, 1993). Broad spectrum antibiotics can be secreted in high levels into the ejaculate (Berger *et al.*, 1990), but the effect on fertility is not known. Phenytoin, used for seizure prevention, interferes with metabolism of 17-ketosteroids and 17-hydroxysteroids by suppressing androgen production. It also reduces semen quality and the percentage of motile sperm. Cimetidine may enhance the secretion of prolactin and block the effects of androgens (Fourcroy, 1993). Cyclophosphamide, used primarily for susceptible malignancies, is also used in some cases for the treatment of benign diseases and may have long-term effects on the testis (Watson *et al.*, 1985). Any medication should be considered suspect and, if possible, should be avoided by the patient.

The current or past use of illicit and street drugs should be considered in the infertile male. There are no scientific data on the long-term reproductive effects of most of these drugs. The use of anabolic steroids to enhance and enable in sports remains a major problem. As many as 10% of high-school boys have used some form of anabolic steroid, many in conjunction with other unknown enhancing compounds. Although anabolic steroids can cause testicular damage, this appears to be reversible. There are, however, reports of long-lasting thyroid change (Jarow, 1990; Deyssig & Weissel, 1993).

Lifestyles

Any evaluation of the infertile male must include an understanding of sexual preferences and risk-taking lifestyles of the patient, in an attempt to understand the risks for STDs and other opportunistic diseases including HIV (Bray *et al.*, 1991). Abused drugs such as cocaine or heroin may alter the mature sperm (El-Gothamy & El-Samahy, 1992).

Genital infections

A complete history of any STDs should include a full history of the disease and treatments. If identified, an STD such as *Chlamydia* or human papilloma virus (HPV) must be appropriately treated, especially if the partner would be at high risk for reproductive damage (Schachter, 1990). When the male is examined, the rectal examination should note tone, fissures, hemorrhoids, or other mass lesions. The groin and inguinal area should be evaluated for enlarged lymph nodes and the penis for condylomata. Evaluation for *E. coli*, *Proteus* species,

Trichomonas vaginalis, *Gardnerella vaginalis* and *Streptococcus faecalis* may be included. Specific testing should be dependent on the risk factors and the specificity and sensitivity of the testing available (Barratt *et al.*, 1990).

Occupational history

Review of current and past occupational exposures must always be an integral part of the history. The review should not be limited to exposures of the workplace but should include hobbies that might affect reproductive health. Ionizing radiation, lead, ethylene oxide dibromochloropropane, and perchloroethylene are regulated because of their effects on the reproductive systems (Dixon, 1986; Eskenazi *et al.*, 1991; Schrader & Kesner, 1993).

Thermal radiation

Heat is known to damage the unprotected testis and alter spermatogenesis and spermiogenesis; there is little evidence, though, that the usual heat of clothing, exercise or hot baths has an adverse effect. The sauna does not appear to alter fertility potential (Horvatta *et al.*, 1988). However, it is reasonable to modify some activities to evaluate the effect on sperm maturation and concentration in the subfertile male without another obvious cause for decreased semen quality.

Surgical history

The surgical history should note any operations, hernia repair and retroperitoneal surgery such as retroperitoneal lymph node dissection that could alter sympathetic controls. Any bladder neck operations such as a Y-V plasty or bladder reconstruction, or any history suggestive of intermittent torsion of the testis with delayed intervention, should be recorded. It is especially important to review any childhood inguinal surgery that might have iatrogenically obstructed the vas deferens. Alteration of normal sympathetic control will result in retrograde ejaculation evidenced by post-ejaculate urine demonstrating sperm, or less than 1 ml volume of ejaculate.

Sexual history

The coital techniques used by the couple should be assessed, including timing, frequency, and coincidence with ovulatory patterns. Coital positions should maximize vaginal deposition of the ejaculate. The contraceptive history of the couple and any possible previous pregnancies or encounters without conception can also be ascertained at this point. Lubricants are not recommended as they may adversely affect the motility of the sperm (Frishman *et al.*, 1992). Saliva has been shown to be spermicidal in concentrations as low as 2% in the semen (Tulandi *et al.*, 1982; Kaye *et al.*, 1991). Both Astroglide and K-Y lubricants (12.5% concentrations) can impair progressive motility. Because their persistence in the vagina has not been evaluated all vaginal lubricants should be avoided throughout the menstrual cycle in patients desiring conception. If lubricants are necessary, the least toxic appear to be light cooking oils and egg white (Tulandi & McInnes, 1984). Of course, spermicidal agents such as nononoxynol are contraindicated.

General examination

The routine evaluation of the male partner should evaluate, in a systematic pattern, the possible causes of the infertility. The examination should include the body habitus, hair distribution, fat distribution, adenopathy, evidence of gynecomastia, thyroid and liver function, penile meatal position, scrotum, testis size and presence of varicocele, as well as evaluation of the entire epididymis, vas deferens and prostate. The examination must follow a consistent pattern so that no portion of it is overlooked. The family and medical history will have identified any additional areas of concern.

The evaluation of the male breast is a crucial part of the examination. Gynecomastia must be differentiated from enlarged pectoralis muscles: it is an area of increased consistency of breast tissue in the male that is distinct from the surrounding soft tissue. Breast enlargement may be normal in the prepubertal male as a result of imbalances in circulating androgens and estrogens. In the older male the prevalence of gynecomastia is between 30% and 60%. To evaluate the breast correctly the physician should compress the subcutaneous tissue of the male breast toward the nipple with the tips of the fingers (Braunstein, 1993). Breast cancer, although rare in the male is an important consideration.

Identification of a eunuchoid physique may be difficult, but is an important marker of inadequate androgens during critical times of male development. An arm span more than 5 cm greater than height, a ratio of upper body segment to lower body segment that is less than 1 (measured from the crown of the head to the pubic symphysis and pubic symphysis to the floor), sparse pubic hair, minimal beard growth, inappropriately small penis and testicles are all consistent with a eunuchoid physique. Kallmann's syndrome and Klinefelter's syndrome are two examples of eunuchoid habitus. The habitus consistent with Kallmann's syndrome is representative of a delay in epiphyseal closure. Men with Klinefelter's syndrome are tall and have long extremities.

The physical examination can continue in sequence with the examination of the scrotum, starting with the normal thin scrotal skin and identifying any lesions. It is crucial that the patient be comfortable and warm for this part of the examination. In addition to identifying any cystic structures on either the testis, epididymis or adnexal area, the size, shape and consistency of both the testes and epididymides should be ascertained. The volume of the testes should be appropriate and they should be approximately symmetrical. The measurement of the testis is the gold standard of andrology (Takihara, 1983; Takihara *et al.*, 1987). To be accurate, calipers, ultrasound, orchiometers or any other consistent measurement method should be used. Ultrasound may be necessary to complete the examination, particularly if there is a hydrocele, and to rule out tumors (Leonhardt & Goodwing, 1992).

Varicocele

The most controversial part of the examination of the infertile male is the evaluation for a possible varicocele. A varicocele is a dilatation of the testicular veins of the pampiniform plexus within the spermatic cord. The chief drainage of the testis is by way of the internal spermatic or testicular vein, which is thought to be the primary vein involved in the varicocele. The varices are not often in the pampiniform plexus. It is difficult to distinguish between the dilated tortuous varicocele and the pampiniform plexus of the internal spermatic vein (Hollingshead, 1971). The dense pampiniform plexus can normally consist of some 10 or 12 veins, primarily situated anterior to the vas.

The incidence of palpable varicocele is higher among infertile men, and ranges from 21% to 41%, compared with 4.4–22.6% in the general population (Centola *et al.*, 1987; Peng *et al.*, 1990; Takihara *et al.*, 1991; Dhabuwala *et al.*, 1992). In the majority of cases (up to 90%), the varicocele is found on the left side, although bilateral varicoceles are frequently present. It is not clear whether there are ethnic differences in the incidence of varicoceles, or any associated effects on fertility. In one study, no differences in the ethnic predisposition for varicocele were found (Alcalay *et al.*, 1986). A varicocele is not usually palpated until puberty, the incidence rising dramatically at 10–14 years of age, presumably because of increasing testosterone activity. A varicocele is thought to be present with an incidence of 15% by the age of 13 years. In the adolescent a dilated pampiniform plexus, associated with decreasing growth of the ipsilateral testis, is an indicaton for varicocelectomy (Buch & Cromie, 1985; Kass & Belman, 1987).

The relationship of the varicocele to fertility potential is unclear, although there is a higher incidence of varicocele in the infertile male population. There is no correlation between the volume of the varicocele and the fertility outcome after surgery. It has been suggested that histological evaluation identifying Leydig cell changes would improve identification of patients for treatment (Hadziselimovic *et al.*, 1989). Recent use of gonadotropin-releasing hormone stimulation testing may also define adolescent patients for early treatment (Kass *et al.*, 1993). A secondary varicocele may be the result of continued venous back-pressure. Possible progressive testicular atrophy and secondary infertility might benefit from earlier varicocelectomy (Lipshultz & Corriere, 1977; Gorelick & Goldstein, 1993).

Heat, increased hydrostatic pressure or increased toxins such as adrenal metabolites have been suggested as effects of varicoceles. Testicular damage, secondary atrophy or increased pressure from a varicocele may result in damage to either the Sertoli cell or the Leydig cell. Men with secondary infertility and varicocele demonstrate a lower mean sperm concentration (30.2 versus 46.10) and more abnormal-shaped sperm (72% vs 40%) than younger men with primary infertility and varicocele (Gorelick & Goldstein, 1993). If the varicocele is a surrogate marker for other existing pathophysiology, then a proportion of the patients will have progressive damage to the testes with age and progression of the disease.

Varicoceles may have adverse outcomes when associated with cofactors. One study looked at the interrelationships between cigarette smoking, testicular varicoceles and seminal fluid indices, and suggested that smokers with varicoceles had 10 times greater incidence of oligozoospermia than that in non-smokers with varicoceles, and 5 times greater incidence than that in men who smoked and did not have varicoceles (Klaiber *et al.*, 1987). Smoking should be discouraged if at all possible, not only for the possible improvement in fertility, but because of the effect of passive smoking on the female partner and the respiratory effects on children (John, 1991). There may be additional cofactors associated with varicocele pathophysiology.

To examine the patient for a possible varicocele he must be palpated in both the standing and supine positions. The spermatic cord above the testis must be palpated. The Valsalva maneuver may confirm the presence of a varicocele on one or both sides, which should decompress in the supine position. The patient is asked to increase abdominal pressure by either coughing or a Valsalva maneuver to enable palpation of the venous trill consistent with retrograde blood flow. The enlarged vessels may be superior to the testis as well as next to or below the testis.

A variety of techniques have been used to document the change in blood flow, change in temperature, or change in diameter of the varices. These have included use of the Doppler technique to identify retrograde blood flow, ultra-

Table 14.2   *Varicocele grading systems*

Grading of a varicocele
Grade 1: palpable only with Valsalva maneuver
Grade 2: moderate enlargement
Grade 3: easily palpated as a large 'bag of worms'

Varicocele grade
Small: distinct dilation of the internal spermatic veins palpable during a Valsalva maneuver in the upright position
Moderate: palpable in the upright position with the aid of a Valsalva maneuver
Large: both palpable and visible through the scrotal skin with the aid of a Valsalva maneuver in the upright position

sound to identify the size of the varicosities, a scrotal scan to identify venous stasis, and scrotal thermography to identify changes in temperature. It is hoped that improved imaging techniques will better allow improved study of the vasculature of the testis. One possible approach may be dynamic enhanced magnetic resonance imaging (Costabile *et al.*, 1993). These methods of examining the varicocele allow grading of the varicocele (Table 14.2).

It is reasonable to do a varicocelectomy for an identified varicocele if there are no other identifiable causes for the infertility. However, the rationale for treating the 'male factor' in men with normal sperm counts is not clear (Howards, 1992). There is probably insufficient evidence to resolve the rationale for treating subclinical varicoceles. Clearly, there are many questions that need to be answered regarding the identification of patients who benefit from treatment. Reliable outcome measurements are needed to assess treatment efficacy (Hirsch *et al.*, 1980).

Laboratory evaluation

The routine laboratory evaluation of the infertile male should include a total or free testosterone level, a chemistry screen to include glucose, a CBC, liver and renal profile and a urinalysis. Glycosylated hemoglobin should be tested in diabetic men. If further endocrine evaluation is indicated, it should include LH, FSH, prolactin, estradiol and thyroid studies. At least one semen analysis, and preferably two or three, done according to WHO standards should be obtained (see Chapter 3).

Further evaluations should be done if there is pyospermia (white blood cells in semen), clumping or agglutination of sperm or isolated motility disorders. A urinalysis, and expressed prostatic secretions (EPS), will identify the possibility of infection (Jequier & Cruch, 1986). Infections of the genitourinary tract are possible causes of impaired fertility and should be treated. The presence of up to five white blood cells per high-power field is considered normal (Jequier & Cruch, 1986).

Electroejaculation and semen recovery

Electrostimulation (EE) using a rectal probe has provided a new method for recovery of semen from men who are anejaculatory. This includes an increasing number of men of reproductive age with disabilities such as spinal cord injuries (SCI), multiple sclerosis and spina bifida, cancer survivors and post-surgical dissections (Bennett *et al.*, 1987, 1988; Haseltine *et al.*, 1993). Parenting remains an important consideration and desire for these men that now can be fulfilled. Between 1988 and 1991 there were more than 65 pregnancies in part-ners of men with SCI using these retrieval techniques (Hamer & Bain, 1986; Bennett *et al.*, 1988; Halstead & Seager, 1993). Anyone contemplating pro-viding these procedures should be specially trained in the treatment and safety issues (Stephen & Avila 1991). A significant proportion of semen samples obtained by EE have spermatogenic abnormalities (Hirsch *et al.* 1992). Temperature and voltage must not exceed certain limits and must be carefully controlled (Halstead & Seager, 1993). All the devices currently used have been developed from animal models and need continual and careful monitoring.

References

Aboul-Azm, T.E. (1979). Anatomy of the human seminal vesicles and ejaculatory ducts. *Arch. Androl.*, **3**, 287–92.

Alcalay, J., Kedem, R., Kornbrot, B. & Sayfan, J. (1986). The ethnic distribution of varicocele. *Military Med.*, **151**, 327–8.

American Fertility Society (AFS) (1993). Guidelines for gamete donation: 1993. *Fertil. Steril.*, **59** (Suppl.), 1s–9s.

Anguiano, A., Oates, R.D., Amos, J.A., Dean, M., Gerrard, B. & Stewart, C. (1992). Congenital bilateral absence of the vas deferens: a primary genital form of cystic fibrosis. *JAMA*, **267**, 1994–7.

Arnold, S.J. (1993). Unrecognized congenital posterior urethral minivales in men. *Urology*, **41**, 554–6.

Averett, H.E., Borke, G.M. & Jarrell, M.A. (1990). Effects of cancer chemotherapy on gonadal function and reproductive capacity. *Cancer*, **40**, 199.

Barratt, C.L.R., Chauhan, M. & Cooke, I.D. (1990). Donor insemination: a look to the future. *Fertil. Steril.*, **54**, 375–85.

Bennett, C.J., Seager, S.W.J. & McQuire, E.J. (1987). Electroejaculation for recovery of retrograde ejaculation. *J. Urol.*, **137**, 513–15.

Bennett, C.J., Seager, S.W.J., Vasher, E.A., McGuire, E.J. (1988). Sexual dysfunction and electroejaculation in men with spinal cord injury: a review. *J. Urol.*, **139**, 453–7.

Berger, S.A., Yavetz, H., Paz, G., Gorrea, A. & Homonnai, Z. (1990). Concentration of ofloxacin and ciprofloxacin in human semen following a single oral dose. *J. Urol.*, **144**, 683–4.

Braunstein, G.D. (1993). Gynecomastia. *N. Engl. J. Med.*, **328**, 490.

Bray, M.A., Minkoff, H., Solte, B., Sierra, M.P., Clarke, L. & Reyes, F.I. (1991). Human immunodeficiency virus-1 infection in an infertile population. *Fertil. Steril.*, **56**, 16–19.

Buch, J.P. & Cromie, W.J. (1985). Evaluation and treatment of the preadolescent varicocele. *Urol. Clin. North Am.*, **12**, 312.

Centola, G.M., Lee, K. & Cockett, A.T.K. (1987). Relationship between testicular volume and presence of varicocele. *Urology*, **30**, 479–81.

Chapman, R.M. (1983). Gonadal injury resulting from chemotherapy. *Am. J. Ind. Med.*, **4**, 149–61.

Christenson, P.J., Fourcroy, J.L. & O'Connell, K.J. (1987). A case of bilateral absence of the vas deferens and the body and tail of the epididymis in association with multiple congenital anomalies. *J. Androl.*, **3**, 326–8.

Clark, R.V. & Sherins, R.J. (1983). Clinical trial of testolactone for treatment of idiopathic male infertility (abstract). *J. Androl.*, **4**, 31.

Clifton, D.K. & Bremner, W.J. (1983). The effect of testicular x-irradiation on spermatogenesis in man: a comparison with the mouse. *J. Androl.*, **4**, 387–92.

Cockett, A.T.K., Urry, R.L. & Dougherty, K.A. (1979). The varicocele and semen characteristics. *J. Urol.*, **121**, 435.

Conley, G.R., Sant, G.R., Ucci, A.A. & Mitcheson, H.D. (1983). Seminoma and epididymal cysts in a young man with known diethylstilbestrol exposure *in utero*. *JAMA*, **249**, 1325–6.

Cortes, D., Muiller, J. & Skakkeback, N.E. (1987). Proliferation of Sertoli cells during development of the human testis assessed by stereological methods. *Int. J. Androl.*, **10**, 589–96.

Cosentino, M.J., Chey, W.Y., Takihara, H. & Cockett, A.T.K. (1984). The effects of sulfasalazine on human male fertility and seminal prostaglandins. *J. Urol.*, **132**, 682–6.

Costabile, R.A., Choyke, P.L., Frank, J.A., Girton, M.E., Diggs, R., Billups, K.L., Moonen, C. & Desjardins, C. (1993). Dynamic enhanced magnetic resonance imaging of testicular perfusion in the rat. *J. Urol.*, **149**, 1195–7.

DaCunha, M.F., Meistrich, M.L., Fuller, L.M., *et al.* (1984). Recovery of spermatogenesis after treatment for Hodgkin's disease: limiting dose of MOPP chemotherapy. *J. Clin. Oncol.*, **2**, 571–7.

Damewood, M.D. & Grochow, L.B. (1986). Prospects for fertility after chemotherapy or radiation for neoplastic disease. *Fertil. Steril.*, **45**, 443–59.

Deyssig, R. & Weissel, M. (1993). Ingestion of androgenic-anabolic steroids induces mild thyroidal impairment in male body builders. *J. Clin. Endocrinol. Metab.*, **76**, 1069–71.

Dhabuwala, B., Hamid, S. & Moghissi, K.S. (1992). Clinical versus subclinical: varicocele improvement in fertility after varicocelectomy. *Fertil. Steril.*, **57**, 854–7.

Dixon, R. (1986). Toxic responses of the reproductive system. In *Casarrett and Doull's Toxicology*, 3rd edn, ed. C.D. Klaassen, M.O. Amdur & J. Doull, pp. 453–4. New York: Macmillan.

Dobs, A.S., Sarma, P.S., Guarnieri, T. & Griffith, L. (1991). Testicular dysfunction with amiodarone use. *J. Am. Coll. Cardiol.*, **18**, 1328–32.

Dostal, I.A., Chapin, R.E., Stefanski, S.A., Harris, M.W. & Schwetz, B.A. (1988). Testicular toxicity and reduced Sertoli cell numbers in neonatal rats by di(2-ethylbexyl)phthalate and the recovery of fertility in adults. *Toxicol. Appl. Pharmacol.*, **95**, 104–21.

Einhorn, L.H., Richie, J.P. & Shipley, W.V. (1993). Cancer of the testis. In *Cancer: Principles and Practice of Oncology*, ed. J.R. Vincent, T. DeVita, S. Herllman & S. Rosenberg, pp. 1126–51. Philadelphia: J.B. Lippincott.

El-Gothamy, Z. & El-Samahy, M. (1992). Ultrastructure sperm defects in addicts. *Fertil. Steril.*, **57**, 699–702.

Eliasson, R. (1976). Clinical examination of infertile men. In *Human Semen and Fertility Regulation*, ed. by E.S.E. Hafez, pp. 321–31. St Louis: C.V. Mosby.

Eliasson, R. & Lindholmer, C. (1976). Functions of male accessory genital organs. In *Human Semen and Fertility Regulation*, ed. E.S.E. Hafez, pp. 44–50. St Louis: C.V. Mosby.

Eliasson, R., Mossberg, B., Camner, P. & Afzelius, B.A. (1977). The immotile cilia syndrome. *N. Engl. J. Med.*, **297**, 1–6.

Eskenazi, B., Fenster, L., Hudes, M., Wyrobek, A.J., Katz, D., Gerson, J. & Rempel, D. (1991). A study of the effect of perchloroethylene exposure on the reproductive outcomes of wives of dry-cleaning workers. *Am. J. Ind. Med.*, **20**, 593–600.

Farthing, M.J.R., Rees, L.H., Edwards, C.R.W. & Dawson, A.M. (1983). Male gonadal dysfunction in coeliac disease. *Clin. Endocrinol.*, **19**, 127–35.

Fourcroy, J.L. (1993). Effects of medications on fertility in males with physical disabilities with sexually transmitted disease. In *Reproductive Issues for Persons with Physical Disabilities*, ed. F.P. Haseltine, S.S. Cole & D.B. Gray, pp. 265–73. Baltimore: Paul H. Brookes.

Fourcroy, J.L. & Belman, A.B. (1982). Transverse testicular ectopia with persistent mullerian duct. *Urology*, **19**, 536–8.

Fourcroy, J.L., Popek, E.J., Sesterhenn, I., *et al.* (1994). Cystic dysgenesis of the testis. Abstract presentation at the ASA.

Frishman, G.N., Luciano, A.A. & Maier, D.B. (1992). Evaluation of Astroglide, a new vaginal lubricant: effects of length of exposure and concentration on sperm motility. *Fertil. Steril.*, **58**, 630–2.

Gill, W.B., Schumacher, G.F.B. & Bibbo, M. (1977). Pathological semen and anatomical abnormalities of the genital tract in human male subjects exposed to diethylstilbestrol *in utero*. *J. Urol.*, **117**, 477–80.

Gorelick, J.I. & Goldstein, M. (1993). Loss of fertility in men with varicocele. *Fertil. Steril.*, **59**, 613–16.

Hadziselimovic, F., Herzog, B., Liebundgut, B., Jenny, P. & Buser, M. (1989). Testicular and vascular changes in children and adults with varicocele. *J. Urol.*, **142**, 583–5.

Hahn, E.W., Feingold, S.M., Simpson, L. & Batata, M. (1983). Recovery from aspermia induced by low-dose radiation in seminoma patients. *Cancer*, **50**, 337–40.

Halstead, L. & Seager, W.J. (1993). Electroejaculation and its techniques in males with neurologic impairments. In *Reproductive Issues for Persons with Physical Disabilities*, ed. F.P. Haseltine, S.S. Cole & D.B. Gray, pp. 311–30. Baltimore: Paul H. Brooke.

Hamer, P.M. & Bain, J. (1986). Ejaculatory incompetence and infertility. *Fertil. Steril.*, **45**, 384–7.

Handelsman, D.J. & Turtle, J.R. (1983). Testicular damage after therapy for thyroid cancer. *Clin. Endocrinol.*, **18**, 465–72.

Handelsman, D.J., Conway, A.J., Boylan, L.M. & Turtle, J.R. (1984). Young's syndrome: obstructive azoospermia and chronic sinopulmonary infection. *N. Engl. J. Med.*, **310**, 3–9.

Haseltine, F.P., Cole, S.S. & Gray, D.B. (1993). *Reproductive Issues for Persons with Disabilities*. Baltimore: Paul H. Brooke.

Hellerstein, D.K., Meacham, R.B. & Lipshultz, L.I. (1992). Transrectal ultrasound and partial ejaculatory duct obstruction in male infertility. *Urology*, **39**, 449–58.

Hendry, W.F. (1981). The long term results of surgery for obstructive azoospermia. *Br. J. Urol.*, **53**, 664–71.

Hendry, W.E., A'Hearn, E.P.A. & Cole, P.J. (1993). Was Young's syndrome caused by exposure to mercury in childhood? *BMJ*, **307**, 1579–82.

Hirsch, A.V., Kellet, M.J., Robertson, J.E., *et al.* (1980). Doppler flow studies, venography, and thermography in the evaluation of varicoceles of fertile and subfertile men. *Br. J. Urol.*, **52**, 560–5.

Hirsch, I.H., Sedor, J., Jeyendran, R.S. & Staas, W.E. (1992). The relative distribution of viable sperm in the antegrade and retrograde portions of ejaculates obtained after electrostimulation. *Fertil. Steril.*, **57**, 399–408.

Hollingshead, W.H. (1971). *Anatomy for Surgeons*, vol. 2. New York: Harper & Row.

Horvatta, O., Back, L., Kaukoranta-Tolvanen, S. & Huhtaniemi, I. (eds.) (1988). The Finnish sauna does not disturb testicular function. In *Molecular and Cellular Endocrinology of the Testis*, Fifth European Workshop. Serono Symposia Publications. New York: Raven Press.

Howards, S.S. (1992). Subclinical varicocele. *Fertil. Steril.*, **57**, 725–6.

Hudson, E., Dore, C., Sowter, C., Toovey, S. & Levi, A.J. (1982). Sperm size in patients with inflammatory bowel disease on sulfasalazine therapy. *Fertil. Steril.*, **38**, 77–84.

Hudson, R.W. (1988). The endocrinology of varicoceles. *Fertil. Steril.*, **49**, 199–208.

Jaffe, N., Sullivan, M.P., Ried, H., Boren, H., Marshall, R., Meistrich, M., Maor, M. & da-Cunha, M. (1988). Male reproductive function in long-term survivors of childhood cancer. *Med. Pediatr. Oncol.*, **16**, 241–7.

Jarow, J.P. (1990). Anabolic steroid-induced hypogonadotropic hypogonadism. *Am. J. Sports Med.*, **18**, 429–31.

Jequier, A.M. (1985). Obstructive azoospermia: a study of 102 patients. *Clin. Reprod. Fertil.*, **3**, 21–36.

Jequier, A.M. & Cruch, J.P. (1986). *Semen Analysis*. Oxford: Blackwell Scientific.

John, E.M. (1991). Prenatal exposure to parents' smoking and childhood cancer. *Am. J. Epidemiol.*, **133**, 123–32.

Johnson, L., Zane, R.S., Petty, C.S. & Neave, W.B. (1984). Quantification of the human Sertoli cell population: its distribution, relation to germ cell number, and age-related decline. *Biol. Reprod.*, **31**, 785–95.

Jonsson, M.S., McCormick, J.R., Gillie, C.G. & Gondos, B. (1982). Kartagener's syndrome with motile spermatozoa. *N. Eng. J. Med.* **307**, 1121–33.

Jouannet, P., Ducot, B., Feneux, D. & Spira, A. (1988). Male factors and the likelihood of pregnancy in infertile couples. *Int. J. Androl.*, **11**, 379–94.

Kallmann, F.J., Schonfeld, W.A. & Barron, S.E. (1944). The genetic aspects of primary eunuchoidism. *Am. J. Ment. Defic.*, **48**, 203.

Kaplan, E., Swachman, H., Perlmutter, A.D., Rule, A., Khaw, K.-T. & Holsclaw, D. (1968). Reproductive failure in males with cystic fibrosis. *N. Engl. J. Med.*, **279**, 65–9.

Kass, E.J. & Belman, A.B. (1987). Reversal of testicular growth failure by varicocele ligation. *J. Urol.*, **137**, 475–6.

Kass, E.J., Freitas, J.E., Salisz, J.A. & Steinert, B.W. (1993). Pituitary gonadal dysfunction in adolescents with varicocele. *Urology*, **42**, 179–81.

Kaye, M.C., Schroeder-Jenkins, M. & Rothman, S.A. (1991). Impairment of sperm motility by water-soluble lubricants as assessed by computer assisted sperm analysis. *J. Androl.*, **12**, P52.

Klaiber, E.L., Broverman, D.M., Pokoly, T.B., Albert, A.J., Howard, P.J. & Sherer, J.F. (1987). Interrelationships of cigarette smoking, testicular varicoceles and seminal fluid indexes. *Fertil. Steril.*, **47**, 481–6.

Krieger, J.N. (1990). Prostatitis, epididymitits and orchitis. In *Sexually Transmitted Diseases*, 2nd edn, ed. K.K. Holmes, P. Mardh, P.F. Sparling, P.J. Wener, W. Cates, S.M. Lemon & W.E. Stamm, p. 571. New York: McGraw-Hill Information Services.

Kulin, H.E. & Santner, S.J. (1986). The assessment of diminished testicular function in boys of pubertal age. *Clin. Endocrinol.*, **25**, 283–92.

Leonhardt, W.C. & Goodwing, G. (1992). Sonography of intrascrotal adenomatoid tumor. *Urology*, **39**, 90–2.

Lione, A. (1987). Ionizing radiation and human reproduction. *Reprod. Toxicol.*, **1**, 3–16.

Lipshultz, L.I. & Corriere J.N. Jr (1977). Progressive testicular atrophy in the varicocele patient. *J. Urol.*, **117**, 175–6.

Lubinsky, M.S. (1983). Cataracts and testicular failure in three brothers. *Am.J. Med. Genet.*, **16**, 149–52.

Matwijiw, I. (1987). Aplasia of nasal cilia with situs inversus, azoospermia and normal sperm flagella: a unique variant of the immotile cilia syndrome. *J. Urol.*, **137**, 522–3.

Meistrich, M.L. (1986). Critical components of testicular function and sensitivity to disruption. *Biol. Reprod.* **34**, 17–28.

Morrish, D., Venner, P., Sly, O., Barron, G., Bhardwaj, D. & Outhet, D. (1990). Mechanisms of endocrine dysfunction in patients with testicular cancer. *J. Natl. Cancer Inst.*, **82**, 412–18.

Nieschlag, E., Lammers, V. & Freichem, C.W. (1982). Reproductive function in young fathers and grandfathers. *J. Clin. Endocrinol. Metab.*, **55**, 676–81.

O'Morain, C., Smethurst, P., Dore, C.J. & Levi, A.J. (1984). Reversible male infertility due to sulphasalazine studies in man and rat. *Gut*, **25**, 1078–84.

Oates, R.D. & Lipshultz, L.I. (1989). Fertility and testicular function in patients after chemotherapy and radiotherapy. In *Advances in Urology*, ed. B. Lytton, pp. 55–83. Chicago: Year Book Medical.

OTA (1988). *Infertility: Medical and Social Choices*. Office of Technology Assessment, Congress of the US, OTA-BA-358.

Paterson, L. & Jarow, J.P. (1990). Transrectal ultrasonography in the evaluation of the infertile man: a report of 3 cases. *J. Urol.*, **144**, 1469–71.

Peng, B.C.H., Tomashefsky, P. & Nagler, H.M. (1990). The co-factor effect: varicocele and infertility. *Fertil. Steril.*, **54**, 143–8.

Physician's Desk Reference (PDR) (1994). Finasteride (Proscar) Merck; testosterone (Testoderm) Alza. Montvale, NJ: Medical Economics Data Production Co.

Porch, P.P. (1978). Aspermia owing to obstruction of distal ejaculatory duct and treatment by transurethral resection. *J. Urol.*, **119**, 141–2.

Pryor, J.P. & Hendry, W.F. (1991). Ejaculatory duct obstruction in subfertile males: analysis of 87 patients. *Fertil. Steril.*, **56**, 725–30.

Ratcliffe, J.M., Schraeder, S.M., Steenland, K., Clapp, D.E., Turner, T. & Hornung, W.R. (1987). Semen quality in papaya workers with long term exposure to ethylene dibromide. *Br. J. Ind. Med.*, **44**, 317–26.

Rigot, J.M., Lafitte, J.J., Dumur, V., Gervai, R., Manouvrier, S., Biserte, J., *et al.* (1991). Cystic fibrosis and congenital absence of the vas deferens. *N. Engl. J. Med.*, **325**, 64–5.

Riley, S.A. (1987). Sulfasalazine induced seminal abnormalities in ulcerative colitis: results of mesalazine substitution. *Gut*, **28**, 1009–12.

Rivkees, S.A., Hall, D.A., Boepple, P.A. & Crawford, J.D. (1987). Accuracy and reproducibility of clinical measures of testicular volume. *J. Pediatr.*, **110**, 914–17.

Russell, L.D. & Griswold, M.D. (1993). *The Sertoli Cell*. Clearwater, Florida: Cache River Press.

Saez, J.M. (1994). Leydig cells: endocrine, paracrine, and autocrine regulation. *Endocr. Rev.*, **15**, 574–626.

Salbenblatt, J.A., Bender, B.G., Puck, M.H., Robinson, A., Faiman, C. & Winter, J.S.D. (1985). Pituitary–gonadal function in Klinefelter syndrome before and during puberty. *Pediatr. Res.*, **19**, 82–6.

Sanders, J.E., Buckner, C.D., Leonard, J.M., *et al.* (1983). Late effects on gonadal function of cyclophosphamide, total body irradiation and marrow transplantation. *Transplantation*, **36**, 252–5.

de Santi, M.M., Gordic, M. & Lungarella, G. (1985). Severe teratospermia in an infertile man with bronchiectasis. *Fertil. Steril.*, **44**, 849–52.

Schachter, J. (1990). Chlamydial infections. *Western J. Med.*, **153**, 523–34.

Schellen, T.M. & van Stratten, A. (1980). Autosomal recessive hereditary congenital aplasia of the vasa deferentia in four siblings. *Fertil. Steril.*, **35**, 401–4.

Schlegel, P.N., Chang, T.S.K. & Marshall, F.F. (1991). Antibiotics: potential hazards to male fertility. *Fertil. Steril.*, **55**, 235–42.

Schrader, S.M. & Kesner, J.S. (1993). Male reproductive toxicology. In *Occupational and Environmental Reproductive Hazards*, ed. M. Paul, pp. 3–17. Baltimore: Williams & Wilkins.

Schrader, S.M., Turner, T.W. & Ratcliffe, J.M. (1988). The effects of ethylene dibromide on semen quality: a comparison of short-term and chronic exposure. *Reprod. Toxicol.*, **2**, 191.

Scorer, G. & Farrinton, G.H. (1971). *Congenital Deformities of the Testis and Epididymis*. New York: Appleton-Century-Crofts.

Sokol, R.Z., Petersen, G., Steiner, B.S., *et al.* A controlled comparison of the efficacy of clomiphene citrate in male infertility. *Fertil. Steril.*, **49**, 865–70.

Speroff, L., Glass, A. & Kase (1989). The ovary. In *Clinical Gynecology: Endocrinology and Infertility*, 4th edn. Baltimore: Williams & Wilkins.

Stephen, J.M. & Avila, J.A. (1991). Letter to the editor. *N. Engl. J. Med.*, **324**, 993.

Takihara, H. (1983). Significance of testicular size measurement in andrology. I. A new orchiometer and its clinical application. *Fertil. Steril.*, **33**, 836–40.

Takihara, H., Cosentino, M.J., Sakatoku, J. & Cockett, A.T.K. (1987). Significance of testicular size measurement in urology. II. Correlation of testicular size with testicular function. *J. Urol.*, **137**, 416–19.

Takihara, H., Akatoku, J. & Cockett, A.T.K. (1991). The pathophysiology of varicocele in male infertility. *Fertil. Steril.*, **55**, 861–8.

Taussig, L.M., Lobeck, C.C., Sant'Agnese, P.A., Ackerman, D.R. & Kauttwinkel, J. (1972). Fertility in males with cystic fibrosis. *N. Engl. J. Med.*, **325**, 64–5.

Tulandi, T. & McInnes, R.A. (1984). Vaginal lubricants: effect of glycerin and egg white on sperm motility and progression *in vitro*. *Fertil. Steril.*, **41**, 151–3.

Tulandi, T., Plouffe, L. & McInnes, R.A. (1982). Effect of saliva on sperm motility and activity. *Fertil. Steril.*, **38**, 721–3.

Turek, P.J., Eqalt, D.H., Snyder, H.M. III & Duckett, J.W. (1994). Normal epididymal anatomy in boys. *J. Urol.*, **151**, 726–7.

Van Thiel, D.H., Gavalet, J.S., Lester, R., *et al.* (1975). Alcohol induces testicular atrophy. *Gastroenterology*, **69**, 326.

Van Thiel, D.H., Gavalet, J.S., Smith, W.O., *et al.* (1979). Hypothalamic–pituitary–gonadal dysfunction in men using cimetidine. *N. Engl. J. Med.*, **300**, 1012.

Viviani, S., Santoro, A., Ragni, G., Bonfante, V., Bestetti, O. & Bonadonna, G. (1985). Gonadal toxicity after combination chemotherapy for Hodgkin's disease: comparative results of MOPP vs ABVD. *Eur. J. Cancer Clin. Oncol.*, **21**, 601–5.

Wang, C., Chan, C., Wong, K.-K., *et al.* (1983). Comparison of the effectiveness of placebo, clomiphene citrate, mesterolone, pentoxifylline, and testosterone, rebound therapy for the treatment of idiopathic oligospermia. *Fertil. Steril.*, **40**, 358–65.

Watson, A.R., Rance, C.P. & Bain, J. (1985) Long-term effects of cyclophosphamide on testicular function. *BMJ*, **291**, 1457–60.

Werner, C.A. (1950). Mumps orchitis. *Ann. Intern. Med.*, **32**, 1066.

Whitehead, E.D. & Leiter, E. (1981). Genital abnormalities and abnormal semen analyses in males exposed to diethylstilbestrol (DES) *in utero*. *J. Urol.*, **125**, 47–50.

Whitehead, E., Morris, S.M., Jones, P.H., Beardwell, C.G., & Deskin, D.P. (1982). Gonadal function after combination chemotherapy for Hodgkin's disease in childhood. *Arch. Dis. Child.* **47**, 287–91.

Whorton, D., Krauss, R.M., Marshall, S. & Milby, T.H. (1979). Infertility in male pesticide workers. *Lancet*, **ii**, 1259–61.

Wilson, J.D. (1992). Syndromes of androgen resistance. *Biol. Reprod.*, **46**, 168–73.

World Health Organization (1987). *WHO Laboratory Manual for the Examination of Human Semen and Semen–Cervical Mucus Interaction*. Cambridge: Cambridge University Press.

15

Azoospermia: the diagnosis and treatment

HARRIS M. NAGLER

Introduction

Although obstruction of the reproductive tract leading to azoospermia is not the major cause of infertility, accurate diagnosis of its cause and its anatomic location is essential and may permit successful reconstruction. The diagnostic, laboratory, and surgical procedures utilized to arrive at the appropriate diagnosis and the available therapeutic modalities will be discussed.

Approach to the azoospermic male

A thorough reproductive, developmental, medical, surgical, and exposure history is essential for the accurate assessment of the azoospermic male. Male reproduction is dependent upon the normalcy of the hypothalamic–pituitary–gonadal axis, the testicle, the anatomic reproductive tract, and sexual function.

Azoospermia is defined as the absence of sperm from the ejaculate. There must be a normal conduit system and normal sexual function to allow for delivery of the sperm. The azoospermic individual has, by definition, an abnormality within one of these loci, and the appropriate evaluation should identify the site of the abnormality. The couple's reproductive, sexual, developmental, medical, and surgical histories should be elicited in an attempt to identify abnormalities within each of these processes necessary for normal reproductive function. A sexual and reproductive history may define the problem and its duration.

The developmental history attempts to define the normalcy of pubertal development, which is dependent on a normally functioning hypothalamic–pituitary–gonadal axis. The medical and surgical histories should identify potential risk factors which may contribute to an individual's infertility. Emphasis must be placed on developmental abnormalities, medical

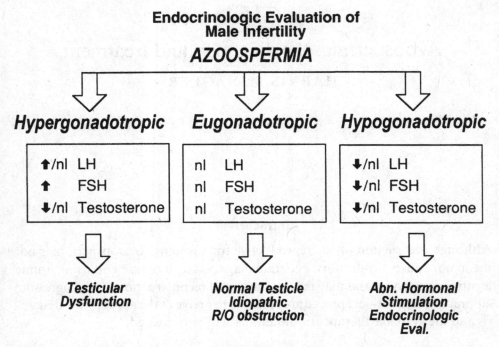

Endocrinologic Evaluation of
Male Infertility

AZOOSPERMIA

Hypergonadotropic	Eugonadotropic	Hypogonadotropic
↑/nl LH ↑ FSH ↓/nl Testosterone	nl LH nl FSH nl Testosterone	↓/nl LH ↓/nl FSH ↓/nl Testosterone
Testicular **Dysfunction**	**Normal Testicle** **Idiopathic** **R/O obstruction**	**Abn. Hormonal** **Stimulation** **Endocrinologic** **Eval.**

Fig. 15.1. Algorithm: endocrinologic evaluation of the azoospermic male. The endocrinologic evaluation of the azoospermic male is outlined. The diagnostic groupings and suggested evaluation are provided.

conditions, and surgical procedures relating to or affecting testicular development, descent, or the reproductive tract.

Gonadotropin determination has allowed the practitioner to characterize male infertility as (1) hypogonadotropic, (2) hypergonadotropic, or (3) normal gonadotropic (eugonadotropic) (Nagler & Thomas, 1987). Clinical studies have resulted in the establishment of three major etiologic categories of male infertility: (1) prestesticular, (2) testicular, and (3) post-testicular causes. Pretesticular causes of infertility are the result of inadequate hormonal stimulation of spermatogenesis. Testicular causes of infertility are the result of intrinsic testicular dysfunction and are characterized by elevated gonadotropins (hypergonadotropic). Post-testicular abnormalities are the result of obstruction or dysfunction of the reproductive tract, and are characterized by normal gonadotropins (eugonadotropic).

A *pretesticular* cause of azoospermia, characterized by abnormally low gonadotropins (hypogonadotropism) requires thorough endocrinologic evaluation (Fig. 15.1). Hypogonadotropism may be the result of congenital abnormalities, such as Kallmann's syndrome, or acquired abnormalities of the pituitary or hypothalamus. Endocrine replacement therapy of pretesticular azoospermia may be quite successful (Paulsen *et al.*, 1970; Sherins, 1984).

Testicular dysfunction which causes azoospermia is characterized by elevated gonadotropins (hypergonadotropism) (Fig. 15.1). The testicle is not capable of responding appropriately, and the gonadotropins rise secondary to the disruption of the negative feedback loop. FSH reflects the integrity of the germ cell–Sertoli cell functional unit. Marked elevation of FSH (>2.5 times normal) in the azoospermic individual is indicative of severe testicular dysfunction which is not amenable to conventional intervention. The exception to this dictum may be the individual with marked atrophy of one testis and a normal contralateral testis with findings consistent with obstruction. These patients may have surgically correctable obstruction. Patients with marked elevations of the gonadotropins and azoospermia do not require further evaluation; they have *testicular azoospermia*. Isolated elevations of FSH may be observed in patients with Sertoli cell only syndrome, orchitis, cryptorchidism, idiopathic dysfunction, maturation arrest, and toxic effects of radiation or chemotherapy. Many testicular abnormalities associated with azoospermia cause elevation of both LH and FSH. Elevation of the LH indicates disordered Leydig cell function. Entities associated with elevations of both gonadotropins include Klinefelter's syndrome, vanishing testes syndrome, bilateral cryptorchidism, and idiopathic causes.

The azoospermic patient with normal gonadotropins (eugonadotropic) may have an obstructive cause of azoospermia (Figs. 15.1, 15.2). Primary testicular abnormalities such as Sertoli cell only syndrome and maturation arrest may also result in azoospermia associated with normal gonadotropins. Patients with these testicular abnormalities can be differentiated from the azoospermic patient with obstruction only by performing testicular biopsies. Testicular biopsy should be done to evaluate the azoospermic patient with normal gonadotropins and normal ejaculate volumes (Fig. 15.1).

Testicular biopsy

Testicular biopsy has been utilized in the evaluation of male infertility since its introduction in the 1940s (Charny, 1940; Hotchkiss, 1942). Although it has been employed to evaluate patients with low sperm counts, it is used primarily in the diagnostic evaluation of the eugonadotropic azoospermic patient to differentiate between testicular and post-testicular (obstructive) causes of infertility (Nagler & Thomas, 1987; Fig. 15.2). The volume of ejaculate should be normal and fructose should be present in the ejaculate prior to proceeding with testicular biopsies, since an abnormal volume or the absence of fructose may

NORMAL LH
NORMAL FSH
NORMAL TESTOSTERONE

OBSTRUCTION
MATURATION ARREST
SERTOLI CELL ONLY SYNDR.
EJACULATORY DYSFUNCTION
SEXUAL DYSFUNCTION

Fig. 15.2. The differential diagnosis of eugonadotropic azoospermia.

indicate an abnormality of ejaculation or the ejaculatory duct apparatus. Biopsies should only be performed when the information which may be obtained will alter the therapy that may be offered to a patient.

Silber & Rodriguez-Rigau (1981) demonstrated that partial (subclinical) epididymal obstruction could result in *severe* oligozoospermia. Patients with severe oligozoospermia (i.e., <1 million sperm/ml) should be evaluated as though they were azoospermic. The diagnosis of partial epididymal obstruction requires detailed analysis of testicular biopsy material. Testicular biopsy of the oligozoospermic man should not be done unless the physical examination or history indicates that there may have been processes which may have caused partial or unilateral obstruction of the reproductive system.

Many authors feel that testicular biopsy need not be done bilaterally. Posinovec (1976) suggests that an adequate assessment of testicular function can be made by unilateral biopsy when the testes are not dissimilar. Others have advocated bilateral biopsies when there is a suggestion that an asymmetric lesion exists (Ibrahim *et al.*, 1977). Differences in testicular size, a palpably absent vas deferens, or epididymal induration also suggest the need for bilateral biopsies, although we believe that *both* testes should be biopsied under all circumstances. Testicular histologic heterogeneity and asymmetry in apparently similar testes warrants routine biopsy of both testes unless one is severely abnormal (Lipshultz *et al.*, 1990; Krause & Nagler, 1992).

A limitation of the testicular biopsy as a diagnostic technique is its reliance on conventional pathologic interpretation of spermatogenesis. Histologic reporting is generally limited by subjective analysis and is, therefore, often observer and experience dependent (Kaufman & Nagler, 1987).

Window technique

The 'window' technique is widely employed for open testicular biopsy. The delicate testicular architecture is protected by using 'no touch' technique. This requires the surgeon to lift and excise the testicular tissue as it is extruded through an incision in the tunica albuginea. The specimen is then fixed in either

Bouin's solution or Zenker's without touching the biopsy; formalin or formaldehyde is destructive to the testicular architecture.

Two new techniques for assessing spermatogenesis based on the cytologic analysis of the germinal epithelium from the incisional testis biopsy specimens have recently been developed. These are the touch imprint and cytocentrifuge preparations (Coburn *et al.*, 1986). In the former, a portion of testicular parenchyma obtained during an open biopsy is touched to or gently moved across a microscope slide. The specimen is stained with the Papanicolaou or hematoxylin–eosin stain following fixation. If spermatogenesis is complete, tailed spermatozoa will be readily identified. This technique permits the differentiation of late maturation arrest from normal spermatogenesis. The preparation of a testicular cytology specimen by cytocentrifugation of a testicular biopsy has also been described. This technique is more cumbersome and does not appear to offer advantages over the touch preparation.

These techniques permit immediate and accurate assessment of spermatogenesis, allowing the surgeon to make intraoperative decisions. Frozen section analysis of testicular histology is extremely difficult and unreliable, and, therefore, has not been advocated. Furthermore, because mature, intact spermatozoa are clearly identified by these cytologic techniques, they are extremely useful in distinguishing late maturation arrest from normal biopsy specimens. A testicular biopsy should not be done without a concurrent cytologic preparation.

Needle biopsy

Recently, needle biopsy has been advocated in the evaluation of male infertility (Cohen & Warner, 1979; Cohen *et al.*, 1984). This technique has the advantage of being quick and simple, since it does not require an operating room and can easily be performed with a local anesthetic in the office. In 1989, Rajfer & Binder reported on the use of a spring-loaded biopsy gun (Biopty gun) to perform testicular biopsies. Limitations associated with this technique include the small size of the sample and the potential distortion of tubular histology (Kaufman & Nagler, 1987). Because of these limitations, standard open biopsy continues to be the most widely utilized technique for definitive histologic diagnosis of testicular biopsies.

Flow cytometry

Routine histologic evaluation of testicular biopsy specimens is time-consuming, subjective, and permits only qualitative assessment of cellular defects. DNA flow cytometry is a rapid and reproducible technique which allows quantitative assessment of spermatogenesis from specimens obtained by needle aspiration or standard biopsy techniques (Thorud *et al.*, 1980; Pfitzer *et al.*, 1982; Chan *et al.*, 1984; Kaufman & Nagler, 1987; Hellstrom *et al.*, 1990). The method objectively distinguishes and quantitates cell populations on the basis of the DNA content of individual cells. Normal spermatogenesis includes cells which have diploid (2N), tetraploid (4N), and haploid (1N) chromosomal content. Normal spermatogenesis can, therefore, be defined on the basis of an optimal ratio between populations of cells with each of these ploidy counts – a determination that can be made with flow cytometry. Alteration in these ploidy relationships may indicate disordered spermatogenesis. Although flow cytometers are becoming more available in hospital pathology departments, and may provide the clinician with accurate information upon which to make a clinical decision, this technology has not been widely employed in the evaluation of the azoospermic individual (Hellstrom *et al*, 1990).

Vasography

When testicular biopsy demonstrates normal spermatogenesis in the azoospermic individual, obstruction is likely to exist. Formal scrotal exploration and vasography are required to permit an accurate diagnosis of obstruction. Diagnostic seminal vesiculography or vasography was initially carried out by Belfield in 1913. Vasography provides excellent delineation of the vas deferens, seminal vesicles and ejaculatory ducts, and allows identification of obstruction anywhere within these sites. The risks of iatrogenic damage to the vas deferens, seminal vesicles and ejaculatory ducts have been minimized by the advent of microsurgical techniques and less caustic (hydrophilic) contrast material (Nagler & Thomas, 1987).

Utilization of the touch preparation has permitted the clinician to make accurate assessments of spermatogenesis and appropriate intraoperative therapeutic decisions. In cases where there is a clear indication of obstruction on the basis of physical examination and/or history, the surgical procedure may include biopsy and vasography for confirmation followed by surgical reconstruction, all at the same sitting. Since vasography may result in adhesion formation and scarring complicating subsequent reconstructive surgery, it is best to perform vasography at the time of anticipated reconstruction. Vasography should be performed utilizing microsurgical techniques (Fig. 15.3) to prevent subsequent sperm leakage and possible iatrogenic scarring and obstruction. Direct vas puncture may be the least traumatic technique for vasography (Nagler & Thomas, 1987). However, multiple punctures may be required to

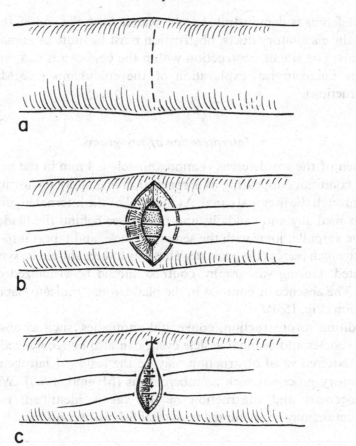

Fig. 15.3. Vasotomy. (a) A vasotomy is made perpendicular to the long axis of the vas deferens under the operating microscope. This should just enter the vasal lumen. (b) After the vasal fluid has been examined and vasography completed, the vasotomy is closed. In this illustration a two-layer technique is demonstrated. Sutures are placed in the mucosa. They are then tied. (c) Additional sutures are placed in the muscular layer of the vas closing the vasotomy.

enter the vasal lumen, with subsequent tissue damage and possible obstruction. In this regard direct puncture vasography has been reported to cause scarring and obstruction in experimental animals (Paulson *et al.*, 1974; Gordon & Clahassey, 1978; Wagenknecht *et al.*, 1982; Thomas, 1984). If operative vasography is performed, the presence or absence of fluid must be noted. The presence of sperm in the fluid indicates obstruction distal (abdominal) to the vasotomy site (see Microsurgical Reconstruction).

Obstruction within the epididymis can be ascertained only by exploration and examination of tubular contents. Attempts to visualize the epididymis radiographically may result in disruption of the delicate epididymal tubule. If the vas deferens is demonstrated to be patent from the site of the vasotomy through the ejaculatory ducts, obstruction must be more proximal within the epididymis. The site of obstruction within the epididymis can only be determined by microsurgical exploration of the epididymis (see Microsurgical Reconstruction).

Interpretation of vasograms

The lumen of the vas deferens is approximately 0.4 mm in the normal unobstructed condition, appearing as a pencil-thin line along its normal anatomic course through the inguinal canal. At the level of the internal inguinal ring, the vas turns medially and caudally, and progresses behind the bladder where it forms the ampulla, joins with the seminal vesicle, and tapers into the ejaculatory duct which pierces the prostate. These structures should be symmetric and non-dilated. During vasography, contrast should be visualized entering the bladder. The absence of contrast in the bladder may indicate ejaculatory duct obstruction (Fig. 15.4).

In addition to obstruction, congenital anomalies, such as absence of the seminal vesicles and seminal vesicle cysts, can also be recognized from vasograms. Acquired vasal obstruction may be the result of iatrogenic injury or inflammatory processes such as tuberculosis (Mygind, 1960). When normal spermatogenesis and obstruction in the vas is identified, microsurgical reconstruction may be attempted to re-establish vasal continuity.

Vasal obstruction: microsurgical reconstruction

One of the more common causes of azoospermia is vasectomy. Approximately 1 million men undergo vasectomy (voluntary sterilization) in the United States annually. It is among the most common of all urologic procedures performed there (Montie & Stewart, 1974), with more than 15% of all couples who use contraception relying on sterilization of the male partner (Pratt *et al.*, 1985). The widespread utilization of microsurgical techniques and the awareness of microsurgical principles has made vasectomy reversal a highly successful procedure in up to 90% of individuals (Silber, 1977). The microsurgical techniques used for vasectomy reversal are the same techniques utilized in the reconstruction of iatrogenic, inflammatory, and congenital causes of obstruction.

Initial attempts at vasovasostomy were carried out using macroscopic (non-magnified) techniques. Results were generally disappointing, since macroscopic vasovasostomies did not allow for reliable juxtaposition of the mucosa. This recognition led to widespread utilization of loupes for magnification, with

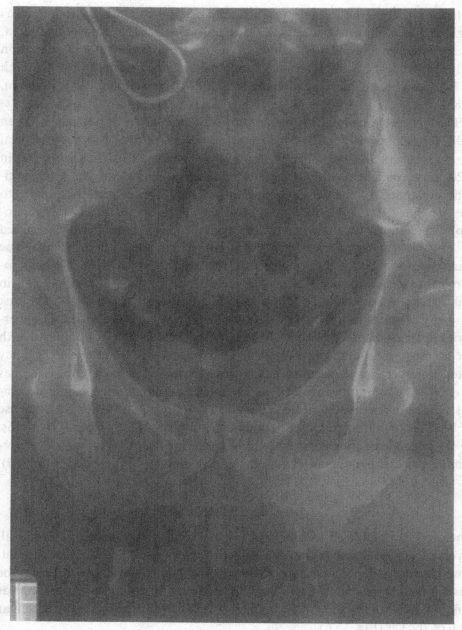

Fig. 15.4. Vasography. Operative vasography demonstrating obstruction of both the left and right vas within the pelvis. No contrast is seen entering the bladder. The obstruction appears to be congenital in origin. The problem is not amenable to a reconstructive procedure.

patency rates ranging from 63% to 92% and pregnancy rates reported to be as high as 57% (Amelar & Dubin, 1975; Fallon *et al.*, 1981; Kessler & Freiha, 1981). Patency rates as high as 84% have been reported with a combination loupe magnification and internal stenting procedures; pregnancy rates as high as 70% have been achieved with these techniques (Shessel *et al.*, 1981; Redman, 1982).

The true modern era of vasovasostomy was heralded by the reports of Owen (1977) and Silber (1977) who concurrently developed a two-layer microsurgical vasovasostomy. Silber (1977) reported a 91% patency rate in 42 patients. Lee, in a 20 year experience with 624 patients, demonstrated a slight, but not significant, advantage of the two-layer anastomosis in terms of return of sperm to the ejaculate (91% versus 89%) and pregnancy (52% versus 50%). Both microscopic techniques were superior to the macroscopic technique, which resulted in an 84% patency rate and 35% pregnancy rate (Lee, 1986). The Vasovasostomy Study Group recently reported the results of 1469 microsurgical vasovasostomies. The overall success rate for the evaluable patients in this series was 86% with a 52% pregnancy rate (Belker *et al.*, 1991). The vast majority of series utilizing a two-layer anastomosis have confirmed the superiority in terms of patency rates of the microsurgical technique compared with the macrosurgical and loupe-magnified vasovasostomy technique. Pregnancy rates, however, do not seem to reflect these improved patency rates. Whereas macroscopic techniques require no specialized training, microscopic vasovasostomy requires that the surgeon acquire a certain level of expertise in the use of both the operating microscope and microsurgical skills (Yarbro & Howards, 1987), and skill of the operator seems to be the most significant variable determining successful outcome (H.M. Nagler & A. Belker, unpublished data 1987).

Microsurgical technique

The modified one-layer technique involves placing sutures which traverse all layers of the vasal wall (a through-and-through suture). These sutures are followed by intervening seromuscular sutures which purposefully do not enter the vasal lumen (Fig. 15.5). A two-layer technique initially approximates the vas mucosa, followed by a second layer of suture which approximates the muscular wall of the vas (Fig. 15.6).

New techniques

There have been many modifications of the techniques utilized to achieve vasovasostomies. Some are simply 'tricks' which may facilitate the procedure,

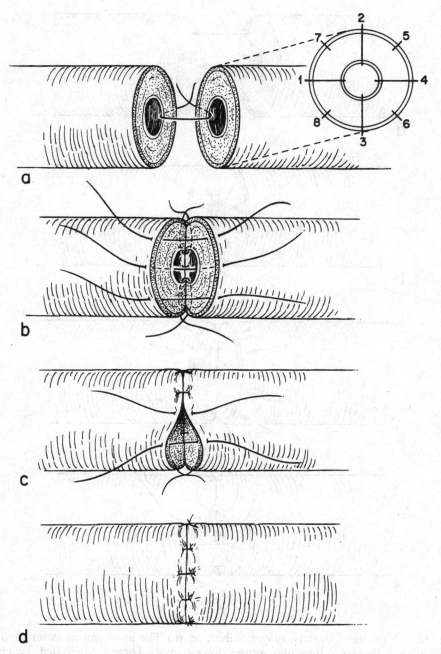

Fig. 15.5. Modified one-layer vasovastomy. (a) The first suture is placed full thickness including the muscular wall of the vas and the mucosa. This approximates the vas allowing the placement of two additional full-thickness sutures. These are demonstrated as 2 and 3 on the cross-section insert. (b) After sutures 2 and 3 have been placed, the last full-thickness suture (4) is placed. This is tied down approximating the mucosa. This is then followed by muscular sutures as indicated. (c) Muscular sutures are placed and tied sequentially. (d) The anastomosis is completed.

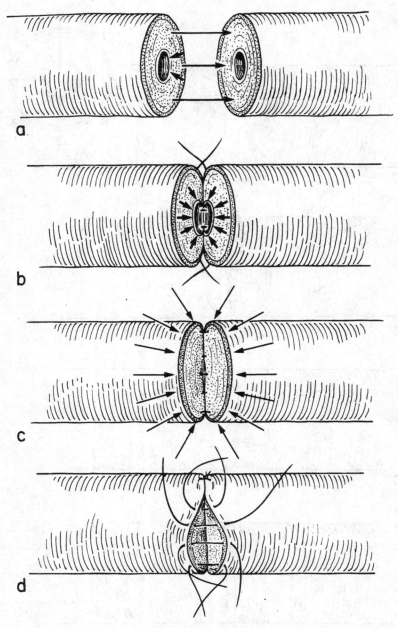

Fig. 15.6. Vasovasostomy: two-layer technique. (a) The anastomosis is initiated by three posteriorly placed muscular sutures (long arrows). These are then tied. Two posterior mucosal sutures are then placed (short arrows). (b) Additional mucosal sutures are placed as indicated by the short arrows. These are then tied. (c) The mucosal anastomosis has been completed. The second (muscular) layer of the anastomosis is continued anteriorly as indicated by the long arrows. (d) The muscular layer (second layer) anastomosis is completed.

whereas others are new approaches to achieving an anastomosis. The feasibility of laser-executed anastomoses has been extensively investigated (Jain & Gorisch, 1979; Quigley *et al.*, 1985) but they have not been widely embraced in clinical practice (Gilbert & Beckert, 1989). Fibrin tissue glue has been suggested as a replacement for sutured anastomosis. This technique does not obviate the need for suture placement, but as in the case of laser it may diminish both the surgical time and operative skill required (Weiss & Mellinger, 1992). This approach had been eschewed because of the requirement for pooled fibrin and the associated risk of transmitted diseases (Neiderberger *et al.*, 1993).

Complications

Vasal reconstructive procedures are well tolerated and often performed on an ambulatory basis. The complications associated with reconstructive procedures are similar to those associated with any scrotal surgery, including scrotal hematoma and swelling or infection. Testicular atrophy, as a result of injury to the spermatic artery, is a rare complication, and is more likely to occur when there has been a previous attempt at microsurgical reconstruction.

Epididymal obstruction: vasoepididymostomy

Epididymal obstruction may be encountered in the azoospermic male undergoing evaluation for infertility. Epididymal obstruction may be suspected because of the patient's history and/or physical examination, and can be the result of congenital anatomic abnormalities of the vas/epididymis, inflammatory processes, or acquired vasal obstruction. Epididymitis from gonorrhea, tuberculosis or *Chlamydia* is frequently cited as a cause of obstructive azoospermia (Bayle, 1952; Hagner, 1955; Hanley, 1955). The diagnosis of epididymal obstruction can only be made at the time of surgical exploration of the azoospermic male. The patient with proven spermatogenesis and the absence of fluid containing sperm in the proximal vasal fluid is likely to have epididymal obstruction. The significance of the fluid characteristics in the proximal vas at the time of vasal reconstruction has been the subject of a recent review by the Vasovasostomy Study Group (Belker *et al.*, 1983; Fuchs *et al.*, 1985). The presence of clear copious sperm-containing fluid indicates patency. The finding of fluid of intermediate quality is less clear, while a poor prognosis is associated with the absence of fluid or the presence of thick pasty fluid. If sperm heads are observed in the proximal vasal fluid, there is probably no epididymal obstruction. Epididymal obstruction may also be found in the patient undergoing a vasectomy reversal (Silber, 1979, 1981, 1984; Thomas, 1987). In this case, obstruction of the vas results in increased intratubular epididymal pressures which may cause the epididymal tubule to rupture or 'blow out'. The extravasation of sperm and the consequent inflammatory response may result in obstruction. The presence of fluid without sperm may or may not be associated with epididymal obstruction.

The epididymis is a poorly understood organ with complex functions related to sperm storage, maturation, and transport (Orgebin-Crist, 1969; Hinrichsen & Blaquier, 1980; Howards, 1983; Moore *et al.*, 1983; Thomas, 1987; Silber, 1989). In spite of the fact that sperm maturation occurs within the epididymis, sperm from the most proximal portions of the epididymis and efferent tubules may be able to fertilize an ovum *in vitro* (Silber *et al.*, 1990). The results of microsurgical reconstruction procedures indicate that sperm function better as they traverse a greater length of epididymis (Silber, 1978; Wagenknecht, 1985; Schoysman & Bedford, 1986; Blaquier *et al.*, 1989; Cooper, 1990). Therefore, at the time of microsurgical reconstruction of the obstructed epididymis, the surgeon should attempt to preserve as much of the epididymis as possible.

Technique

The advent of microsurgical techniques has resulted in the abandonment of macrosurgical vasoepididymostomy (Thomas, 1987). Macrosurgical vasoepididymostomy relied on the creation of a fistula between incised epididymal tubules and a spatulated vas deferens.

Currently, vasoepididymostomy is performed utilizing either of two microsurgical techniques which allow the anastomosis of the vasal mucosa to the epididymal tubule. Silber (1978) is generally credited with the popularization of the tubule-specific vasoepididymostomy. The reliability of this technique, when compared with macroscopic techniques, has resulted in its widespread utilization and modification (Ozdiler & Kelami, 1981; McLoughlin, 1982; Fogdestam & Fall, 1983; Wagenknecht, 1985; Fogestam *et al.*, 1986).

End-to-end vasoepididymostomy

In end-to-end vasoepididymostomy the obstructed epididymis is transected from the distalmost portion proceeding to the caput until a tubule on the cut surface effluxes sperm containing fluid. This effluxing tubule is proximal to the obstruction. Although the cut surface of the epididymis will have many 'lumina', only the proximal one (i.e., the lumen that is in continuity with the proximal aspect of the epididymal tubule) will continue to drain sperm-containing fluid. The vasal mucosa is sutured to the identified epididymal tubule, and the vasal muscular wall is sutured in a second layer to the epididymal tunica.

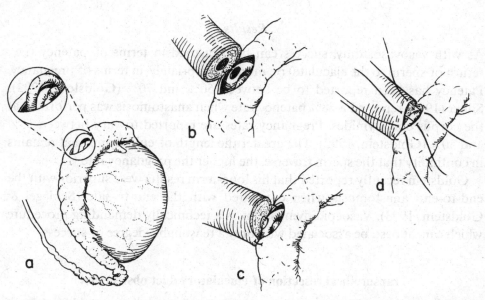

Fig. 15.7. Vasoepididymostomy: end-to-side technique. (a) The tunica overlying the epididymis has been incised exposing the underlying dilated epididymal tubule. The magnified view demonstrates the site of incision of the tubule. (b) The vas has been approximated to the tunica of the epididymis. This suture will initiate the formation of the posterior aspect of the anastomosis. (c) Additional outer layer sutures have been placed. This completes the posterior aspect of the outer layer of the anastomosis. The mucosal anastomosis has been started. (d) After completion of the mucosal anastomosis, the second layer of the anastomosis is completed.

End-to-side vasoepididymostomy (Fig. 15.7)

The epididymis is examined under the operating microscope to identify the presumed point of obstruction. When dilated, tubules are visualized beneath the epididymal tunic, after which a small window is created allowing the surface of the tubule to be clearly identified and incised. If fluid is encountered, it is examined for the presence of sperm. If no sperm are found, a more proximal tubule is exposed. When an appropriate tubule is identified, the anastomosis is performed in two layers. The epididymal tubule is sutured to the vas mucosa, and a second layer of sutures approximates the muscular wall of the vas to the tunica of the epididymis. This approach avoids transection of the epididymis, hemostasis is not problematic, and identification of sperm-containing epididymal tubules is facilitated. Furthermore, one can be certain that the anastomosis is carried out to the 'proximal' tubule because this technique does not disrupt the epididymal tubule.

Results

As with vasovasostomy, success can be measured in terms of patency (i.e., return of sperm to the ejaculate) or, more appropriately, in terms of pregnancy. Patency has been reported to be between 50% and 70% (Goldstein, 1992). Silber (1989) reported a 78% patency rate when anastomosis was performed at the corpus epididymides. Pregnancy rates are reported to vary between 15% and 30% (Goldstein, 1992). The greater the length of epididymis that remains in continuity that the sperm traverse, the higher the pregnancy rate.

Goldstein recently reported that his long-term results were superior with the end-to-end anastomosis when compared with the end-to-side (Schlegel & Goldstein, 1993). Vasoepididymostomy is a technically demanding procedure which can, at best, be associated with only a reasonable degree of success.

Transurethral resection of ejaculatory duct obstruction

Ejaculatory duct obstruction, an uncommon but easily treatable cause of obstruction of the male reproductive tract, is reported to occur in 3–7.4% of infertile men (Dubin & Amelar, 1971; Wagenknecht, 1982). Bilateral ejaculatory duct obstruction should be suspected in any patient with a low ejaculate volume and fructose-negative azoospermia (Fig. 15.8). The vas must be palpated to insure the patient does not have congenital vasal agenesis (CAV), since in CAV there is a coexistent absence of the seminal vesicles. Retrograde ejaculation should be ruled out by demonstrating the absence of sperm from a post-ejaculatory urine specimen (Keiserman *et al.*, 1974).

Patients with severe oligozoospermia and a low ejaculate volume may have incomplete or partial ejaculatory duct obstruction. Transrectal ultrasonography has given urologists the ability to detect abnormalities of the ejaculatory duct apparatus which previously could be detected only by invasive vasography. Ejaculatory duct obstruction is readily amenable to transurethral surgery and, therefore, must be part of the differential diagnosis of the azoospermic individual (Lipshultz & Howards, 1983).

Diagnosis

When the diagnosis of ejaculatory duct obstruction is suspected, transrectal ultrasonography is performed allowing for the accurate assessment of the size of the seminal vesicles and ejaculatory ducts. Abnormalities such as cystic structures or dilatation of the ejaculatory duct can be assessed (Fig. 15.9).

Obstruction of the ejaculatory duct apparatus may be the result of either

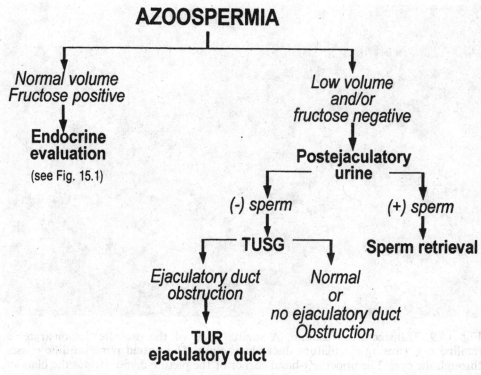

Fig. 15.8. Algorithm for the diagnostic evaluation of low-volume or fructose-negative azoospermia. TUR, transurethral resection; TUSG, transrectal ultrasound (also TRUS or TRUSP).

congenital, embryologic or acquired abnormalities (Shabsigh *et al.*, 1989). Acquired obstructions are more common, and may account for a significant proportion of patients with ejaculatory duct obstruction. This form of obstruction is the result of inflammatory processes of the posterior urethra, such as prostatitis, tuberculosis, and urethritis (Pomerol, 1978; Amelar & Dubin, 1982). Urethral trauma or instrumentation can also produce ejaculatory duct obstruction (Carson, 1984).

Preoperative transrectal ultrasonography will establish the diagnosis of the site of obstruction and will determine whether the obstruction is amenable to transurethral resection. In some cases, the site of obstruction is beyond the confines of the prostate and transurethral resection of the prostate would be of no benefit.

Although vasography has traditionally been utilized to make the diagnosis of ejaculatory duct obstruction, with the advent of ultrasound it is rarely required if the diagnosis is suspected. The utilization of transrectal seminal vesiculography in the diagnosis of ejaculatory duct obstruction is currently being studied (Katz *et al.*, 1994).

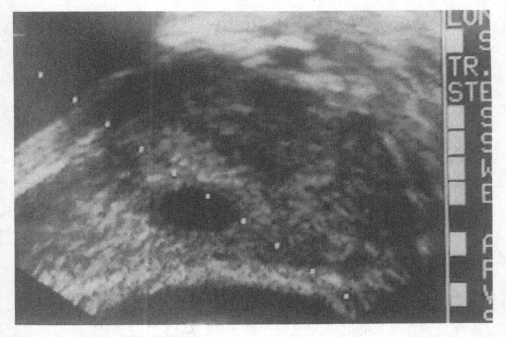

Fig. 15.9. Transrectal ultrasound. A sagittal view of the prostate demonstrates a midline cyst causing ejaculatory duct obstruction. The dotted puncture line passes through the cyst. The upper left-hand corner of the picture demonstrates the bladder (black).

Technique

Transurethral resection (TUR) will remove the obstructed distal ends of the ejaculatory ducts within the posterior portion of the prostate gland lateral to the verumontanum. Although earlier reports describe two separate incisions lateral and proximal to the verumontanum, currently only the proximal portion of the verumontanum is resected (Fig. 15.10) (Carson, 1984; Goldwasser *et al.*, 1985). If the obstruction is distal, the dilated ejaculatory ducts may be entered immediately (Fig. 15.11). If not, the resection is continued toward the bladder neck and posteriorly, until efflux of seminal fluid is seen from the unobstructed ejaculatory ducts.

Complications

The major complications of TUR of the ejaculatory ducts involve injury to adjacent structures. Since most patients undergoing this procedure are young men with small prostates, great care must be taken to avoid injury to the bladder neck, external sphincter or rectal wall. Epididymitis may result from any

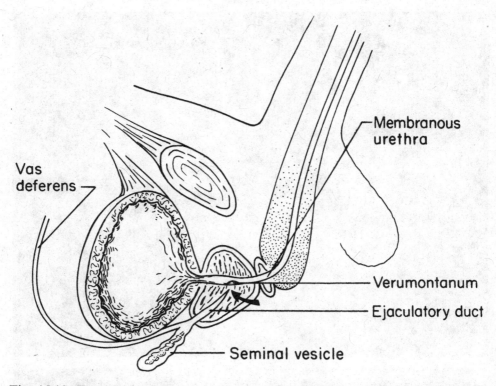

Fig. 15.10. Transurethral resection of ejaculatory duct obstruction. The patient is demonstrated in the lithotomy position. The dilated ejaculatory duct is seen traversing the substance of the prostate and tapering to a point of obstruction proximal to the verumontanum.

urethral instrumentation. Although the incidence of epididymitis after TUR of the ejaculatory ducts has not been reported, it is anticipated that disruption of the normal ejaculatory duct apparatus may be associated with an increased incidence of epididymitis. Many patients experience transient postoperative difficulty with urination. Patients are routinely treated with terazosin for 1 week after surgery. Since there is the potential for fibrosis and reobstruction of the ejaculatory duct, the oligozoospermic patient should be fully apprised of therapeutic options prior to undergoing TUR of the ejaculatory ducts. In the oligozoospermic individual, cryopreservation of semen should be offered.

Results

The prognosis for patients with ejaculatory duct obstruction has been reported to vary with its etiology (Goldwasser *et al.*, 1985). Congenital obstruction treated by transurethral surgery has resulted in normal sperm counts in 71% of

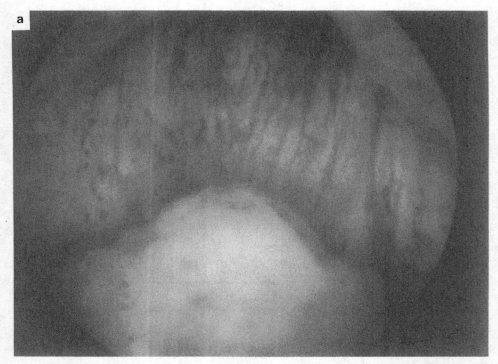

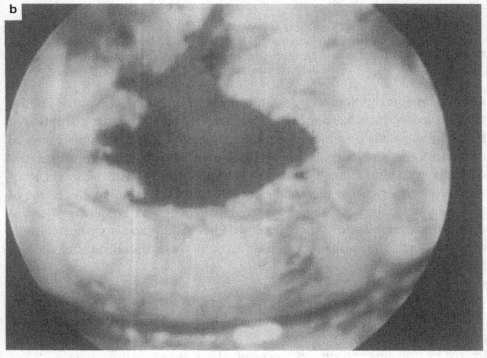

patients, and pregnancies in 57%. Correction of acquired obstruction not associated with genital tract infection has resulted in normal sperm counts in 50%, although no pregnancies resulted.

Of 24 patients treated with TUR of the ejaculatory ducts, 22 have experienced either an increase in semen volume, concentration and/or count (E.I. Mitchnick, N.E. Medley & H.M. Nagler, unpublished data 1994).

Although the response to TUR of ejaculatory duct obstruction is variable it can also be quite dramatic. The patient with low-volume ejaculate and fructose-negative azoospermia may have essentially normal semen parameters postoperatively. Semen parameters may improve sufficiently to allow other therapies to be employed.

Approach to non-reconstructable obstruction

Non-remedial obstructive azoospermia may be due to congenital vasal agenesis, vasal atresia and failed prior reconstruction. These conditions have been particularly troubling to patients and physicians because there is usually normal spermatogenesis (Ross & Prins, 1986). Possible treatment options in these circumstances include creation of an alloplastic spermatocele and microscopic epididymal sperm aspiration.

Alloplastic spermatocele

Sperm may be retrieved from naturally forming spermatoceles which occur in approximately 1% of all men (Ludvik, 1990). There have been many attempts to create a spermatocele utilizing both artificial material and autologous tissues, with minimal success (Kelami *et al.*, 1977; Jimenez-Cruz, 1980; Marmar *et al.*, 1984; Ross & Prins, 1985; Yoshida *et al.*, 1986; Belker *et al.*, 1986).

Recently, Moni & Lalitha (1992) described a procedure called a 'Moni's window'. This procedure created a window between the obstructed epididymal tubule and the tunica vaginalis space. Sperm accumulated in this potential space and were then aspirated for insemination. Four patients underwent a Moni procedure; all had sperm on aspiration and one couple achieved a pregnancy.

Fig. 15.11. Ejaculatory duct obstruction. (a) Cystoscopic view of the verumontanum in a patient with ejaculatory duct obstruction. The bladder neck is visualized beyond the verumontanum. (b) A midline obstructing cyst has been unroofed by transurethral resection. The irregular margin is the edge of prostatic tissue. The resection loupe is seen at the lower margin of the photograph. Courtesy of Anthony J. Thomas, Jr, MD, and Harris M. Nagler, MD from *Atlas of Surgical Management of Male Infertility*, Igaku-Shoin Medical Publishers, New York, 1995.

A pregnancy rate of 7.7% and a term delivery rate of 4.4% after 130 artificial spermatocele implantations in 91 patients was reported by Belker *et al.* (1986) in a review of the literature. Clearly, other techniques are necessary to achieve conception for men with non-remedial obstruction.

Microscopic epididymal sperm aspiration (MESA)

Congenital absence of the vas deferens accounts for approximately 10% of non-iatrogenic obstructive azoospermia (Belker *et al.*, 1986). This anatomic abnormality precludes reconstructive procedures. An alternative approach to creation of an alloplastic spermatocele in these cases is microsurgical epididymal sperm aspiration (MESA), first described in 1985. Although initially utilized in the treatment of patients with secondary obstructive azoospermia (Temple-Smith *et al.*, 1985), Silber *et al.* (1988) reported application of MESA to the treatment of males with bilateral vasal agenesis.

Congenital agenesis of the vas (CAV) has been associated with cystic fibrosis. Kaufman *et al.* (1986) reported an apparently healthy adult with bilateral vasal agenesis who was subsequently diagnosed as having cystic fibrosis. Following this report it was suggested that men with bilateral vasal agenesis should be evaluated for cystic fibrosis (Kaufman *et al.*, 1986). Oates *et al.* (1991) found that 55% of men with CAV were carriers of cystic fibrosis, whereas only 4% of control patients were heterozygous for cystic fibrosis. Recently, Patrizio *et al.* (1992) reported the genetic testing of the parents and offspring of patients with CAV. They demonstrated that 56% of the patients were positive for at least one of the cystic fibrosis mutations, and six of 18 parents of the index cases were also found to be positive. Three of ten offspring born to positive index cases were found to be carriers of cystic fibrosis mutations. These observations emphasize the importance of genetic screening in this group of patients, with genetic evaluation and counseling being essential prior to use of MESA.

Technique

MESA requires the cooperation of the reproductive endocrinologist and urologic surgeon. Oocyte retrieval should precede sperm retrieval since an unnecessary epididymal aspiration when oocyte retrieval fails may cause damage precluding subsequent aspirations. Eleven percent of attempted aspirations yielded no sperm or sperm inadequate for ovum insemination (Belker *et al.*, 1994).

A micropipette system is used to retrieve sperm from the epididymis. Following exposure of the distal epididymis a micropipette, preloaded with

Hepes buffer or a suitable culture medium, is used to puncture the epididymal tubule and aspirate sperm (Schlegel, 1991). Sufficient motile sperm must be retrieved. If motile sperm are not identified, more proximal aspirations are sequentially performed. Standard ovum insemination or micromanipulation is then carried out depending on the characteristics of the sperm recovered. Microsurgical closure of the epididymal tubules minimizes scarring which would perhaps preclude repeat MESA procedures; Belker *et al.* (1994) reported that 12% of 193 MESA attempts were repeat MESA procedures.

Results

The recent results of MESA indicate that epididymal sperm are capable of fertilization *in vitro* (Temple-Smith *et al.*, 1985; Silber *et al.*, 1988, 1990). Silber *et al.* (1990) reported a fertilization rate of 60%, and a clinical pregnancy rate of 31% with MESA. Seven deliveries and three miscarriages were reported for a live birth rate of 21.9% per cycle. Belker *et al.* (1994) reviewed MESA in 219 patients at 22 centers. The overall fertilization rate of this collaborative report was only 33%; the pregnancy rate per center ranged from 9% to 33%.

Micromanipulation techniques have shown that epididymal sperm lacking motility may have fertilization capacity (Olar *et al.*, 1990). Intracytoplasmic sperm injection has currently been applied to MESA procedures and may be useful when only non-motile sperm are recovered.

MESA is an exciting, extremely expensive, labor-intensive new technique which provides a form of therapy for couples with a previously untreatable condition. Couples must undergo appropriate genetic counseling and be aware of the emotional and financial risks before embarking on this form of therapy.

Ejaculatory dysfunction

Ejaculatory failure or the inability to ejaculate may be the consequence of injury from trauma, surgery or medical illnesses to sympathetic pathways involved in ejaculation. Although these abnormalities do not result in anatomic obstruction, they do result in a functional obstruction. Both allo-plastic spermatoceles and sperm aspiration techniques have been employed in the treatment of these individuals (Berger *et al.*, 1985; Bustillo & Rajfer, 1986). Attention has also been directed to the induction of ejaculation by either vibra-tory stimulation (Brindley, 1981) or transrectal electroejaculation techniques (Thomas, 1983; Bennett *et al.*, 1987; Ohl *et al.*, 1989). Sperm may be ejaculated in either an antegrade or retrograde fashion and utilized for insemination or *in vitro* fertilization.

Conclusion

The evaluation and treatment of male factor infertility due to azoospermia relies on the utilization of appropriate diagnostic and therapeutic techniques. A thorough and organized approach will result in the correct diagnosis and the appropriate treatment of the azoospermic male.

References

Amelar, R.D. & Dubin, L. (1975). Vasovasostomy: how effective is it? *Contemp. Gynecol.*, **6**, 36.

Amelar, R.D. & Dubin, L. (1982). Ejaculatory duct obstruction. In *Current Therapy of Infertility*, ed. R.D. Amelar & L. Dubin, p. 80. Trenton: B.C. Decker.

Bayle, H. (1952). Les azoospermies d'origine excretoire. *Bull. Fed. Soc. Gynecol. Obstet.*, **4**, 481.

Belfield, W.T. (1913). Vasotomy: radiography of the seminal duct. *JAMA*, **61**, 1867.

Belker, A.M., Konnak, J.W., Sharlip, I.D. & Thomas, A.J. Jr (1983). Intraoperative observation during vasovasostomy in 334 patients. *J. Urol.*, **129**, 524.

Belker, A.M., Jimenez-Cruz, D.J., Kelami, A. & Wagenknect, L.V. (1986). Alloplastic spermatocele: poor sperm motility in intraoperative epididymal fluid contraindicates prosthesis implantation. *J. Urol.*, **136**, 408.

Belker, A.M., Thomas, A.J. & Fuchs, E.F. (1991). Results of 1469 microsurgical vasovasostomy reversals by the Vasovasostomy Study Group. *J. Urol.*, **145**, 505.

Belker, A.M., Oates, R.D., Goldstein, M., *et al.* (1994). Results in the United States with sperm microaspiration retrieval techniques and assisted reproductive technologies. The sperm microaspiration retrieval techniques study group. *J. Urol.*, **151**, 1255–9.

Bennett, C.J., Ayers, J.W.T., Randolph, J.F., *et al.* (1987). Electroejaculation of paraplegic males followed by pregnancies. *Fertil. Steril.*, **48**, 1070.

Berger, R.E., Muller C., MacIntosh, R., *et al.* (1985). Operative recovery and insemination of vasal sperm: a new and repeatable procedure for the treatment of the anejaculatory infertile male. Abstract 195, AUA meeting, Atlanta, May 1985.

Blaquier, J.A., Cameo, M.S., Dawidowski, A., *et al.* (1989). On the role of epididymal factors in sperm maturation in man. In *Perspectives in Andrology*, ed. M. Serio. New York: Raven Press.

Brindley, G.S. (1981). Reflex ejaculation under vibrancy stimulation in paraplegic men. *Paraplegia*, **19**, 299.

Bustillo, M. & Rajfer, J. (1986). Pregnancy following insemination with sperm aspirated directly from the vas deferens. *Fertil. Steril.*, **46**, 144.

Carson, C.C. (1984). Transurethral resection for ejaculatory duct stenosis and oligospermia. *Fertil. Steril.*, **41**, 482.

Chan, S.L., Lipshultz, L.I. & Schwartzendruber, D. (1984). DNA flow cytometry: a new modality for quantitative analysis of testicular biopsies. *Fertil. Steril.*, **41**, 485.

Charny, C.W. (1940). Testicular biopsy: its value in male sterility. *JAMA*, **115**, 1429.

Coburn, M., Wheeler, T.M. & Lipshultz, L.I. (1986). Cytological examination of testis biopsy specimens. Abstract of American Fertility Society Annual Meeting, Birmingham, Alabama, p. 122. American Fertility Society.

Cohen, M.S. & Warner, R.S. (1979). Needle biopsy of testes: a safe outpatient procedure. *Fertil. Steril.*, **29**, 279.

Cohen, M.S., Frye, S., Warner, R.S. *et al.* (1984). Testicular needle biopsy in diagnosis of infertility. *Urology*, **24**, 439.

Cooper, T.G. (1990). In defense of a function for the human epididymis. *Fertil. Steril.*, **54**, 965.

Dubin, L. & Amelar, R.D. (1971). Etiologic factors in 1294 consecutive cases of male infertility. *Fertil. Steril.*, **22**, 496.

Fallon, B., Miller, R.K. & Gerber, W. (1981). Nonmicroscopic vasovasostomy. *J. Urol.*, **126**, 361.

Fogdestam, I. & Fall, M. (1983). Microsurgical end-to-end and end-to-side epididymovasostomy to correct occlusive azoospermia. *Scand. J. Reconstr. Surg.*, **17**, 137.

Fogdestam, I., Fall, M. & Nilsson, S. (1986). Microsurgical epididymovasostomy in the treatment of occlusive azoospermia. *Fertil. Steril.*, **46**, 925.

Fuchs, E.F., Sharlip, I.D., Belker, A.M. *et al.* (1985). the significance of bilateral proximal vas deferens azoospermia during vasovasostomy. Presented at the American Urology Association 80th Annual Meeting.

Gilbert, P.T. & Beckert, R. (1989). Laser-assisted vasovasostomy. *Lasers Surg. Med.*, **9**, 42.

Goldstein, M. (1992). Surgery of male infertility and other scrotal disorders. In *Campbell's Urology*, vol. 6, ed. P.C. Walsh, A. B. Retik, T.A. Stamey *et al.*, p. 3114. Philadelphia: W.B. Saunders/Harcourt, Brace, Yovanovich.

Goldwasser, B.Z., Weinerth, J.L. & Carson, C.C. III (1985). Ejaculatory duct obstruction: the case for aggressive diagnosis and treatment. *J. Urol.*, **134**, 964.

Gordon, J.A. & Clahassey, E.B. (1978). Evaluation of stricture formation as a complication of vasopuncture and vasography in the guinea pig. *Fertil. Steril.*, **29**, 180.

Hagner, F.R. (1955). The operative treatment of sterility in the male. *JAMA*, **107**, 1851.

Hanley, H.G. (1955). The surgery of male infertility. *Ann. R. Coll. Surg.*, **17**, 159.

Hellstrom, W.J., Tesluk, H., Deitch, A.D., *et al.* (1990). Comparison of flow cytometry to routine testicular biopsy in male infertility. *Fertil. Steril.*, **35**, 321.

Hinrichsen, M.J. & Blaquier, J.A. (1980). Evidence supporting the existence of sperm maturation in the human epididymis. *J. Reprod. Fertil.*, **60**, 291.

Hotchkiss, R.S. (1942). Testicular biopsy in the diagnosis and treatment of sterility in the male. *Bull. N.Y. Acad. Med.*, **18**, 600.

Howards, S.S. (1983). The epididymis, sperm maturation and capacitation. In *Infertility in the Male*, ed. L.I. Lipshultz & S.S. Howards. New York: Churchill Livingstone.

Ibrahim, A.A., Awad, H.A., El-Haggar, S., *et al.* (1977). Bilateral testicular biopsy in men with varicocele. *Fertil. Steril.*, **28**, 663.

Jain, K.K. & Gorisch, W. (1979). Repair of small vessels with the neodymium-YAG laser: a preliminary report. *Surgery*, **85**, 684.

Jiminez-Cruz, J.F. (1980). Artificial spermatocele. *J. Urol.*, **123**, 885.

Katz, D., Mieza, M. & Nagler, H.M. (1994). Ultrasound guided transrectal seminal vesiculography: a new approach to the diagnosis of male reproductive tract abnormalities. Abstract presented at the AUA Annual Meeting, San Francisco, May 1994.

Kaufman, D.G. & Nagler, H.M. (1987). Aspiration flow cytometry of the testes in the evaluation of spermatogenesis in the infertile male. *Fertil. Steril.*, **48**, 287.

Kaufman, D., Schulman, I.I. & Nagler, H.M. (1986). Cystic fibrosis presenting in a 45-year old man with infertility. *J. Urol.*, **136**, 1081.

Keiserman, W.M., Dubin, L. & Amelar, R.D. (1974). A new type of retrograde ejaculation: report of three cases. *Fertil. Steril.*, **25**, 1071.

Kelami, A., Rohloff, D., Affeld, K., *et al.* (1977). Alloplastic spermatocele: insemination from epididymal reservoir. *Urology*, **10**, 310.

Kessler, R. & Freiha, F. (1981). Macroscopic vasovasostomy. *Fertil. Steril.*, **36**, 531.

Krause, I. & Nagler, H.M. (1992). The role of bilateral testicular biopsies in the evaluation of infertile males. Valentines Essay Contest, New York Academy of Medicine.

Lee, H.Y. (1986). A 20-year experience with vasovasostomy. *J. Urol.*, **136**, 413.

Lipshultz, L.I. & Howards, S.S. (1983). Surgical treatment of male infertility. In *Infertility in the Male*, p. 343. New York: Churchill Livingstone.

Lipshultz, L.I., Howards, S.S., McClure, R.D., *et al.* (1990). When and how to do a testis biopsy and vasogram. *Contemp. Urol.*, **7**, 45.

Ludvik, W. (1990). Artificial spermatocele persisting for 14 years. *J. Urol.*, **144**, 992.

Marmar, J.L., DeBenedictis, T.J. & Praiss, D.E. (1984). Clinical experience with an artificial spermatocele. *J. Androl.*, **5**, 304.

McLoughlin, M.G. (1982). Vasoepididymostomy: the role of the microscope. *Can. J. Surg.*, **25**, 41.

Moni, V.N. & Lalitha, P.A. (1992). Moni's window operation: a new surgical technique to create a sperm reservoir in congenital vasal agenesis. *J. Urol.*, **148**, 843.

Montie, J.E. & Stewart, B.H. (1974). Vasovasostomy: past, present, and future. *J. Urol.*, **112**, 111.

Moore, H.D.M., Hartman, T.D. & Pryor, J.P. (1983). Development of the oocyte-penetrating capacity of spermatozoa in the human epididymis. *Int. J. Androl.*, **6**, 310.

Mygind, H.B. (1960). Urogenital tuberculosis in the human male: vesiculographic and urethrographic studies. *Dan. Med. Bull.*, **7**, 13.

Nagler, H.M. & Thomas, A.J. (1987). Testicular biopsy and vasography in the evaluation of male infertility. *Urol. Clin. North Am.*, **14**, 167.

Neiderberger, C., Ross, L.S., Mackenzie, B. Jr, *et al.* (1993). Vasovasostomy in rabbits using fibrin adhesive prepared from a single human source. *J. Urol.*, **149**, 183.

Oates, R.D., Anguiano, A., Milunsky, A., *et al.* (1991). Bilateral congenital absence of the vas (CAV) and cystic fibrosis (CF): a genetic association? Forty-seventh Annual Meeting of the American Fertility Society (Suppl.), abstract 0–008, p. S4.

Ohl, D.A., Bennett, C.J., McCabe, M., *et al.* (1989). Predictors of success in electroejaculation of spinal cord injured men. *J. Urol.*, **142**, 1483.

Olar, T.T., La Nassa, J. & Dickey, R.P. (1990). Fertilization of human oocytes by microinjection of human sperm aspirated from the caput epididymis of an individual with obstructive azoospermia. *J. In Vitro Fertil. Embryo Transf.*, **7**, 160.

Orgebin-Crist, M.C. (1969). Studies of the function of the epididymis. *Biol. Reprod.*, **1**, 155.

Owen, E.R. (1977). Microsurgical vasovasostomy: a reliable vasectomy reversal. *Aust. N.Z. J. Surg.*, **47**, 305.

Ozdiler, E. & Kelami, A. (1981). Microscopical split epididymovasostomy. *Eur. Urol.*, **7**, 81.

Patrizio, P., Asch, R.H., Handelin, B., *et al.* (1992). American Fertility Society Meeting, abstract 0–083.

Paulson, C.A., Espeland, D.H. & Michals, E.L. (1970). Effects of HCG, HMG, HLH and HGH administration on testicular function. In *The Human Testis*, ed. E. Rosenberg & C.A. Paulsen, p. 547. New York: Plenum Press.

Paulson, D.F., Lindsey, C.M. & Anderson, E.E. (1974). Simplified technique for vasography. *Fertil. Steril.*, **25**, 906.

Pfitzer, P., Gilbert, P., Rolz, G., *et al.*, (1982). Flow cytometry of human testicular tissue. *Cytometry*, **3**, 116.

Pomerol, J.M. (1978). Obstruction of the seminal duct. *Int. J. Androl.*, **50** (Suppl. 1).

Posinovec, J. (1976). The necessity for bilateral biopsy in oligo- and azoospermia. *Int. J. Fertil.*, **21**, 189.

Pratt, W.F., Mosher, W.D., Bachrach, C.A., *et al.* (1985). Understanding US fertility: findings from the National Survey of Family Growth, Cycle III. *Pop. Bull.*, **39**, 1.

Quigley, M.R., Bailes, J.E., Kwaan, H.C., Cerullo, L.J., Brown, J.T., Lastre, C. & Monma, D. (1985). Microvascular anastomosis using the milliwatt CO_2 laser. *Laser Surg. Med.*, **5**, 357.

Rajfer, J. & Binder, S. (1989). Use of Biopty gun for transcutaneous testicular biopsies. *J. Urol.*, **142**, 1021.

Redman, J.F. (1982). Clinical experience with vasovasostomy utilizing absorbable intravasal stent. *Urology*, **20**, 59.

Ross, L.S. & Prins, G.S. (1985). Alloplastic spermatoceles: five year experience. *J. Androl.*, **6** (Suppl. 1), 102.

Ross, L.S. & Prins, G. (1986). Alloplastic spermatoceles: a 5-year experience. *J. Urol.*, **136**, 410.

Schlegel, P. (1991). Post Graduate Course, American Urologic Association Meeting, Toronto.

Schlegel, P.N. & Goldstein, M. (1993). Microsurgical vasoepididymostomy: refinements and results. *J. Urol.*, **150**, 1165.

Schoysman, R.J. & Bedford, J.M. (1986). The role of human epididymis in sperm maturation and sperm storage as reflected in the consequences of epididymovasostomy. *Fertil. Steril.*, **476**, 293.

Shabsigh, R., Lerner, S., Fishman, I., *et al.* (1989). The role of transrectal ultrasonography in the diagnosis and management of prostatic and seminal vesicle cysts. *J. Urol.*, **141**, 1206.

Sherins, R.J. (1984). Hypogonadotropic hypogonadism. In *Current Therapy of Infertility 1984–1985*, ed. C.R. Garcia, L. Mastroianni Jr, R.D. Amelar *et al.*, p. 147. Philadelphia: B.C. Decker.

Shessel, F.S., Lynne, C.M. & Politano, V.A. (1981). Use of exteriorized stents in vasovasostomy. *Urology*, **17**, 163.

Silber, S.J. (1977). Microscopic vasectomy reversal. *Fertil. Steril.*, **28**, 11.

Silber, S.J. (1978). Microscopic vasoepididymostomy: specific microanastomosis to the epididymal tubule. *Fertil. Steril.*, **30**, 565.

Silber, S.J. (1979). Epididymal extravasation following vasectomy as a cause for failure of vasectomy reversal. *Fertil. Steril.*, **31**, 309.

Silber, S.J. (1981). Reversal of vasectomy and the treatment of male infertility: role of microsurgery, vasoepididymostomy and pressure-induced change of vasectomy. *Urol. Clin. North Am.*, **8**, 53.

Silber, S.J. (1984). Microsurgery for vasectomy reversal and vasoepididymostomy. *Urology*, **23**, 505.

Silber, S.J. (1989). Results of microsurgical vasoepididymostomy: role of epididymis in sperm maturation. *Hum. Reprod.*, **4**, 298.

Silber, S.J. & Rodriguez-Rigau, L.J. (1981). Quantitative analysis of testicular biopsy: determination of partial obstruction and prediction of sperm count after surgery for obstruction. *Fertil. Steril.*, **36**, 480.

Silber, S.J., Balmaceda, J., Borrero, C., *et al.* (1988). Pregnancy with sperm aspiration from the proximal head of the epididymis: a new treatment for congenital absence of the vas deferens. *Fertil. Steril.*, **50**, 525.

Silber, S.J., Ord, T., Balmaceda, J., Patrizio, P. & Asch, R.H. (1990). Congenital absence of the vas deferens: the fertilization capacity of human epididymal sperm. *N. Engl. J. Med.*, **323**, 1788.

Temple-Smith, P.D., Southwick, G.J., Yates, C.A., *et al.* (1985). Human pregnancy by *in vitro* fertilization (IVF) using sperm aspiration from the epididymis. *J. In Vitro Fertil. Embryo Transf.*, **2**, 119.

Thomas, A.J. (1983). Ejaculatory dysfunction. *Fertil. Steril.*, **14**, 527.

Thomas, A.J. (1984). Vasography. In *Current Therapy of Infertility, 1984–1985*, ed. C.-R. Garcia, L. Mastroianni, R.D. Amelar, *et al.* St Louis: C.V. Mosby.

Thomas, A.J. (1987). Vasoepididymostomy. *Urol. Clin. North Am.*, **14**, 527.

Thorud, E., Clausen, O.P.F. & Abyholm, T. (1980). Fine-needle aspiration biopsies from human testes evaluated by DNA flow cytometry. In *Flow Cytometry IV*, Proceedings of the Fourth International Symposium on Flow Cytometry, Voss, 4–8 June 1979. New York: Columbia University Press.

Wagenknecht, L.V. (1982). Obstruction in the male reproductive tract. In *Treatment of Male Infertility*, ed. J. Brain, W.B. Schill & L. Schwarzstein, p. 221. Berlin: Springer.

Wagenknecht, L.V. (1985). Ten years experience with microsurgical epididymostomy: results and proposition of a new technique. *J. Androl.*, **6**, 26.

Wagenknecht, L.V., Becker, H., Langendorff, H.M., *et al.* (1982). Vasography: clinical and experimental investigations. *Andrologia*, **14**, 182.

Weiss, J.N. & Mellinger, B.C. (1992). Fertility rates with delayed fibrin glue vasovasostomy in rats. *Fertil. Steril.*, **57**, 908.

Yarbro, E.S. & Howards, S.S. (1987). Vasovasostomy. *Urol. Clin. North Am.*, **14**, 515.

Yoshida, H., Miyamoto, K., Yoshida, T., Ogawa, H. & Imamura, K. (1986). Implantation of artificial spermatocele with cup-shaped silicone prosthesis to excretory azoospermia and chemical management of aspirated spermatozoa. *J. Androl.*, **7**, 220–3.

16

White blood cells in semen and their impact on fertility

DEBORAH J. ANDERSON and JOSEPH A. POLITCH

Definition and prevalence of leukocytospermia

Leukocytospermia, also known as leukospermia, pyospermia or pyosemia, is a term used to designate abnormally high concentrations of white blood cells (WBC) in semen (WHO, 1992). The prevalence of leukocytospermia in male infertility patients has varied from 2% to 40%, dependent on the patient population examined and the detection method and threshold value used (Table 16.1). The concentration of seminal WBC used to diagnose leukocytospermia has varied from $\geq 5 \times 10^5$/ml to $\geq 5 \times 10^6$/ml. Comhaire *et al.* (1980) established a cutoff of 1×10^6/ml peroxidase positive polymorpho-nuclear (PMN) leukocytes for diagnosis of male adnexitis. Currently, the World Health Organization (WHO, 1992) recommends the same cutoff for total seminal WBC concentration (PMN leukocytes, macrophages and lymphocytes). When WBC detection techniques are used that measure only a subset of WBC types in semen, underestimation of total WBC numbers in seminal plasma may result. For example, peroxidase tests detect PMN leukocytes but not mononuclear cells. Since these comprise 50–80% of total seminal WBC the total number of leukocytes may be up to twice the number of PMNs detected. Lowering the leukocytospermia threshold value to 5×10^5 PMNs/ml semen provides comparable data to using 1×10^6 total WBC/ml (Politch *et al.*, 1993). Although some studies have demonstrated that individuals with specific seminal WBC concentrations greater than 1×10^6/ml have reduced semen quality and other characteristics associated with subfertility, no study has demonstrated that this seminal WBC threshold (or any other) is critical to human fertility, or to detection of subclinical infection.

Table 16.1 *Prevalence of leukocytospermia in male infertility patients*

Percent prevalence (n)[a]	Detection/ staining method	Type of WBC	Threshold	Country	Reference
24 (300)	Peroxidase	PMN	5×10^5/ml	Netherlands	Endtz (1974)
13 (500)	Peroxidase	PMN	1×10^6/ml	Belgium	Comhaire et al. (1980)
11 (420)	Morphology	All	5×10^6/ml	Germany	Reidel & Semm (1995)
16 (500)	Morphology	All	5×10^6/ml	Germany	Haidl (1990)
23 (179)	Immunohistology	All	1×10^6/ml	USA	Wolff et al. (1990)
38 (280)	Morphology	All	1×10^6/ml	Argentina	Gonzales et al., (1992)
5 (351)	Immunohistology	All	1×10^6/ml	UK	Tomlinson et al. (1992b)
2 (49)	Immunohistology	All	1×10^6/ml	Hong Kong	Kung et al. (1993)
3 (512)	Immunohistology	all	1×10^6/ml	UK	Tomlinson et al. 1993
8 (101)	Immunohistology	All	1×10^6/ml	China	Wang et al. (1994)
7 (1710)	Peroxidase	PMN	1×10^6/ml	USA	Yanushpolsky et al. (1995)

Notes:
[a] *n*, number of subjects in the study.

Characteristics of leukocytospermia

Composition of WBC in semen

The median WBC count in semen from healthy fertile men is 170 000, with a wide range (9000 to over 20 million: Wolff & Anderson, 1988*a*; Harrison *et al.*, 1991). Data from the first quantitative study of WBC populations in semen are shown in Table 16.2. PMNs generally predominate, but numerous macrophages and T lymphocytes can be detected in most semen samples. Studies of leukocytospermia in healthy infertile men and sperm donors demonstrate that elevated numbers of predominantly PMN leukocytes were accompanied by elevated numbers of macrophages and lymphocytes (Wolff & Anderson, 1988*a*). Furthermore, T lymphocytes and macrophages in some leukocytospermic samples express the interleukin 2 (IL-2) receptor or tumor necrosis factor-alpha, respectively, indicating that they are in an activated state (Takahashi *et al.* 1989). WBC in the male urogenital tract may become activated by sperm antigens or products of microorganisms and viruses. Once activated, the WBC could secrete factors that affect reproductive function. Elevated levels of cytokines and reactive oxygen species (ROS), both products of activated WBC, have been detected in semen of infertile men, with adverse effects on sperm function (described below).

Origin of WBC in semen

Semen from vasectomized men usually contains less than one-tenth the number of WBC in normal semen (Olsen & Shields, 1984; Anderson *et al.*, 1991). These data suggest that a majority of WBC in normal semen originate in the testis, rete testis, efferent ducts or epididymis. Few intraepithelial lymphocytes and macrophages have been detected in the normal human prostate (Anderson & Pudney, 1992) although prostatic secretions can contain high levels of WBC in cases of prostatitis (Schaeffer *et al.*, 1981). High levels of WBC ($>10^6$/ml) have also been observed in semen of some vasectomized men, presumably due to subclinical prostatitis or vesiculitis (Anderson *et al.*, 1991). The male genital tract may be differentially affected by the production of immunomodulating factors at various sites within the urogenital tract when inflammation is present (reviewed by Alexander & Anderson, 1987), a function of both the site of inflammation and the activation status of WBC at these various sites. For example, activated WBC and their products when present in the epididymis could have a larger impact on sperm viability and function than activated WBC in the prostate, because sperm are exposed to the epididymal

Table 16.2 *White blood cell subpopulations in the semen of fertile donors and infertility patients*

		Fertile donors	Infertility patients
All white blood cells[a,b]	Detectable in:	17 (100%)	51 (100%)
	Median:	1.7×10^5	1.035×10^6
	Mean±SD:	$1.6 \times 10^6 \pm 4.96 \times 10^6$	$7.2 \times 10^6 \pm 19.6 \times 10^6$
	Range:	$0.09 \times 10^5 - 20.5 \times 10^6$	$0.43 \times 10^5 - 140.6 \times 10^6$
Granulocytes[a]	Detectable in:	17 (100%)	51 (100%)
	Median:	1×10^5	5.4×10^5
	Mean±SD:	$1.35 \times 10^6 \pm 4.8 \times 10^6$	$5.4 \times 10^6 \pm 16.4 \times 10^6$
	Range:	$0.06 \times 10^5 - 19.95 \times 10^6$	$0.32 \times 10^5 - 91.5 \times 10^6$
Monocytes/macrophages	Detectable in:	17 (100%)	51 (100%)
	Median:	0.5×10^5	2.3×10^5
	Mean±SD:	$1.8 \times 10^5 \pm 2.9 \times 10^5$	$9.8 \times 10^5 \pm 1.8 \times 10^6$
	Range:	$0.03 \times 10^5 - 0.998 \times 10^6$	$0.1 \times 10^5 - 8.1 \times 10^6$
CD4+T lymphocytes	Detectable in:	12 (71%)	40 (78%)
	Median:	0.04×10^5	0.14×10^5
	Mean±SD:	$0.09 \times 10^5 \pm 0.13 \times 10^5$	$1.56 \times 10^5 \pm 5.56 \times 10^5$
	Range:	$ND - 0.52 \times 10^5$	$ND - 3.9 \times 10^6$
CD8+T lymphocytes	Detectable in:	9 (53%)	36 (71%)
	Median:	0.02×10^5	0.17×10^5
	Mean±SD:	$0.06 \times 10^5 \pm 0.14 \times 10^5$	$0.86 \times 10^5 \pm 2.1 \times 10^5$
	Range:	$ND - 0.57 \times 10^5$	$ND - 1.3 \times 10^6$
B lymphocytes	Detectable in:	4 (24%)	30 (59%)
	Median:	ND	0.06×10^5
	Mean±SD:	$0.03 \times 10^5 \pm 0.07 \times 10^5$	$0.89 \times 10^5 \pm 4.2 \times 10^5$
	Range:	$ND - 0.25 \times 10^5$	$ND - 2.96 \times 10^6$

Notes:

Adapted from Wolff & Anderson (1988a).

[a] Numbers significantly different between fertile and infertile groups.

[b] Numbers represent cell counts per ejaculate.

ND, not detectable.

environment for extended periods of time and at a different time in their maturation, whereas they are exposed to prostatic factors for a brief period during and after ejaculation.

Etiology of leukocytospermia

Subclinical genital tract infection

The principal etiology of leukocytospermia is subclinical genital tract infection. Primary infections of the reproductive tract enter through the urethra, and can ascend to other sites within the reproductive tract. Systemic infections can spread to the genital tract via WBC (i.e. cytomegalovirus, HIV-1 infection) where they may persist due to the immunologically privileged status of this site (reviewed in Alexander & Anderson, 1987). The most common infections of the male genital tract are *Neisseria gonorrhoea*, *Chlamydia trachomatis*, *Trichomonas vaginalis*, *Ureaplasma urealyticum*, gram-negative enteric bacilli (especially *E. coli*) and the viruses cytomegalovirus (CMV), herpes simplex virus type 2 (HSV-2), human papilloma viruses (HPV), Epstein–Barr virus (EBV), hepatitis B virus (HBV) and the human immunodeficiency viruses (HIV-1 and -2) (Holmes *et al.*, 1990).

Isolation of specific bacterial pathogens associated with leukocytospermia has been unsuccessful (Berger *et al.*, 1982; Hillier *et al.*, 1990). It is technically difficult to culture microorganisms from semen due to toxic effects of seminal plasma, and the high background due to the presence of commensal organisms. New molecular methods such as the polymerase chain reaction are now being applied to quantitate pathogens in semen (Van Voorhis *et al.*, 1991; Witkin *et al.*, 1993; Van den Brule *et al.*, 1993).

Abnormal spermatogenesis

Phagocytic macrophages that have engulfed sperm are common in the male reproductive tract and semen. For many years it has been suggested that these cells scavenge abnormal or dead sperm and play an important role in the normal maintenance of the genital tract. Barratt *et al.* (1990*a*) suggested that leukocytospermia may reflect, in at least some cases, enhanced WBC recruitment and activity in the male urogenital tract as a result of abnormal spermatogenesis or poor sperm viability. Therefore leukocytospermia may be associated with poor semen parameters, but may be a result rather than a cause of male infertility. Abnormally low numbers of WBC are associated with poor fertilizing capacity of sperm in human *in vitro* fertilization attempts (Branigan *et al.*, 1990; Tomlinson *et al.*, 1992*c*).

Other clinical and environmental factors

Close *et al.* (1990) demonstrated that use of cigarettes, alcohol or marijuana can be associated with an increase in WBC concentrations in semen. Cigarette use was significantly associated with increases in seminal WBC, whereas marijuana and alcohol use showed marginally significant elevations of WBC counts in semen. Other factors that could contribute to increased seminal WBC include sexual behavior (especially with anal intercourse), frequency of ejaculation, hygiene practices, partner's use of potentially irritating vaginal products (i.e. nonoxynyl-9), hot baths, vasovasostomy and varicocele.

Methods of detection and quantification of WBC in semen

Round cell counts

The non-sperm cells in the ejaculate are either immature germ cells or WBC (Smith *et al.*, 1989), which must be differentiated by specific stains (see below). These cells, collectively known as 'round cells', can be counted using phase contrast microscopy. Because WBC cannot be distinguished from immature germ cells, and because there is no clear relationship between these types of cells, total round cell counts are of no value for approximating WBC in semen (Politch *et al.*, 1993; Sigman & Lopes, 1993).

Bryan–Leishman or Papanicolaou stains

The Bryan–Leishman and Papanicolaou stains (cf. WHO, 1992), performed on semen smears, are intended to separate WBC from immature germ cells. In particular, PMN leukocytes can be differentiated from spermatids, and lymphocytes/monocytes from secondary spermatocytes. However, these techniques involve a lengthy laboratory preparation and numerous steps, require a highly trained technician to ensure proper assessment of seminal round cells, and do not permit *precise* quantification of WBC.

Immunohistology

Immunohistology (El-Demiry *et al.*, 1986a; Wolff & Anderson, 1988a) enables quantitation of total WBC in semen. Individual subtypes can be enumerated by detecting WBC phenotypic antigens with specific monoclonal antibodies. This approach is considered the 'gold standard' of semen WBC techniques; however, it requires training, and is time-consuming and expensive.

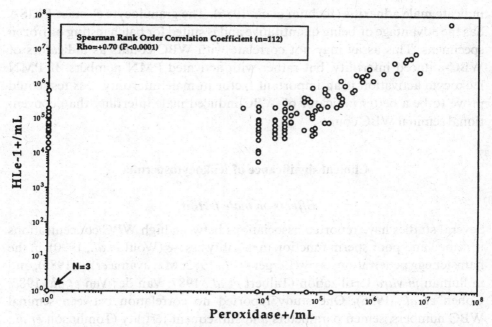

Fig. 16.1. Correlation of concentrations of HLe-1-positive cells and peroxidase-positive cells in semen of 112 men. HLe-1-positive cells were determined by immunohistology and peroxidase-positive cells by a modification of the method of Endtz (1974). (Adapted from Politch *et al.*, 1993.)

Peroxidase tests

Tests of peroxidase (Endtz, 1974; Nahoum & Cardozo, 1980) are easy to perform on wet mounts, inexpensive and reliable. These assays detect the peroxidase enzyme present in PMN leukocytes, but do not detect other WBC in semen. Because PMN leukocytes are the predominant WBC in semen, peroxidase-positive cell concentrations correlate with total WBC counts as detected by immunohistology tests (Fig. 16.1). Different thresholds for leukocytospermia should be used with this test (Politch *et al.*, 1993).

Granulocyte elastase test

Granulocyte elastase, an enzyme specific to PMN leukocytes, is released from activated leukocytes. It has been quantified in human seminal plasma by an enzyme-linked immunosorbent assay (ELISA). Wolff & Anderson (1988*b*) demonstrated good correlation (*r*=0.70) with total WBC concentrations in semen determined by immunohistology. PMN elastase levels above 1000 ng/ml were shown to be diagnostic for leukocytospermia. High levels reportedly indicate male adnexitis (Jochum *et al.*, 1986). The granulocyte elastase ELISA has the advantage of being quantitative and is suited for batch testing of frozen specimens. This assay may not correlate with WBC counts as indicators of WBC-induced infertility, but rather with activated PMN numbers. If PMN leukocyte activation is an important factor in male infertility, this test could prove to be a better indicator of WBC-induced male infertility than conventional seminal WBC counts.

Clinical significance of leukocytospermia

Effects on male fertility

Several studies have reported associations between high WBC concentrations in semen and poor sperm function in motility assays (Wolff *et al.*, 1990), in the hamster egg penetration assay (Berger *et al.*, 1982; Maruyama *et al.*, 1985), and in human *in vitro* fertilization (Talbert *et al.*, 1987; Van der Ven *et al.*, 1987; Cohen *et al.*, 1985). One study reported no correlation between seminal WBC numbers, semen parameters and subsequent fertility (Tomlinson *et al.*, 1993). Most of the specimens included in this study were within the normal range for WBC counts and it did not have adequate power for the leukocytospermia category to conclude that seminal WBCs have no effect on fertility (Yanushpolsky *et al.*, 1994). Additional studies that evaluate WBC groups, and WBC-associated factors (activation markers, cytokines) in conjunction with various markers of sperm function, are clearly needed.

Several WBC products have been shown to be toxic to sperm. Hydrogen peroxide (H_2O_2), free oxygen radicals and reactive nitrogen intermediates are produced by activated macrophages and granulocytes, and are highly toxic to sperm (reviewed in Anderson & Hill, 1988). Cytokines, including gamma-interferon produced by activated T cells, and tumor necrosis factor-alpha produced by activated macrophages, have been shown to adversely affect sperm motility (Hill *et al.*, 1987; Eisermann *et al.*, 1989) and penetration of hamster eggs (Hill *et al.*, 1989). The degree of sperm damage by WBC products could depend on the location of the inflammatory reaction (affecting when the sperm are exposed in their life cycle) and the duration of exposure of sperm to these products. Little is known about cytokine levels in reproductive tissues or semen, or about the effects of these cytokines, tested alone or in combination, on sperm viability and function. Furthermore, cytokines or other WBC products could affect the function of the testis, epididymis, ducts or accessory glands, thereby affecting fertility (Cooper *et al.*, 1990; Wolff *et al.*, 1991; Gonzales *et al.*, 1992).

Relationship with antisperm antibodies

The relationship between seminal WBC and antisperm antibodies is controversial and complex. The presence of antisperm antibodies in both semen and serum of male infertility patients has been associated with infections of the genital tract (Quesada *et al.*, 1968; Witkin & Toth, 1983; Ingerslev *et al.*, 1986; Shahmanesh *et al.*, 1986; Close *et al.*, 1987). However, an association of male genital tract inflammation and antisperm antibodies has not been consistently established. Wolff *et al.* (1990) found no relationship between leukocytospermia (>1 × 10^6 WBC/ml) and the presence of antisperm antibodies. Gonzales *et al.* (1992), and Kortebani *et al.* (1992) reported an increase in the incidence of antisperm antibodies in leukocytospermic men, when accompanied by hypofunction of the seminal vesicles. The incidence of antisperm antibodies in leukocytospermic men with normal seminal vesicles did not differ from that of non-leukocytospermic men. Tomlinson *et al.* (1993) found no relationship between the presence of, or titers of, antisperm antibodies and various WBC types in semen. El-Demiry *et al.* (1986*b*) reported a significant correlation between seminal PMN concentrations and IgG antisperm antibodies in 19 infertility patients. The most consistent relationship between seminal WBC and antisperm antibodies has been demonstrated in men who have undergone vasovasostomy for vasectomy reversal. Witkin & Goldstein (1988) reported a decrease in T suppressor cytotoxic lymphocytes in vasovasostomized men that may be associated with local antisperm antibody production. Under normal conditions, T suppressor cytotoxic lymphocytes are thought to reduce the immune response to sperm in the male genital tract. Vasectomy may disturb T cell regulation, allowing the production of antisperm antibodies. Although this observation has been demonstrated several times in semen (Barratt *et al.*, 1990*b*; Tomlinson *et al.*, 1993) as well as in the testis (El-Demiry *et al.*, 1987), Barratt *et al.* (1990*b*) have shown that antisperm antibodies can be associated with a predominance of seminal T suppressor cytotoxic lymphocytes in men with either vasovasostomy or an undetermined cause of antisperm antibodies.

Treatment of leukocytospermia

Numerous investigators have used antibiotic treatment for leukocytospermia. Sokol *et al.* (1975) administered antibacterial therapy to men with high seminal WBC concentrations, resulting in an improvement in semen quality and fertility after treatment. Haidl (1990) found that combined antiphlogistic and antibiotic treatment improved sperm motility, reduced seminal WBC concentrations, and reduced the number of bacteria in male infertility patients with chronic non-specific genital infection. Branigan *et al.* (1992) reported resolution of leukocytospermia following administration of doxy-cycline, followed by treatment with trimethoprim-sulfamethoxazole. A number of studies have found antibiotic therapy to concomitantly decrease seminal WBC concentrations and improve sperm function in the hamster egg penetration test (Berger *et al.*, 1982; Stenchever *et al.*, 1982; Maruyama *et al.*, 1985). Berger *et al.* (1982) also reported an increase in conceptions with leukocytospermic men treated with antibiotics. Comhaire *et al.* (1986) and Yanushpolsky *et al.* (1995) reported no significant beneficial effect of either doxycycline or trimethoprim–sulfamethoxazole treatment after correcting for the high rate of spontaneous resolution in untreated leukocytospermic men. The acute versus chronic (possibly intermittent) nature of leukocy-tospermia, its relationship to male fertility, and the effects of antibiotic therapy need further study.

Newer strategies to improve sperm function in men with leukocytospermia involve reactive oxygen species (ROS) or reactive nitrogen species (RNS) intermediates. Clinical trials are under way with vitamin E, a ROS scavenger, in patients with high free radical levels in their semen (Tomlinson *et al.*, 1992*a*). Pentoxifylline, a phosphodiesterase inhibitor which increases intra-cellular cAMP levels, has recently been used to enhance sperm motility in asthenozoospermic men (Yovich *et al.*, 1990). This drug may be useful in the treatment of men with leukocytospermia since reactive nitrogen inter-mediates produced by activated granulocytes and macrophages have been shown to decrease cyclic nucleotide levels in spermatozoa (Tomlinson *et al.*, 1992*a*).

Summary

Leukocytospermia, increased concentrations of WBC in seminal plasma, can alter sperm function and lead to infertility. These leukocytes, especially when activated, are capable of releasing cytokines and reactive oxygen species that affect sperm motility, capacitation and fusogenic events, as well as influencing the generation of antisperm antibodies. Diagnosis requires observation of leukocytes in seminal plasma using differential stains, or qualitative or quanti-tative assay of their unique secretory products.

Empirical antibiotic therapy has been recommended by some investigators, with variable reports of efficacy. In addition to removing the WBC from seminal plasma, other recently suggested treatment strategies involve attempts to neutralize their secretory products which have a deleterious effect on sperm function.

References

Aitken, R.J. & West, K.M. (1990). Analysis of the relationship between reactive oxygen species production and leucocyte infiltration in fractions of human semen separated on Percoll gradients. *Int. J. Androl.*, **13**, 433–51.

Alexander, N.J. & Anderson, D.J. (1987). Immunology of semen. *Fertil. Steril.*, **47**, 192–205.

Anderson, D.J. & Hill, J.A. (1988). Cell-mediated immunity and infertility. *Am. J. Reprod. Immunol. Microbiol.*, **17**, 22–30.

Anderson, D.J. & Pudney, J. (1992). Mucosal immune defense against HIV-1 in the male urogenital tract. *Vaccine Res.*, **1**, 143–50.

Anderson, D.J., Politch, J.A., Martinez, A., *et al.* (1991). White blood cells and HIV-1 in semen from vasectomized seropositive men. *Lancet*, **388**, 573–4.

Barratt, C.L.R., Bolton, A.E. & Cooke, I.D. (1990*a*). Functional significance of white blood cells in the male and female reproductive tract. *Hum. Reprod.*, **5**, 639–48.

Barratt, C.L.R., Harrison, P.E., Robinson, A. & Cooke, I.D. (1990*b*). Antisperm antibodies and lymphocyte subsets in semen: not a simple relationship. *Int. J. Androl.*, **13**, 50–8.

Berger, R.E., Karp, L.E., Williamson, R.A., Koehler, J., Moore, D.E. & Holmes, K.K. (1982). The relationship of pyospermia and seminal fluid bacteriology to sperm function as reflected in the sperm penetration assay. *Fertil. Steril.*, **37**, 557–64.

Berger, R.E., Smith, W.D., Critchlow, C.W., Stenchever, M.A., Moore, D.E., Spadoni, L.R. & Holmes, K.K. (1983). Improvement in the sperm penetration (hamster ova) assay (SPA) results after doxycycline treatment of infertile men. *J. Androl.*, **4**, 126–30.

Branigan, E.F., Politch, J.A. & Anderson, D.J. (1990). Correlation of white blood cells (WBC) and immature germ cells (IGC) in human semen with fertilization of mature human oocytes *in vitro*. Presented at the 1990 meeting of the American Fertility Society.

Branigan, E.F., Zarutskie, P.W. & Muller, C.H. (1992). Efficacy of identifying and treating leukocytospermia in couples with idiopathic infertility. Proceedings of the Pacific Coast Fertility Society Meeting, Palm Springs, California.

Close, C.E., Wang, S.P., Roberts, P.L. & Berger, R.E. (1987). The relationship of infection with *Chlamydia trachomatis* to the parameters of male fertility and sperm autoimmunity. *Fertil. Steril.*, **48**, 880–3.

Close, C.E., Roberts, P.L. & Berger, R.E. (1990). Cigarettes, alcohol and marijuana are related to pyospermia in infertile men. *J. Urol.*, **144**, 900–3.

Cohen, J., Edwards, R., Fehilly, C., Fishel, S., Hewitt, J., Purdy, J., Rowland, G., Steptoe, P. & Webster, J. (1985). *In vitro* fertilization: a treatment for male infertility. *Fertil. Steril.*, **43**, 422–32.

Comhaire, F., Verschraegen, G. & Vermeulen, L. (1980). Diagnosis of accessory gland infection and its possible role in male infertility. *Int. J. Androl.*, **3**, 32–4.

Comhaire, F.H., Rowe, P.J. & Farley, T.M. (1986). The effect of doxycycline in infertile couples with male accessory gland infection: a double blind prospective study. *Int. J. Androl.*, **9**, 91–8.

Cooper, T.G., Weidner, W. & Nieschlag, E. (1990). The influence of inflammation of the human male genital tract on secretion of the seminal markers alpha-glucosidase, glycerophosphocholine, carnitine, fructose and citric acid. *Int. J. Androl.*, **13**, 329–36.

Eisermann, J., Register, K.D., Strickler, R.C. & Collins, J.L. (1989). The effect of tumor necrosis factor on human sperm motility *in vitro. J. Androl.*, **10**, 270–4.

El-Demiry, M.I.M., Hargreave, T.B., Busuttil, A., James, K. & Chisholm, G.D. (1986*a*). Identifying leukocytes and leukocyte subpopulations in semen using monoclonal antibody probes. *Urology*, **28**, 492.

El-Demiry, M.I.M., Young, H., Elton, R.A., Hargreave, T.B., James, K. & Chisholm, G.D. (1986*b*). Leucocytes in the ejaculate from fertile and infertile men. *Br. J. Urol.*, **58**, 715–20.

El-Demiry, M.I.M., Hargreave, T.B., Busuttil, A., Elton, R., James, K. & Chisholm, G.D. (1987). Immunocompetent cells in human testis in health and disease. *Fertil. Steril.*, **48**, 470–9.

Endtz, A.W. (1974). A rapid staining method for differentiating granulocytes from 'germinal cells' in Papanicolaou-stained semen. *Acta Cytol.*, **18**, 2–7.

Gonzales, G.F., Kortebani, G. & Mazzolli, A.B. (1992). Leukocytospermia and function of the seminal vesicles on seminal quality. *Fertil. Steril.*, **57**, 1058–65.

Haidl, G. (1990). Macrophages in semen are indicative of chronic epididymal infection. *Arch. Androl.*, **25**, 5–11.

Harrison P.E., Barratt, C.L.R., Robinson, A.J., Kessopoulou, E. & Cooke, I.D. (1991). Detection of white blood cell populations in the ejaculates of fertile men. *J. Reprod. Immunol.*, **19**, 95–8.

Hill, J.A., Haimovici, F., Politch, J.A. & Anderson, D.J. (1987). Effects of soluble products of activated lymphocytes and macrophages (lymphokines and monokines) on human sperm motion parameters. *Fertil. Steril.*, **47**, 460–5.

Hill, J.A., Cohen, J. & Anderson, D.J. (1989). The effects of lymphokines and monokines on human sperm fertilizing ability in the hamster egg penetration test. *Am. J. Obstet. Gynecol.*, **160**, 1154–9.

Hillier, S.L., Rabe, L.K., Muller, C.H., Zarutskie, P., Kurzan, F. & Stenchever, M. (1990). Relationship of bacteriologic characteristics to semen indices in men attending infertility clinic. *Obstet. Gynecol.*, **75**, 800–4.

Holmes, K.K., March, P., Sparling, P.F. & Wiesner, P.J. (eds.) (1990). *Sexually Transmitted Diseases.* New York: McGraw-Hill Information Services Company.

Ingerslev, H.J., Walter, S., Anderson, J.T., Brandenhoff, P., Eldrup, J., Geerdsen, J.P., Scheibel, J., Tromholt, N., Jensen, H.M. & Hjort, T. (1986). A prospective study of antisperm antibody development in acute epididymitis. *J. Urol.*, **136**, 162–4.

Jochum, M., Papst, W. & Schill, W.B. (1986). Granulocyte elastase as a sensitive diagnostic parameter of silent male genital tract inflammation. *Andrologia*, **18**, 415.

Kortebani, G., Gonzales, G.F., Barrera, C. & Mazzolli, A.B. (1992). Leucocyte populations in semen and male accessory gland function: relationship with antisperm antibodies and seminal quality. *Andrologia*, **24**, 197–204.

Kovalski, N.N., deLamirande, E. & Gagnon, C. (1992). Reactive oxygen species generated by human neutrophils inhibit sperm motility: protective effect of seminal plasma and scavengers. *Fertil. Steril.*, **58**, 809–16.

Kung, A.W., Ho, P.C. & Wang, C. (1993). Seminal leucocyte subpopulations and sperm function in fertile and infertile Chinese men. *Int. J. Androl.*, **16**, 189–94.

Maruyama, D.K., Hale, R.W. & Rogers, D.J. (1985). Effects of white blood cells on the *in vitro* penetration of zona-free hamster eggs by human spermatozoa. *J. Androl.*, **6**, 127–35.

Nahoum, C.R.D. & Cardozo, D. (1980). Staining for volumetric count of leukocytes in semen and prostate-vesicular fluid. *Fertil. Steril.*, **34**, 68–9.

Olsen, G.P. & Shields, J.W. (1984). Seminal lymphocytes, plasma and AIDS. *Nature*, **309**, 116.

Politch, J., Wolff, H., Hill, J.A. & Anderson, D.J. (1993). Comparison of methods to enumerate white blood cells in semen. *Fertil. Steril.*, **60**, 372–5.

Quesada, E.M., Dukes, C.D., Deen, G.H. & Franklin, R.R. (1968). Genital infection and sperm agglutinating antibodies in infertile men. *J. Urol.*, **99**, 106–8.

Reidel, H.-H. & Semm, K. (1995). Leucospermia and male fertility. *Arch. Androl.*, **4**, 51–6.

Schaeffer, A.J., Wendel, E.F., Dunn, J.K. & Grayhack, J.T. (1981). Prevalence and significance of prostatic inflammation. *J. Urol.*, **125**, 215–19.

Shahmanesh, M., Stedronska, J. & Hendry, W.F. (1986). Antispermatozoal antibodies in men with urethritis. *Fertil. Steril.*, **46**, 308–11.

Shimoya, K., Matsuzaki, N., Tsutsui, T., Tanighuchi, T., Saji, F. & Tanizawa, O. (1993). Detection of interleukin-8 (IL-8) in seminal plasma and elevated IL-8 in seminal plasma of infertile patients with leukospermia. *Fertil. Steril.*, **59**, 885–8.

Sigman, M. & Lopes, L. (1993). The correlation between round cells and white blood cells in the semen. *J. Urol.*, **149**, 1338–40.

Smith, D.C., Barratt, C.L. & Williams, M.A. (1989). The characterization of non-sperm cells in the ejaculates of fertile men using transmission electron microscopy. *Andrologia*, **21**, 319–33.

Sokol, S., Jacobson, C.B. & Derrick, F.C. (1975). Use of methenamine hippurate in male infertility. *Urology*, **6**, 59–62.

Stenchever, M.A., Spadoni, L.R., Smith, W.D., Karp, L.E., Shy, K.K., Moore, D.E. & Berger, R. (1982). Benefits of the sperm (hamster ova) penetration assay in the evaluation of the infertile couple. *Am. J. Obstet. Gynecol.*, **143**, 91–6.

Takahashi, K., Wolff, H. & Anderson, D.J. (1989). Immunohistologic detection of cytokine production by white blood cells in leukocytospermia semen samples. Presented at American Society for Andrology Annual Meeting, New Orleans, LA, 13–16 April.

Talbert, L.M., *et al.* (1987). Semen parameters and fertilization of human oocytes *in vitro*: a multivariate analysis. *Fertil. Steril.*, **48**, 270–8.

Teague, N.S., Boayarsky, S. & Glenn, J.F. (1971). Interference of human spermatozoa motility by *E. coli*. *Fertil. Steril.*, **22**, 281–92.

Tomlinson, M.J., East, S.J., Barratt, C.L.R., Bolton, A.E. & Cooke, I.D. (1992a). Preliminary communication: possible role of reactive nitrogen intermediates in leucocyte-mediated sperm dysfunction. *Am. J. Reprod. Immunol.*, **27**, 89–92.

Tomlinson, M.J., White, A., Barratt, C.L., Bolton, A.E. & Cooke, I.D. (1992b). The removal of morphologically abnormal sperm forms by phagocytes: a positive role for seminal leukocytes? *Hum. Reprod.*, **7**, 517–22.

Tomlinson, M.J., Barratt, C.L.R., Bolton, A.E., Lenton, E.A., Roberts, H.B. & Cooke, I.D. (1992c). Round cells and sperm fertilizing capacity: the presence of immature germ cells but not seminal leukocytes are associated with reduced success of *in vitro* fertilization. *Fertil. Steril.*, **58**, 1257–9.

Tomlinson, M.J., Barratt, C.L.R. & Cooke, I.D. (1993). Prospective study of leukocytes and leukocyte subpopulation in semen suggest they are not a cause of male infertility. *Fertil. Steril.*, **60**, 1069–75.

Van den Brule, A.J., Hemrika, D.J., Walboomers, J.M., *et al.* (1993). Detection of *Chlamydia trachomatis* in semen of artificial insemination donors by polymerase chain reaction. *Fertil. Steril.*, **59**, 1098–104.

Van der Ven, H.H., Jeyendran, R.S., Perez-Palaez, M., Al-Hasani, S., Diedrich, K. & Krebs, D. (1987). Leukocytospermia and the fertilizing capacity of spermatozoa. *Eur. J. Obstet Gynecol. Reprod. Biol.*, **24**, 49–52.

Van Voorhis, B.J., Martinez, A., Meyer, K. & Anderson, D.J. (1991). Detection of HIV-1 in semen from seropositive men using culture and polymerase chain reaction DNA amplification techniques. *Fertil. Steril.*, **55**, 588–94.

Wang, A.W., Politch, J.A. & Anderson, D.J. (1994). Leukocytospermia in male infertility patients in China. *Andrologia*, **26**, 167–72.

Witkin, S.S. & Goldstein, M. (1988). Reduced levels of T suppressor/cytotoxic lymphocytes in semen from vasovasostomized men: relationship to sperm autoantibodies. *J. Reprod. Immunol.*, **14**, 283–90.

Witkin, S.S. & Toth, A. (1983). Relationship between genital tract infections, sperm antibodies in seminal fluid, and infertility. *Fertil. Steril.*, **40**, 805–8.

Witkin, S.S., Jeremias, J., Grifo, J.A. & Ledger, W.J. (1993). Detection of *Chlamydia trachomatis* in semen by the polyermase chain reaction in male members of infertile couples. *Am. J. Obstet. Gynecol.*, **168**, 1457–62.

Wolff, H. & Anderson, D.J. (1988*a*). Immunohistological characterization and quantitation of leukocyte subpopulations in human semen. *Fertil. Steril.*, **49**, 497–504.

Wolff, H. & Anderson, D.J. (1988*b*). Evaluation of granulocyte elastase as a seminal plasma marker for leukocytospermia. *Fertil. Steril.*, **50**, 129–32.

Wolff, H., Politch, J.A., Martinez, A., Haimovici, F., Hill, J.A. & Anderson, D.J. (1990). Leukocytospermia is associated with poor semen quality. *Fertil. Steril.*, **53**, 523–36.

Wolff, H., Bezold, G., Zebhauser, M. & Mauver, M. (1991). Impact of clinically silent inflammation on male genital tract organs as reflected by biochemical markers in semen. *J. Androl.*, **12**, 331–4.

WHO (1992). *WHO Laboratory Manual for the Examination of Human Semen and Sperm–Cervical Mucus Interaction*, 3rd edn, pp. 8–50. Cambridge: Cambridge University Press.

Yanushpolsky, E.T., Politch, J.A., Hill, J.A. & Anderson, D.J. (1995). Antibiotic therapy and leukocytospermia: a prospective randomized controlled study. *Fertil. Steril.*, **63**, 142–7.

Yovich, J.M., Edirisinghe, W.R., Cummins, J.M. & Yovich, J.L. (1990). Influence of pentoxifylline in severe male factor infertility. *Fertil. Steril.*, **53**, 715.

17

Psychological aspects of male infertility: lifting the shroud of shame

THE LATE BARBARA J. BERG and SUSAN G. MIKESELL

Introduction

Infertility has predominantly been viewed as a female infliction (Menning, 1988). In some cultures, when a couple is unable to conceive the man may be granted a divorce so he can remarry, on the basis of the automatic assumption of female factor infertility (Greil, 1991). The notion that the problem might originate in man is not even entertained. In our own culture, most infertility research has focused on the female reproductive system, resulting in a greater array of diagnostic and treatment alternatives for women than for men (Office of Technology Assessment, 1988). Yet, approximately 35% of infertile couples have trouble conceiving due to male factor infertility and another 20% due to combined male and female factor problems (Menning, 1988). In this chapter we will first address the societal context of male infertility and masculinity, then discuss gender and couple patterns of distress and treatment, how health care professionals can reduce the shame response, secrecy in donor insemination, and male sexual dysfunction.

The male response to infertility

Historically and across cultures, there has been difficulty in accepting the existence of male infertility. The individual and collective denial of male factor infertility may occur for a variety of reasons. Since it takes two to create a pregnancy, the assumption of who is defective may be guided by which gender is easier to label as abnormal. Historically, women have been viewed as being less valuable, less intelligent, and less capable in our male-dominated society (Tavris, 1992). Since the characteristics of the more powerful groups in a society will be viewed as more positive than those of the non-dominant groups (Steinem, 1983), when problems exist they are more likely to be attributed to the less powerful non-dominant group.

The societal inability to assign responsibility for infertility to men reflects both the level of importance that men have in society and the importance that fertility holds for men. Men are valued in most cultures and there are very high standards of behavior they are expected to meet; any signs of weakness or defectiveness are viewed with great concern. The traditional components of male role norms include avoiding femininity, restrictive emotionality, non-relational attitudes toward sexuality, self-reliance, aggression, homophobia, and seeking achievement and status (Levant *et al.*, 1992). There is discomfort when men possess traits typically assigned to women, such as emotionality (e.g., crying), sensitivity, and vulnerability. In the military, new recruits are humiliated by being referred to as 'girls'. In these types of settings, the feminine noun is equated with weakness and defectiveness.

The sexual and fertile capabilities of men are viewed as synonymous. It is not uncommon to hear a layperson refer to an infertile man as being 'impotent', even though sexual functioning and the reproductive quality of the sperm are separate functions. Men are expected to exhibit sexual readiness and prowess at all times (Zilbergeld, 1978), and the most overt indicator of sexual competence is the ability to impregnate a woman. Thus, sexual virility and reproductive capacity are essential to the male's self-image, termed the 'masculine mandate' by Levant (1992). Although conception is dependent upon a certain level of sexual proficiency in the man, male infertility is rarely the result of impaired sexual functioning (Bents, 1985). Clearly, a man who suffers from sexual dysfunctions such as impotence may have difficulty impregnating a female partner. But sexual problems only account for 5–10% of all infertility (Amelar *et al.*, 1977). Indeed, many men can suffer from sexual difficulties yet possess normal fertility.

The closely intertwined image of sexual and fertile capabilities is further woven into our societal views of masculinity. Masculinity is viewed as dependent upon both sexual virility and the ability to impregnate women. If a man suffers from infertility he may also be portrayed as less masculine, and the diagnosis of infertility thus depreciates his masculine self-image. The threat of a male infertility diagnosis can shatter the man's basic sense of self-esteem. Although parenting is less central to the male identity than to the female identity (Chodorow, 1978), fertility or the *ability to reproduce* is very central to the masculine mandate. When men are infertile the sudden realization of this fertility disorder and its perceived effect on masculinity can initiate a shame response which includes feeling deficient and ashamed. Shame can be triggered when a routine sperm count turns into a statement about one's limited capacity to reproduce, a condition that is known by his partner, the doctor, and the laboratory and office personnel. Even if a man has succeeded in previous tests of masculinity, when he is confronted with the test of impregnating his wife, this failure can leave him with a sense of disgrace and shame. The shame can be so profound that men can compensate by fabricating tales of their accomplishments. The bragging about imagined sexual exploits commonly heard among male adolescents attests to the intense need to create a masculine image, even if it is based on fiction. Relevant myths about fertility which evolve from cultural expectations are highlighted in the Appendix.

Many infertile men feel some sense of shame. Men who have had little previous experience with feelings of inadequacy are at greater risk, as are men who are locked into traditional role behavior or who come from families that place a high value on masculinity and progeny. If the man comes from a family in which shame was already present or has experienced an early loss such as a divorce or death of a parent, he may have fewer, or maladaptive coping mechanisms with which to address the feelings of shame. Interpersonal trust as well as one's internal sense of well-being can be powerfully disrupted by the experience of shame. In providing these men with diagnostic and treatment options, it is important to realize that the masculine mandate can make them more vulnerable. Knowing these vulnerabilities can limit the level of shame that infertile men will have to confront. Men who have had the option to express feelings and doubts about their ability or desire to live up to the masculine mandate, and have been supported by other men in their developmental years, will probably experience less shame when exposed to infertility.

Patterns of male and female distress

The infertile man, similar to his female counterpart, finds himself bombarded at times with the same unexpectedly intense feelings. Infertility can represent multiple losses: control over one's life, individual genetic continuity between one's past and future, the joint conception of a child with one's life partner, the physical and emotional satisfactions associated with pregnancy and birth, and the opportunity to parent (Johnston, 1992). These losses are comparable to death and divorce, yet there are no rituals to help men and women cope with this kind of grief (Mahlstedt, 1985). Infertility can negatively interfere with the marriage and other social relationships, especially in advanced stages of treatment (Berg & Wilson, 1991). The person's body image, sexual functioning and basic self-esteem can be disrupted. As detailed above, men, in particular, may perceive that infertility is a threat to their masculinity and their sexual virility which can cause them to lose status. They may feel they have lost the ability to carry on the family name, the genetic lineage, and the achievement of a sense of immortality (Baran & Pannor, 1993). Men worry about their wive's emotional and physical health as well as their own, and may feel the need to be constantly supportive while downplaying their own emotional needs. Infertile men can also experience threats to the typical roles they assume. Men are not accustomed to the role of needing or asking for help since they are often viewed as the one who provides the help. A tendency to be solution-oriented can also quickly become deflated when medical treatment cannot easily provide a solution.

Although most infertility treatment is focused on women, men have found many components of treatment to be stressful, including the semen analysis (Camilleri, 1980; Kentenich *et al.*, 1992; Lalos *et al.*, 1985c), timed intercourse, the postcoital examination (Mahlstedt *et al.*, 1987), the onset of menses, waiting periods (Kentenich *et al.*, 1992) and the diagnosis of infertility (Berger, 1980). Sometimes procedures such as laparoscopy which are performed on their partners are felt to be more distressing than a procedure involving themselves such as semen analysis (Kentenich *et al.*, 1992). Because much of the available treatment is centered on women, the general exclusion of men from the treatment process can make them feel peripheral, unimportant and unnecessary.

When both infertile men and women have been studied, it has been reported that women find infertility to be a problem of greater significance than men (Freeman *et al.*, 1985; Greil *et al.*, 1988). Infertile women have been shown to experience significantly higher levels of depressive symptoms (Daniluk, 1988; Lalos *et al.*, 1985b,d; Mahlstedt *et al.*, 1987), anxiety (Lalos *et al.*, 1985d; Newton *et al.*, 1990), emotional distress (Daniluk, 1988; Lalos *et al.*, 1985b,d; McEwan *et al.*, 1987), and lower self-esteem in comparison with infertile men (Bernstein *et al.*, 1985; Draye *et al.*, 1988; Lalos *et al.*, 1985d).

Other studies have found similarities in the response to distress among infertile men and women. An absence of gender differences has been noted in personality characteristics (Lalos *et al.*, 1985d), psychiatric symptoms (Adler & Boxley, 1985; Draye *et al.*, 1988; Berg *et al.*, 1991), sexual satisfaction (Bernstein *et al.*, 1985; Daniluk, 1988; Berg *et al.*, 1991), and marital adjustment (Adler & Boxley, 1985; Draye *et al.*, 1988; Berg *et al.*, 1991). For example one study showed that both men and women suffered from symptoms of depression and interpersonal sensitivity at comparable rates (Berg *et al.*, 1991). The methodological concerns such as gender differences in self-disclosure and types of distress displayed may need to be addressed before definite conclusions can be drawn about how infertile women function in comparison with infertile men.

Whether infertile men and women experience comparable levels of distress may be less important than examining potential gender differences in the contextual aspects of distress. Berg and colleagues (1991) found that infertile women and men did not differ in their level of distress, but did experience infertility in different ways and attempted different strategies to alleviate distress. These contextual elements of the experience may ultimately be more important to consider in relation to gender than simply whether one gender is more distressed than the other.

Men with the infertility problem feel a greater sense of personal responsibility which in turn is related to greater emotional distress (Berg *et al.*, 1991). Unlike women, men's feelings of loss, stigma, and lowered self-esteem were not present when the man's fertility remained intact (Nachtigall *et al.*, 1992). Regardless of diagnosis, however, all men felt a sense of role failure (Kedem *et al.*, 1990).

Men and women cope differently with the strain of infertility (Mahlstedt, 1985; Harrison *et al.*, 1986; Draye *et al.*, 1988; Takefman *et al.*, 1990; Berg *et al.*, 1991). Women are more prone to discuss infertility, and to disclose infertility to a wider range of acquaintances (Berg *et al.*, 1991). Women also engage in a greater degree of information-seeking (e.g., reading about infertility) (Berg *et al.*, 1991) and seek solace in support group formats in greater numbers than men (McCartney & Wada, 1990).

Couples out of step: dyadic patterns

Clinicians have noted that differences in coping styles between a husband and wife can be a source of contention in the couple. Men often cope with the strain of infertility by keeping it to themselves, while women are more prone to talk about their distress (Mahlstedt, 1985). Although psychological research on infertile couples has often studied both members of the couple, researchers have failed to analyze dyadic patterns adequately. More commonly, the average male score on a test instrument is compared with the average female score to determine the existence of gender differences.

Berg & Wilson (1993) separated their sample of infertile couples into four groups based upon which spouse(s) experienced distress: (1) both non-distressed (33%), (2) male distressed (18%), (3) female distressed (22%), and (4) both distressed (27%). Most couples (60%) were experiencing parallel functioning, with both partners being either distressed or non-distressed. The remainder of the sample represented couples in complementary patterns with one partner distressed and the other functioning normally. Although it is assumed that the prevalent couple pattern has women distressed while men are not, this assumption leads professionals to ignore the majority of infertile couples.

Infertile women often feel that their husbands are equally interested in having children as they are (van Keep & Schmidt-Elmendorff, 1975; Callan & Hennessey, 1988). It is apparent, however, that the desire to have children is often greater among women (van Keep & Schmidt-Elmendorff, 1975; Johnston *et al.*, 1987; Berg *et al.*, 1991). Those couples who have greater concordance in their desire to have children tend to have more successful marriages (Ulbrich *et al.*, 1990).

Infertile men and the treatment process

Men are more reluctant to enter the treatment process for infertility. When the couple is unable to conceive, it is usually the woman who initiates discussion about the possibility of infertility with her partner (Lalos *et al.*, 1985c; Greil *et al.*, 1988) encouraging an exploration of medical options in her quest to have a biological child (Morse & Dennerstein, 1985; Draye *et al.*, 1988). The initial medical contact is more likely to be the woman's gynecologist (Office of Technology Assessment, 1988). After the initial medical contact, women continue to take the leadership role in treatment (Greil, 1991).

Numerous factors might explain this gender-based pattern of treatment utilization. These may include a closer relationship between the woman and the gynecologist whom she sees on a regular basis, the result of women feeling more comfortable with the patient role, a greater willingness to admit to problems of this nature, or perhaps to assumptions that the infertility problem must be with the woman. Assumptions of female factor infertility can be the result of believing the myth of infertility as a 'female condition' but, more importantly, the primary force behind the focus on the woman may result from an underlying reluctance to uncover a male factor infertility problem.

As described above, men can find the prospect of being diagnosed as infertile to be quite threatening (Shapiro, 1988). One obstetrician-gynecologist reported that 26% of the men who presented with their female partners for an infertility evaluation refused the semen analysis (Camilleri, 1980). Yet, of the men who were examined in this study, 65% had semen that could be considered moderately or severely defective. In another study, a majority of men developed 'impotence' after receiving a male factor diagnosis (Berger, 1980). The stigma and shame associated with male infertility is perceived to be so great that some (fertile) partners of infertile men have been reported to assume a courtesy stigma. In these cases the woman preferred that others believe the infertility was her difficulty instead of her male partner's (Berger, 1980; Miall, 1986). Women may feel they can cope better with the infertility diagnosis.

Table 17.1   *Methods for reducing feelings of shame during the treatment of male infertility*

Collection of the semen sample
1. Make the option of home collection available.
2. Inform the man that it is common to find this process uncomfortable.
3. Provide a private locked collection room.
4. Keep requests for semen specimens to a minimum.

Provision of results
1. Tell the man directly about the results of his semen analysis.
2. Validate his feelings of disappointment and inform him that most people want biological children.
3. Help the couple express disappointment in constructive ways.
4. Assist the woman in being supportive of his loss feelings without negating her desire for a pregnancy.
5. Let the couple have adequate time to absorb the information about his infertility before pursuing donor insemination.
6. Remember that encouragement of secrecy promotes a shame response.

Treatment
1. Make the man feel welcome to attend any medical appointment whether his presence is required or not, especially during his partner's insemination with donor sperm.

Language
1. Avoid any terminology that is derogatory. If discussing sexual dysfunction, use the diagnostic terms 'male erectile disorder' instead of 'impotence' and 'inhibited male orgasm' instead of 'retarded ejaculation' or 'ejaculatory incompetence'.

Reducing the shame response invoked by treatment

If the shame that men are guarding against can be addressed directly in the process of infertility treatment, men may have a more successful experience in managing this challenge to their masculinity. There are four opportunities in the evaluation and treatment of male infertility for reduction of the shame response: the collection of sperm, the provision of results, treatment, and language (Table 17.1). With sperm collection it is important to be aware that the request for a sperm sample is routine only to the medical staff, not to the man. Men need to be informed that other men often find this procedure to be uncomfortable. If home collection is an option, this should be mentioned early, and the man offered a choice of which setting would be more comfortable for him. Men need to have their privacy respected as much as possible by having the collection room located in a place that is not readily observable, particularly by the staff who are most aware of its purpose. Public bathrooms should never be used. Men should also be given the option of having their partners with them instead of having to rely upon pornography. With each additional request for a semen specimen, the potential for anxiety and shame can rise. Thus, requests for sperm samples should be kept to a minimum in order to form a diagnosis and treatment plan.

The man should be told *directly* the results of the semen analysis. It is not uncommon for positive or negative results from the semen analysis to be given to the man's female partner. This circumventing of direct communication to the man about his bodily functions is disrespectful of his feelings and can further marginalize the man's role in the treatment process. Direct communication of the results allows for the opportunity to answer questions, refute misconceptions, and to listen to the man's feelings.

Donor insemination should not be presented as the next step in the treatment process at the time the diagnosis is disclosed, since it involves major emotional, ethical, and moral decision-making, and is not an actual cure for infertility (Johnston, 1992). Nor should donor insemination be encouraged as a method to hide the man's infertility.

Men need to be included as much as possible even if their attendance is not medically necessary. In the case of artificial donor insemination, the man needs to be welcomed and encouraged to attend the inseminations. The majority of couples report that the male partner's presence at the insemination was positive (Klock & Maier, 1991). When the infertile man has been involved in the insemination procedure, it appeared to enhance his subsequent fathering response (Rubin, 1965).

Reassurance needs to be given whether or not the man overtly expresses his emotions and thoughts. It is important to not assume that a calm, unexpressive man is feeling no shame, and to prepare the man for potential reactions to the infertility diagnosis. Phrases that can be used include: 'I know this is difficult to hear', 'This might come as a shock; most people are surprised when they find they have fertility problems' or 'Most people want to have their own biological child and it is natural to be disappointed.' Couples can be helped to express disappointment in constructive ways. The woman's anger about the infertility needs to be directed away from her husband. He might want to share with her his understanding of the disappointment she must feel about being deprived of pregnancy with his child. The woman can be supportive of her partner's pain, loss, and grief, and still desire a pregnancy. The desire for pregnancy does not have to be submerged in order to be supportive.

It is natural for men to want to repress the affect of shame and the experiences that induce it. This makes health care professionals more likely to miss shame when assessing the man's psychological reactions. The affect of shame can be identified through the content of the man's discourse and emotional reactions.

Donor insemination* and the issue of secrecy

'Total secrecy involved in donor insemination inhibits the working through of conflicts about infertility and donor insemination itself' (Berger, 1980, p. 1047)

Since there are comparatively few treatment alternatives available for infertile men (Office of Technology of Assessment, 1988), the option of utilizing donor sperm exists as one of the principal options. Certain male factor problems such as azoospermia, or severe oligozoospermia can be circumvented by inseminating sperm from a fertile donor into the infertile man's female partner. If successful, the infertile couple can proceed to share the pregnancy, delivery, and childrearing experiences similar to fertile couples. The infertile man can become the social father while the woman is both a biological and social parent.

The psychological complexity of donor insemination has been circumvented through the encouragement of secrecy and denial by health care professionals as a means for dealing with the psychological, legal, and ethical ramifications of this form of third party reproduction. With little examination of the consequences, the practice of anonymity was developed in the United States to protect the couple, offspring, donor, and medical profession (Mahlstedt & Probasco, 1991). In a recent survey, 56% of reproductive endocrinologists did not recommend disclosure, even to the offspring (Leiblum & Hamkins, 1992). The infertile couple has often been instructed to rear the donor child as a biological child without sharing the circumstances of the child's conception with anyone, including the child, the woman's obstetrician, or the child's pediatrician. However, this secrecy may avoid the difficult issues raised by the husband's infertility. Assurances that once conception occurs donor involvement will be forgotten or irrelevant may not only be difficult to achieve, but may inhibit examination of how third party reproduction affects all of those concerned (Mahlstedt & Greenfield, 1989).

The majority of heterosexual couples pursuing donor insemination adopt a policy of secrecy (Berger, 1980; Klock, 1993). The reasons for secrecy vary from 'It's no one's business' (Berger, 1980), protecting the child or not complicating their life unnecessarily, 'We don't want the child to feel different' (Berger, 1980; Rowland, 1985; Klock & Maier, 1991), to protecting the father from social stigma and loss of self-esteem (Rowland, 1985; David *et al.*, 1988). Avoiding possible damage to the father–child relationship is also a reason for secrecy (Rowland, 1985; Klock & Maier, 1991). Many couples have intercourse

---

* The term donor insemination will be used instead of therapeutic donor insemination (TDI). Since donor insemination is not therapeutic to the infertile man or his partner, this terminology acts to conceal the true nature of this alternative.

following the insemination, reasoning that the husband could indeed be the biological father (Klock & Maier, 1991). These attempts at intercourse may suggest that the couple is having difficulty accepting the reality of donor insemination as a method of family building. Many of the initial reasons given for secrecy may appear to center on the child's best interests, but upon repeated questioning, couples admitted that secrecy actually served to hide the husband's infertility (Berger, 1980; Brand, 1987). Alternatively, couples who told their offspring, felt the child 'had a right to know' and indicated that they did not want the child to find out from anyone else about their origins – a distinct possibility because most parents tell someone (Klock & Maier, 1991).

Secrecy provides the fertile ground in which to cultivate feelings of shame. The very nature of secretiveness suggests that whatever is held secret has the power to invoke shame or hurt if the secret were known. The encouragement of secrecy with donor insemination is more likely to communicate societal disapproval of male infertility as well as the donor insemination process and lead to a shame response rather than to reduce distress. Secrecy creates unnecessary estrangements, causes the loss of potential support from family, friends, and professionals (Karpel, 1980; Sokoloff, 1987), and makes it all the more difficult for couples to seek appropriate help when the family has later difficulties (Gerstel, 1963). We have discovered that the policies of denial, repression, and secrecy were not only ineffective in reducing distress but can inadvertently lead to increased distress. Alternatively, disclosure about infertility can be therapeutic in that it can help relieve anxiety, restore self-esteem, and help to renegotiate personal perceptions of infertility (Miall, 1986).

If the policy of secrecy were to be abandoned, an unstated fear is the sector of untold numbers of donor offspring searching for their donor parents. Since the donor offspring are related biologically to their social mother, there is probably less likelihood that they would even want to search out their other genetic parent. Interestingly, the majority of sperm donors (60%) who participate on conditions of anonymity, do not object to having the offspring contact them when they have reached age 18 years (Rowland, 1985; Mahlstedt & Probasco, 1991).

Given the far-reaching personal implications of pursuing donor insemination, many have emphasised that couples should allow adequate time to reach the decision removed from the trauma of diagnosis (Berger, 1980; Ledward *et al.*, 1982; Mahlstedt & Greenfield, 1989; Baran & Pannor, 1993). If a couple proceeds with donor insemination immediately after receiving the male factor diagnosis, they may not have had adequate time to assimilate the diagnosis, grieve for their lack of ability to have a biological child together, and make a joint decision about what options to best pursue as a couple. The offer of anonymous donor insemination may be accepted quickly as an alternative because it protects the cultural position for the man. In other words, by all outside appearances he has passed the test of impregnating his wife as long as the secret is kept. Some couples naturally delay their decision for several months and may not even be consciously aware of why they are doing so (Berger, 1980). In his small sample, Berger (1980) found that the couples who delayed pursuing insemination experienced better adjustment than those who pursued it closer to the time of receiving the diagnosis. Enforcing a 3 or 4 months delay before initiating donor insemination may therefore be prudent. There is a need for men to mourn their infertility before attempting donor insemination in order to prevent future adjustment difficulties (Watters & Sousa-Poza, 1966; Berger, 1980; Notman, 1983; Baran & Pannor, 1993). If donor insemination is pursued when the man is ambivalent about this method of having a child, there is the potential that he will withdraw from, or reject, the donor child.

If the infertile man has not resolved his feelings about the impact of infertility upon his masculinity, the donor child can serve as a painful reminder of his perceived 'lack of manhood'. Many men will become over-focused on their work, which can allow them to excel in one area of the masculine mandate, but may also serve to avoid an emotional connection with the donor child (Gerstel, 1963; Watters & Sousa-Poza, 1966). Donor insemination can shift the power balance, thus causing subsequent difficulties in the marital relationship (Rowland, 1985; Sokoloff, 1987; Baran & Pannor, 1993). For some men, having their partner impregnated with another man's sperm is the symbolic equivalent of infidelity (Sokoloff, 1987; Baran & Pannor, 1993). Although they are intellectually cognizant that the procedure is done in a medical office with no sexual contact, the feelings of adultery may be too difficult for the man to overcome. Many of these couples appear to be functioning normally on the surface but many of the unresolved issues around donor insemination can be harmful to family relationships (Baran & Pannor, 1993). Marital counseling may be indicated in these circumstances.

It is the responsibility of medical professionals working in this field to prevent the occurrence of adjustment problems, since couples will have little understanding about the psychological ramifications with this method of reproduction. Couples should have a consultation with a mental health professional who is familiar with the field of the reproductive technologies before beginning donor insemination (Stewart *et al.*, 1982; Micioni *et al.*, 1987; Edelman, 1989; Klock, 1993). There are varying ideas about the purpose of such a consultation, with some emphasizing the need to screen out couples with compromised psychological functioning, while others stress the need to assist couples in the decision-making process, playing an essentially supportive and advocacy role. Some clinics have a mental health professional as an integral part of the treatment team (Nijs & Rouffa, 1975), since it is unusual for reproductive health care professionals to have the time or expertise to assist couples in this difficult decision-making process.

Men and mental health treatment

Although both men (95%) and women (98%) agree that there is a need for psychological assistance with infertility, a much smaller percentage of men (54%) than women (72%) would personally be willing to avail themselves of such services (Daniluk, 1988). Many men (31%) felt that psychological help would be of the greatest benefit immediately following the diagnosis, and most men (76%) preferred couples therapy to individual or group formats. Although the overwhelming majority (91%) of donor insemination couples reported no psychological consultations, most (82%) felt counseling should be available, and 39% even thought a psychological consultation should be mandatory before pursuing donor insemination (Klock & Maier, 1991).

Women are more involved in infertility support groups (Kentenich, *et al.*, 1992). In general, men appear reluctant to attend meetings and feel uncomfortable revealing emotions to others, particularly strangers (Lentner & Glazer, 1991). Participants of support groups find them helpful for a variety of reasons. Women expect to be able to express their emotions to someone who would understand while men anticipated that they would obtain practical information. However, once there, men who attended support groups found them as beneficial as did women (Lentner & Glazer, 1991).

Sexual dysfunction

Sexual problems in infertile couples have been described (Mai *et al.*, 1972; Elstein, 1975; Drake & Grunert, 1979). However, the rates of sexual dysfunction may not be any higher in the infertile than in the normal population (Keye & Deneris, 1982/3). Many investigators have demonstrated that sexual problems are often iatrogenic (Bullock, 1974; Elstein, 1975; Walker, 1978; Drake & Grunert, 1979; Berger, 1980), that is, they are initiated by the discovery of infertility or result from the pressures of treatment. Clearly, most sexual problems are the result of infertility rather than its cause (Drake & Grunert, 1979).

Infertility can mistakenly be confounded with a disorder of sexual functioning. The myth of infertility as reflecting a sexual disorder has been challenged by many researchers and activists (Menning, 1988). In the majority of cases, the presence of infertility does not reflect any difficulties in the couple's ability to maintain a normal sexual relationship. However, there will be a percentage of infertile couples who experience sexual dysfunction. For some, the sexual problem may be a primary determinate of the couple's difficulty achieving conception. Camilleri (1980) found that, among 332 infertile couples, two women were still virgins. In a series of 1294 couples, 5.5% of couples had sexual problems as a primary cause of infertility (Dubin & Amelar, 1971). Sexual dysfunctions such as hypoactive sexual desire disorder, sexual aversion disorder, male erectile disorder, premature ejaculation, inhibited male orgasm, vaginismus, and dyspareunia all have the potential to prevent the normal and frequent heterosexual intercourse which is necessary for conception to occur.

In one study the majority (63%) of 16 couples experienced a temporary period of 'impotence' immediately following the diagnosis of male factor infertility which lasted over a month (Berger, 1980). Drake & Grunert (1979) found that 10% of women scheduled for a routine postcoital examination demonstrated some degree of mid-cycle sexual dysfunction. The stress of a postcoital examination is considerable in that not only is intercourse prescribed at a particular time but the couple's performance is evaluated afterwards. Five couples of 51 experienced acute sexual dysfunctions primarily during the woman's ovulatory period (mid-cycle) but reported no history of sexual problems prior to the diagnosis of infertility. Three of these five couples experienced inhibited male orgasm while two complained of male erectile dysfunction. Keye and Deneris (1982/3) found that women feel an increased desire at mid-cycle, while this increasing demand for coitus corresponded to decreased libido in their husbands.

A detailed sexual history is thus necessary to uncover sexual problems which might be primary or secondary to infertility. During questioning about sexual function, it is ideal to query each partner privately as well as together since this provides each person with an opportunity to raise questions without worrying about the reaction of their partner (Walker, 1978). When sexual problems are present, organic etiological factors must be excluded first. If a man experiences an erectile disorder only with his partner but not during masturbation, this suggests that the erectile disorder is due to psychological factors. Physician's can provide normative information about sexuality in order to refute common myths (Walker, 1978), counsel the patient to avoid harmful substances such as alcohol, alter medications which have a deleterious effect on sexual functioning (Keye, 1984), and provide basic information on the anatomy and physiology of sexual response, reproductive physiology and coital techniques. Flexibility needs to be supported so that the couple's desire for a biological child is balanced with their needs in other areas.

All discussions of sexuality require sympathetic non-judgmental, and unhurried attitude on the part of the health care professional (Elstein, 1975; Walker, 1978). Men who are experiencing mild and acute sexual dysfunction can be reassured that this is common and often the result of pressures involved with treatment, and that the problem will resolve without specific intervention. However, if the presence of a sexual dysfunction has led to pronounced anxiety about future sexual functioning, self-imposed performance pressure might be sufficient to maintain the sexual problem indefinitely (Masters & Johnson, 1970). The couple might want to consider taking a 'vacation' from the treatment process, or trying to re-focus their sexual relations towards the expression of affection rather than 'baby-making' (Drake & Grunert, 1979). The health care professional should make an effort to reduce performance expectations (e.g., semen analyses, postcoital examinations) when sexual functioning is affected by the treatment process (Elstein, 1975). Some psychological-based factors might be more difficult to treat than others, and require referral to a mental health professional. An underlying depression or past sexual trauma will be more complicated to resolve than transitory performance pressure.

When required, referral to a sex therapist can be a difficult process for men, since it is an overt admission that they have a sexual dysfunction. It is important to reassure the couple that sexual dysfunctions are common and often can be resolved with a short period of therapy. Approximately 50% of men will experience transient difficulties with achieving or maintaining an erection in their lifetime (Kaplan, 1974). Some couples may fear that sex therapy will be a lengthy and costly endeavor, with a low likelihood of success. However, the typical length of sex therapy is only 2–6 months, with encouraging rates of success (Kilmann & Mills, 1983). If the man refuses referral to a mental health professional, it may be helpful to suggest reading a book such as *Male Sexuality: A Guide to Sexual Fulfillment* (Zilbergeld, 1978), which discusses common male sexual dysfunctions and gives specific recommendations of helpful exercises to overcome their difficulties. A self-help strategy will probably not be as successful as a tailored treatment approach which is guided by a sex therapist, although it is the best alternative if the man is unwilling to undergo therapy.

Conclusions

Infertility can be a profound and troubling experience for men. Although they may not see parenting as central to their identity, the masculine mandate with which all men are expected to comply is dependent upon the ability to reproduce. When men do not fulfill the requirements of this mandate, they can experience shame and fear rejection from others because of their perceived shortcomings. The confounding of reproductive and sexual potency (Bents, 1985) has furthered the sense of shame that men can feel when diagnosed with infertility because they are often wrongly viewed as sexually inadequate. Recognition of these issues will assist the reproductive health practitioner in best serving the patient with male infertility. Especially important in this regard are the issues involving donor insemination.

Although many of the recommendations made in this chapter may induce some discomfort in medical professionals who have been practicing the policies which were directly questioned, these issues should be carefully reconsidered. While the policies of secrecy and anonymity may be challenged, the good intentions of health care professionals are not. A mental health perspective provides a different way of looking at the issues and understanding the outcomes.

Appendix. Myths about male infertility

Myth 1
Male infertility is an indication of problems in sexual functioning and a loss of masculinity.
Fact 1
Infertility is not synonymous with sexual dysfunction or lessened masculinity. If sexual problems or doubts about masculinity occur, it is more likely a result of anxiety and shame about fear of rejection for not living up to cultural and personal expectations.

Myth 2
Men do not have a need to reproduce that is comparable to women.
Fact 2
Although men may have different reasons from women for wanting biological children, men in our society have a socially proscribed need to beget children. In our culture, fertility is a required part of the masculine mandate.

Myth 3
Most men will be devastated if their infertility is known to others, particularly other men.
Fact 3
The knowledge of infertility is not the cause of the feelings of devastation, it is the sense of rejection by others that is expected to occur.

Myth 4
Men are unable to address the feelings accompanying a diagnosis of male infertility.

Fact 4
Men have the feelings, although they may need help in finding the language to express the feelings they experience. Men will have the capability to deal with loss if they are given the time, opportunity, and assistance needed.

Myth 5
Most infertile men need to maintain secrecy about their diagnosis and the option of donor insemination.
Fact 5
Men want to be authentic. If the environment supports the resolution of infertility loss and the integration of male reproductive dysfunction into the man's redefinition of his masculinity without the induction of shame he will feel less of a need to maintain secrecy.

Myth 6
A pregnancy following donor insemination eliminates the need for the man to mourn his loss of a biological child.
Fact 6
Suggesting that giving birth to a biological child with half the couple's genes is a 'treatment' for male infertility, as opposed to a partial adoption, interferes with the man's mourning for the loss of his biological child and his inherent expectation to reproduce.

References

Adler, J.D. & Boxley, R.L. (1985). The psychological reactions to infertility: sex roles and coping styles. *Sex Roles*, **12**, 271–9.

Amelar, R.D., Dubin, L. & Walsch, P.C. (1977). *Male Infertility*. Philadelphia: W.B. Saunders.

Amuzu, B., Laxova, R. & Shapiro, S.S. (1990). Pregnancy outcome, health of children, and family adjustment after donor insemination. *Obstet. Gynecol.*, **75**, 899–905.

Baran, A. & Pannor, R. (1993). *Lethal Secrets: The Psychology of Donor Insemination*. New York: Amistad.

Bents, H. (1985). Psychology of male infertility: a literature survey. *Int. J. Androl.*, **8**, 325–36.

Berg, B.J. & Wilson, J.F. (1991). Psychological functioning across stages of treatment for infertility. *J. Behav. Med.*, **14**, 11–16.

Berg, B.J., Wilson, J.F. & Weingartner, P.J. (1991). Psychological sequelae of infertility treatment: the role of gender and sex-role identification. *Soc. Sci. Med.*, **33**, 1071–80.

Berger, D.M. (1980). Couples' reactions to male infertility and donor insemination. *Am. J. Psychiatry*, **137**, 1047–9.

Bernstein, J., Potts, N. & Mattox, J.H. (1985). Assessment of psychological dysfunction associated with infertility. *J. Obstet. Gynecol. Neonatal Nursing*, **14**, 63–6.

Brand, H.J. (1987). Complexity of motivation for artificial insemination by donor. *Psychol. Rep.*, **60**, 951–5.

Bullock, J.L. (1974). Iatrogenic impotence in an infertility clinic: illustrative case. *Am. J. Obstet. Gynecol.*, **124**, 476–8.

Callan, V.J. & Hennessey, J.F. (1988). The psychological adjustment of women experiencing infertility. *Br. J. Med. Psychol.*, **61**, 137–40.

Camilleri, A.P. (1980). A realistic approach to infertility. *The Practitioner*, **224**, 835–7.

Chodorow, N. (1978). *The Reproduction of Mothering: Psychoanalysis and the Sociology of Gender*. Berkeley: University of California Press.

Clayton, C.E. & Kovacs, G.T. (1982). AID offspring: initial follow-up study of 50 couples. *Med. J. Aust.*, **1**(8), 338–9.

Daniluk, J.C. (1988). Infertility: intrapersonal and interpersonal impact. *Fertil. Steril.*, **49**, 982–90.

David, D., Soule, M., Mayaux, M.J., Guimard-Moscato, M.L., Czyglik, F., Levy, A., Cahen, F., Bissery, J., Noel, J., Schwartz, D. & David, G. (1988). Insemination artificielle avec donneur. *J. Gynecol. Obstet. Biol. Reprod.*, **17**, 67–74.

Drake, T.S. & Grunert, G.M. (1979). A cyclic pattern of sexual dysfunction in the infertility investigation. *Fertil. Steril.*, **32**, 542–5.

Draye, M.A., Woods, N.F. & Mitchell, E. (1988). Coping with infertility in couples: gender differences. *Health Care Women Int.*, **9**, 163–5.

Dubin, L. & Amelar, R.D. (1971). Etiologic factors in 1294 consecutive cases of male infertility. *Fertil. Steril.*, **22**, 469–74.

Edelman, R.J. (1989). Psychological aspects of artificial insemination by donor. *J. Psychosom. Obstet. Gynecol.*, **10**, 3–13.

Elstein, M. (1975). Effect on infertility and psychosexual function. *BMJ*, **iii**, 296–9.

Freeman, E.W., Boxer, A.S., Rickels, K., Tureck, R. & Mastroianni, L. (1985). Psychological evaluation and support in a program of *in vitro* fertilization and embryo transfer. *Fertil. Steril.*, **43**, 48–53.

Gerstel, G. (1963). A psychoanalytic view of artificial donor insemination. *Am. J. Psychother.*, **17**, 64–77.

Greil, A.L. (1991). *Not Yet Pregnant: Infertile Couples in Contemporary America*. New Brunswick: Rutgers University Press.

Greil, A.L., Leitko, T.A. & Porter, K.L. (1988). Infertility: his and hers. *Gender Soc.*, **2**, 172–99.

Harrison, R.F., O'Moore, R.R. & O'Moore, A.M. (1986). Stress and fertility: some modalities of investigation and treatment in couples with unexplained infertility in Dublin. *Int. J. Fertil.*, **3**, 153–9.

Humphrey, M. & Humphrey, H. (1987). Marital relationships in couples seeking donor insemination. *J. Biosoc. Sci.*, **19**, 209–19.

Johnston, M., Shaw, R. & Bird, D. (1987). 'Test-tube baby' procedures: stress and judgement under uncertainty. *Psychol. Health*, **1**, 25–38.

Johnston, P.I. (1992). *Adopting after Infertility*. Indianapolis, IN: Perspectives Press.

Kaplan, H.S. (1974). *The New Sex Therapy: Active Treatment of Sexual Dysfunctions*. New York: Brunner/Mazel Publication.

Karpel, M.A. (1980). Family secrets. I. Conceptual and ethical issues in the relational context. II. Ethical and practical considerations in therapeutic management. *Family Process*, **19**, 295–306.

Kedem, P., Mikulincer, M. & Nathanson, Y.E. (1990). Psychological aspects of male infertility. *Br. J. Med. Psychol.*, **63**, 73–80.

Kentenich, H., Schmiady, H., Radke, E., Stief, G. & Blankau, A. (1992). The male IVF patient: psychosomatic considerations. *Hum. Reprod.*, **7**, 13–18.

Keye, W.R. (1984). Psychosexual responses to infertility. *Clin Obstet. Gynecol.*, **27**, 760–6.

Keye, W.R., Jr & Deneris, A. (1982/3). Female sexual activity, satisfaction and function in infertile women. *Infertility*, **5**, 275–85.

Kilmann, P.R. & Mills, K.H. (1983). *All About Sex Therapy*. New York: Plenum Press.

Klock, S.C. (1993). Psychological aspects of donor insemination. In *Infertility and Reproductive Medicine Clinics of North America*, vol. 4, ed. D. Greenfeld. Philadelphia: W.B. Saunders.

Klock, S.C. & Maier, D. (1991). Psychological factors related to donor insemination. *Fertil. Steril.*, **56**, 489–95.

Lalos, A., Jacobsson, L., Lalos, O. & von Schoultz, B. (1985a). The wish to have a child: a pilot-study of infertile couples. *Acta Psychiatr. Scand.*, **72**, 476–81.

Lalos, A., Lalos, O., Jacobsson, L. & von Schoultz, B. (1985b). Psychological reactions to the medical investigation and surgical treatment of infertility. *Gynecol. Obstet. Invest.*, **20**, 209–17.

Lalos, A., Lalos, O., Jacobsson, L. & von Schoultz, B. (1985c). A psychosocial characterization of infertile couples before surgical treatment of the female. *J. Psychosom. Obstet. Gynecol.*, **4**, 83–93.

Lalos, A., Lalos, O., Jacobsson, L. & von Schoultz, B. (1985d). The psychosocial impact of infertility two years after completed surgical treatment. *Acta Obstet. Gynecol. Scand.*, **64**, 599–604.

Ledward, R.S., Symonds, E.M. & Eynon, S. (1982). Social and environmental factors as criteria for success in artificial insemination by donor (AID). *J. Biosoc. Sci.*, **14**, 263–75.

Leeton, J. & Backwell, J. (1982). A preliminary psychosocial follow-up of parents and their children conceived by artificial insemination by donor (AID). *Clin. Reprod. Fertil.*, **1**, 307–10.

Leiblum, S.R. & Hamkins, S.E. (1992). To tell or not to tell: attitudes of reproductive endocrinologists concerning disclosure to offspring of conception via assisted insemination by donor. *J. Psycosom. Obstet. Gynaecol.*, **13**, 267–75.

Lentner, E. (1991). Infertile couples' perceptions of infertility support-group participation. *Health Care Women Int.*, **12**, 317–30.

Levant, R.F. (1992). Toward the reconstruction of masculinity. *J. Family Psychol.*, **5**, 379–402.

Levant, R.F., Hirsch, L.S., Celentano, E., Cozza, T.M., Hill, S., MacEachern, M. & Schnedeker, J. (1992). The male role: an investigation of contemporary norms. *J. Mental Health Counseling*, **14**, 325–37.

Mahlstedt, P.P. (1985). The psychological component of infertility. *Fertil. Steril.*, **43**, 335–46.

Mahlstedt, P.P. & Greenfeld, D.A. (1989). Assisted reproductive technology with donor gametes: the need for patient preparation. *Fertil. Steril.*, **52**, 908–14.

Mahlstedt, P.P. & Probasco, K.A. (1991). Sperm donors: their attitudes toward providing medical and psychosocial information for recipient couples and donor offspring. *Fertil. Steril.*, **56**, 747–53.

Mahlstedt, P.P., MacDuff, S. & Bernstein, J. (1987). Emotional factors and the *in vitro* fertilization and embryo transfer process. *J. In Vitro Fertil. Embryo Transf.*, **4**, 232–6.

Mai, F.M., Munday, R.N. & Rump, E.E. (1972). Psychiatric interview comparisons between infertile and fertile couples. *Psychosom. Med.*, **34**, 431–40.

Masters, W.H. & Johnson, V.E. (1970). *Human Sexual Inadequacy*. Toronto: Bantam Books.

Matot, J.P. & Gustin, M.L. (1990). Filiation and secrecy in artificial insemination with donor. *Hum. Reprod.*, **5**, 632–3.

McCartney, C.F. & Wada, C.Y. (1990). Gender differences in counseling needs during infertility treatment. In *Psychiatric Aspects of Reproductive Technology*, ed. N.L. Stotland, pp. 141–54. Washington, DC: American Psychiatric Press.

McEwan, K.L., Costello, C.G. & Taylor, P.J. (1987). Adjustment to infertility. *J. Abnormal Psychol.*, **96**, 108–16.

Menning, B.E. (1988). *Infertility: A Guide for the Childless Couple*, 2nd edn. New York: Prentice Hall.

Miall, C.E. (1986). The stigma of involuntary childlessness. *Soc. Probl.*, **33**, 269–82.

Micioni, G., Jeker, L., Zeeb, M. & Campana, A. (1987). Doubtful and negative psychological indications for AID: a study of 835 couples. Treatment outcome in couples with doubtful indication. *J. Psychosom. Obstet. Gynaecol.*, **6**, 89–99.

Morse, C. & Dennerstein, L. (1985). Infertile couples entering an *in vitro* fertilization programme: a preliminary survey. *J. Psychosom. Obstet. Gynecol.*, **4**, 207–19.

Nachtigall, R.D., Becker, G. & Wozny, M. (1992). The effects of gender-specific diagnosis on men's and women's response to infertility. *Fertil. Steril.*, **57**, 113–21.

Newton, C.R., Hearn, M.T. & Yuzpe, A.A. (1990). Psychological assessment and follow-up after *in vitro* fertilization: assessing the impact of failure. *Fertil. Steril.*, **54**, 879–86.

Nijs, P. & Rouffa, L. (1975). AID-couples: psychological and psychopathological evaluation. *Andrologia*, **7**, 187–94.

Notman, M. (1983). Fertility, infertility, and sexuality. In *Treatment Interventions in Human Sexuality*, ed. C.C. Nadelson & D.B. Marcotte. New York: Plenum Press.

Office of Technology Assessment (1988). *Infertility: Medical and Social Choices* (OTA-BA-358). Washington, DC: US Congress.

Rowland, R. (1985). The social and psychological consequences of secrecy in artificial insemination by donor (AID) programmes. *Soc. Sci. Med.*, **21**, 391–6.

Rubin, B. (1965). Psychological aspects of human artificial insemination. *Arch. Gen. Psychiatry*, **13**, 121–32.

Shapiro, C.H. (1988). The psychological aspects of being infertile. In *Social and Medical Concerns*, vol. 4. Contractor document prepared for the Office of Technology Assessment. Washington, DC: US Congress.

Sokoloff, B.Z. (1987). Alternative methods of reproduction: effects on the child. *Clin. Pediatr.*, **26**, 11–17.

Steinem, G. (1983). *Outrageous Acts and Everyday Rebellions*. New York: Holt, Rinehart, and Winston.

Stewart, C.R., Daniels, K.R. & Boulnois, J.D.H. (1982). The development of a psychosocial approach to artificial insemination of donor sperm. *NZ Med. J.*, **95**, 853–6.

Takefman, J.E., Brender, W., Boivin, J. & Tulandi, T. (1990). Sexual and emotional adjustment of couples undergoing infertility investigation and the effectiveness of preparatory information. *J. Psychosom. Obstet. Gynecol.*, **11**, 275–90.

Tavris, C. (1992). *Mismeasure of Woman*. New York: Simon & Schuster.

Ulbrich, P.M., Coyle, A.T. & Llabre, M.M. (1990). Involuntary childlessness and marital adjustment: his and hers. *J. Sex Marital Ther.*, **16**, 147–58.

van Keep, P.A. & Schmidt-Elmendorff, H. (1975). Involuntary childlessness. *J. Biosoc. Sci.*, **7**, 37–48.

Walker, H.E. (1978). Sexual problems and infertility. *Psychosomatics*, **19**, 477–84.

Watters, W.W. & Sousa-Poza, J. (1966). Psychiatric aspects of artificial insemination (donor). *Can. Med. Assoc. J.*, **95**, 106–13.

Zilbergeld, B. (1978). *Male Sexuality: A Guide to Sexual Fulfillment*. New York: Bantam Books.

18

Evaluation of the female partner

KENNETH A. GINSBURG and KRISTINE E. KLINGER

Introduction

While approximately 40% of infertile couples will be found to have a male factor solely responsible or contributing to their infertility, couples in whom *only* the male partner has an infertility problem are less common. All couples presenting for fertility diagnosis and therapy require careful, coordinated evaluation of both partners. Optimally, this consideration of both partners should begin with the initial contact. The andrologist or urologist should establish a working relationship with a gynecologist or reproductive endocrinologist who can evaluate and treat the female partner. This evaluation should be initiated at the time the male partner is starting to undergo evaluation or early in the course of treatment, so that any factors operative in the female partner can be fully investigated and corrected as the male is reaching optimal fertility potential.

Three factors contribute to the majority of diagnosed fertility disorders in infertile couples. These include male factors, ovulatory abnormalities, and mechanical (organic) factors in a woman's reproductive tract. Evaluation and treatment of female factors comprises the remainder of this book. The ovulatory process, cervical and uterine function, patency of the fallopian tubes, and evaluation of the peritoneal environment to exclude endometriosis and pelvic adhesions comprise the major factors evaluated in the female. While many excellent texts and monographs have been written detailing the evaluation of the female partner, this chapter will review important steps in that evaluation with the goal of providing the andrologist/urologist with the understanding necessary to facilitate coordinated care of both partners.

Causes of female infertility

The incidence of infertility in reproductive age women has been reported to be between 1% and 65%, depending upon the sample population, expertise of the

Table 18.1   *Mechanisms of infertility in the female*

Mechanism	Examples or potential causes
Ovulatory failure	Kallman's syndrome Anorexia nervosa Hyperprolactinemia with pituitary adenoma
Ovulatory dysfunction	Oligo-ovulation due to obesity or stress Polycystic ovarian syndrome Luteal phase defect
Cervical	Absolute dysmucorrhea ('dry cervix') after treatment with laser, cold-knife cone biopsy or electrosurgical excision for cervical dysplasia Relative dysmucorrhea from ovulatory failure/dysfunction with hypoestrogenism, or idiopathic Cervicitis
Uterine	Asherman's syndrome Leiomyomata uteri (fibroids) or endometrial polyp Müllerian defects (septum, bicornuate) with habitual abortion
Tubal	Obstruction due to infection, mechanical compression, endometriosis
Peritoneal	Endometriosis Peritoneal adhesions disturbing tubal motility, tubo-ovarian interaction or oocyte release or capture
Immunologic	Secretion of antibodies into cervical mucus, follicular fluid or other sites in reproductive tract that compromise sperm transport and/or sperm–oocyte interaction

examining physicians, availability of sophisticated diagnostic studies and treatment programs, and other factors (WHO, 1991). Causes of infertility in the female can be broadly classified into disorders of the ovulatory process or mechanical and/or physiologic disorders of the reproductive tract (Table 18.1). Ovulatory problems are found in up to one-third of infertile women. These can be obvious, as in the woman who menstruates only once or twice a year, or they may be subtle and detected only with additional testing such as abnormal luteal phase endometrial maturation demonstrated by the endometrial biopsy. Cervical and uterine abnormalities are encountered less frequently. Their diagnosis is important since effective treatment is available for some conditions. Tubal and peritoneal factors must be excluded, including anatomic obstruction of the tubes, pelvic adhesions with altered tubo-ovarian relationships that interfere with oocyte release or capture, and endometriosis.

The incidence of infertility appears to be increasing, possibly representing an actual increase in infertility or greater demand for services. Some diagnoses clearly are more common today, such as tubal disease resulting from sexually transmitted diseases, pelvic inflammatory disease or endometriosis. Ovulatory dysfunction, failed fertilization, or implantation failure as women delay child-bearing are other examples of underlying mechanisms leading to female infertility that are more common now than previously. Female fertility can also be adversely effected by cigarette smoking, postcoital douching and coital lubricants, prescribed and recreational drug use including marijuana, alcohol and narcotics (which alter hypothalamic–pituitary function), and occupational exposures to ionizing radiation and various chemicals.

History and physical examination of the infertile female

When possible, the couple should be interviewed together at the initial visit. This emphasizes the importance of both partners in the potential pathogenesis of infertility and helps to dispel the myth that infertility is a woman's disorder. Furthermore, discussion of the plan of investigation and treatment options with both partners present helps ensure that the information transfer is accurate and complete. Including both partners initiates and strengthens the communication and support needed for the couple to undergo diagnosis and treatment of infertility.

The historical interview of the female should document age, duration of unprotected intercourse, details of the woman's menstrual cycle including molimina, prior pregnancies and periods of infertility (along with diagnoses and treatment), reproductive history with other partners, previous pelvic surgery or gynecologic conditions, contraceptive history, and coital frequency and habits. Evaluation of the menstrual cycle includes an inquiry into the duration and frequency of menses, and presence or absence of premenstrual molimina including dysmenorrhea. Withdrawal bleeding of the uterine lining every 21–35 days is consistent with regular menses or eumenorrhea, while when menses occurs every 36 or more days the woman is said to be oligomenorrhic. The absence of regular menses may not only reflect ovulatory problems, but may also be indicative of other medical or endocrine disorders. The examiner should inquire about medical or surgical conditions, nutritional status, weight change, habits such as cigarette smoking, ethanol use or use of prescribed and illicit drugs. A family history concentrating on known infertility factors in first-degree relatives (e.g., female siblings with endometriosis), multiple gestation, congenital anomalies, genetic disease and medical conditions is also obtained. Conditions which could contraindicate pregnancy, such as severe cardiac disease, must obviously be identified. Previous infertility records, radiographs and videotapes, if available, are requested for review.

Physical examination of the potentially infertile female serves to reinforce the health status of the woman by documenting a normal general examination, while attempting to identify signs of underlying reproductive endocrine or pelvic disease. In particular, the skin is carefully examined for evidence of acne or seborrhea, hirsutism, alopecia, striae or acanthosis nigricans, while the head and neck examination excludes signs of intracranial or thyroid disease. The breasts should be examined for evidence of galactorrhea. Speculum examination looks for lower genital tract abnormalities such as a vaginal septum or cervicitis. At the time of bimanual examination, the uterus is examined for size, consistency, mobility and direction, while unilateral or bilateral adnexal enlargement and fixation may be associated with ovarian neoplasms, inflammatory conditions or endometriosis. The severity and distribution of tenderness is documented. Nodularity, induration or tenderness in the posterior cul-de-sac of Douglas on vaginal or rectal examination can be associated with endometriosis or adhesions.

When warranted, routine laboratory tests such as urinalysis, complete blood cell count, serologic test for syphilis and rubella immunity are obtained. Some centers advocate routine culture of both partners for *Ureaplasma urealyticum* and *Mycoplasma* and *Chlamydia* species, although the cost-effectiveness of such screening has not been demonstrated. In certain ethnic groups, sickle cell, Tay–Sachs or thalassemia screening are indicated.

Diagnostic procedures

Because more than one factor may contribute to a fertility problem, a complete evaluation demonstrating apparently normal fertility potential in the male, documenting normal ovulation, and excluding problems in the female reproductive tract should be planned for all couples. The typical tests proceed from relatively inexpensive and non-invasive tests first to more invasive and expensive diagnostic procedures (Table 18.2). However, if the initial history and examination suggests an obvious problem, it is appropriate to perform tests out of sequence and initially concentrate the diagnostic effort on these problems.

Tests of the ovulatory process

In initiating the thorough infertility investigation of the female, it is most appropriate to begin with an ovulatory assessment. Beyond the menstrual history, there are five tests which will assist in this evaluation. These include basal body temperature (BBT) charting, serial cervical mucus examination, blood and urine hormonal evaluation, follicular ultrasound and luteal phase

Table 18.2   *Diagnostic tests employed in the evaluation of the infertile female*

Factor evaluated	Tests employed
Ovulation	Basal body temperature (BBT) charts
	Serum sampling of steroid, gonadotropin, prolactin, thyroid hormone levels
	Urinary luteinizing hormone test kits
	Serial evaluation of cervical mucus characteristics
	Evaluation of luteal phase adequacy by endometrial biopsy or serum progesterone concentration
Cervical function	Postcoital (Sims–Huhner) test
	In vitro tests of mucus biochemistry, antibody production and sperm–mucus interaction
Uterus	Hysterosalpingography
	Endoscopy (hysteroscopy and laparoscopy)
	Ultrasonography
Tubal patency	Hysterosalpingography
	Dye perfusion during laparoscopy
Peritoneal factor	Laparoscopy

evaluation. Ovulation should be assessed for several cycles before a diagnosis can be made and treatment initiated.

BBT charting is a simple and inexpensive way of attempting to determine whether a woman is ovulating. The hypothalamic regulation of basal temperature is influenced by progesterone, secreted after ovulation by the corpus luteum. Basal temperature increases by approximately 0.5°C when progesterone concentrations exceed 4 ng/ml (Luciano *et al.*, 1990). Recorded daily after 4–6 hours of uninterrupted sleep, a rise in temperature is thought to occur approximately 24 hours after ovulation. The temperature must be taken prior to arising out of bed, since any activity will raise the BBT and introduce inaccuracies. A sustained rise in temperature during the luteal phase is further evidence that ovulation and corpus luteum formation have occurred. The duration of increased temperature should be approximately 14 days, after which the temperature falls preceding the onset of menses. A sustained rise in basal temperature beyond 16 days is a good indicator of early pregnancy. However, because the temperature rise follows ovulation, BBT charts are useful only for retrospective cycle review. There are no prospective indicators of ovulation on the BBT chart, nor is the method foolproof. Ovulation has been reported in up to 20% of women with monophasic temperature charts, while some women with biphasic BBT charts are anovulatory (Jaffe & Jewelewicz, 1991). Despite this, assessment of the probable day of ovulation and the length of the luteal phase are important data obtained by reviewing the BBT chart at the end of the cycle. Further, a consistent pattern of temperature charts provides the information needed to schedule tests or therapy at the expected time of ovulation in the following months.

Several aspects of female reproductive function display rheologic properties which are bioassays of relative estrogen level. Once such function is the cervical mucus, which increases in quantity and quality in response to the rise in estrogen levels which occur as ovulation is approaching (Moghissi, 1966). Low estrogen levels or the presence of progestogen result in poor-quality cervical mucus which is scant, thick, tacky and very cellular. Preovulatory cervical mucus is abundant, clear, thin and watery, with demonstrable elasticity (termed 'Spinnbarkeit') and ferning when dried and examined under the microscope. This mucus facilitates sperm survival, transport into the upper genital tract, and capacitation. Several scoring systems of cervical mucus have been devised (Insler *et al.*, 1972; Moghissi, 1977). Serial examinations of cervical mucus which show an increasing score followed by an abrupt fall are consistent with an increasing estrogen effect followed by the secretion of progesterone, together indicative of ovulation. Evaluation of cervical mucus quality in the periovulatory phase following coitus is an integral part of the Sims–Huhner (postcoital) test, as discussed below.

Evaluation of blood or urinary hormone levels is important not only in the documentation of ovulation, but in establishing the etiology of ovulatory dysfunction. In the anovulatory patient, thyroid stimulating hormone and serum prolactin levels should be measured even in the absence of symptoms or signs of thyroid disease or galactorrhea. Measurement of serum gonadotropins excludes gonadal failure and may confirm the impression of chronic anovulation due to polycystic ovarian syndrome when the LH:FSH ratio is reversed and at least 2:1. If the history or physical examination suggests androgenic abnormalities, serum total testosterone, dehydroepiandrosterone sulfate and 17-hydroxyprogesterone should be measured.

Midcycle changes in serum LH concentration in the late follicular phase (the LH surge) are correlated with the actual time of ovulation; however, frequent sampling several times each day with timely (and expensive) radioimmunoassay is required to utilize this information. More common in clinical use are tests for the detection of LH in the urine (Quagliarello & Arny, 1986). These double-antibody tests are marketed as kits of five to ten tests, allowing repetitive daily sampling until the LH surge is detected. Once the serum LH surge begins, LH is excreted in increasing amounts in the urine for several days; the first day that this increased urinary concentration of LH is detected correlates well with the onset of the serum LH surge, and with subsequent ovulation. Several days prior to the expected day of ovulation, patients begin testing with the homebased predictor kits. The presence of a certain amount of LH will yield a positive result on the test matrix, and ovulation can be expected to occur approximately 24–36 hours after LH is first detected in the urine. Often LH predictor kits are used in combination with BBT charting, since each tests a unique attribute of the ovulatory process. Because they are easy to use, relatively inexpensive and provide rapid results, ovulation predictor kits are also recommended when scheduling timed diagnostic or therapeutic procedures such as postcoital tests (Corsan *et al.*, 1993), endometrial biopsies and inseminations.

Ultrasonography is yet another way of assessing the ovulatory process (Ritchie, 1985). Transvaginal ultrasonography offers well-defined images of the ovaries with little discomfort to the patient. By serially monitoring follicular development beginning several days prior to expected ovulation and determining whether there is a dominant follicle, the precise day of ovulation can be detected. Disappearance of the dominant follicle, significant decrease in size, alteration of the follicular borders, change in echogenic texture or appearance of fluid in the posterior cul-de-sac are indicators of ovulation, especially when seen after documented follicular growth and a urinary LH surge. Good correlation between follicular size and oocyte maturity allows use of follicular ultrasound to assess the *quality* of ovulation, i.e., when follicles are likely to contain mature, fertilizable oocytes. Ultrasonography is also used to count the follicles developing and help predict the occurrence of multiple gestation, especially in pharmacologic ovulation induction cycles (Tal *et al.*, 1985). The ultrasonographic appearance of the endometrium has been evaluated by some investigators and found to yield information indicative of the quality of ovulation (Ueno *et al.*, 1991; Dickey *et al.*, 1993). Although highly accurate when used in conjunction with BBTs and LH testing, transvaginal ultrasonography can be time-consuming and costly for the patient.

The final factor to consider relative to the detection of ovulation is evaluation of the adequacy of the luteal phase of the cycle (Wentz *et al.*, 1990) and hence exclusion of a luteal-phase defect (LPD). Controversy exists regarding both the existence of this clinicopathologic entity and how best to diagnose and treat it. Since the pathogenesis of LPD can involve both deficient progesterone *production* and deficient progesterone *action* in the endometrium, several strategies have been reported to evaluate the luteal phase. Progesterone levels 5–10 ng/ml or greater in the luteal phase are evidence that ovulation and luteinization has occurred. However, it is important to note that because progesterone is released in pulsatile fashion, a single determination may not reflect mean values (Wathen *et al.*, 1984). Serial and/or pooled progesterone samples are often recommended.

Further evaluation of the luteal phase is completed by performing an endometrial biopsy (Balasch *et al.*, 1992) late in the cycle several days before anticipated menses. Although used also to confirm ovulation, endometrial biopsy is an invasive test which is considerably more expensive than BBT or urinary LH testing and hence is not routinely used for this purpose alone. Many practitioners time the acquisition of the specimen to be approximately 10 days after the LH surge or BBT shift, which not only tells when to do the test but confirms that it is being done in an ovulatory cycle. The couple should use barrier contraception to avoid inadvertent interruption of an early pregnancy, but otherwise continue whatever medications are currently used to induce ovulation. The endometrial specimen is dated using Noyes' criteria (Noyes *et al.*, 1950), and compared with the actual cycle day based on onset of subsequent menses. A discrepancy of greater than 2 days in two consecutive cycles is required to establish the diagnosis of LPD, since nearly a third of cycles in ovulatory fertile women will have an inadequate luteal phase (Jaffe & Jewelewicz, 1991). These disorders may rarely be primary defects of the endometrial receptor; more often luteal phase dysfunction is due to abnormal folliculogenesis (Jacobs *et al.*, 1987), hyperprolactinemia or endometriosis.

Evaluation of cervical function

The quality of cervical mucus secretion and its ability to promote sperm survival are crucial factors to assess in evaluating the fertility of a couple. Cervical mucus forms a reservoir for normal spermatozoa that can subsequently migrate into the upper reproductive tract, while filtering abnormal sperm and retarding their progress. In addition, sperm within cervical mucus begin the capacitation process leading to acquisition of the ability to bind, penetrate and fertilize the oocyte. Ejaculated sperm optimally reach the cervical mucus soon after ejaculation. The quality and quantity of cervical mucus change in response to the stimulation of the cervix by steroid hormones. Several days before expected ovulation, correlated with increasing serum estradiol levels, there is an increase in the production of cervical mucus which is copious, clear, thin, acellular and very elastic ('Spinnbarkeit') with a slightly alkaline pH (Gibor *et al.*, 1970). These ideal characteristics (which allow sperm to survive in and penetrate through the cervical mucus) continue for only 1–2 days after ovulation, after which time the mucus becomes impenetrable because of the antiestrogenic effect of circulating progestogens secreted by the corpus luteum.

The standard test to assess cervical mucus function and the interaction between cervical mucus and sperm is the postcoital test (PCT) (Griffith & Grimes, 1990), also called the Sims–Huhner test. Correct timing of the PCT is

Table 18.3 *Determinants of cervical mucus quality and the cervical score*

Factor	Score
Amount	0=None
	1=0.1 ml
	2=0.2 ml
	3=0.3 ml or greater
Viscosity	0=Thick, highly viscous, premenstrual mucus
	1=Intermediate, still viscous
	2=Mildly viscous
	3=Normal preovulatory mucus, fluid
Ferning pattern	0=No crystallization
	1=Atypical ferning
	2=Primary and secondary stems
	3=Tertiary and quarternary stems
'Spinnbarkeit'	0=Less than 1 cm
	1=1–4 cm
	2=5–8 cm
	3=9 cm or greater
Cellularity	0=11 or more leukocytes/hpf
	1=6–10 leukocytes/hpf
	2=1–5 leukocytes/hpf
	3=No leukocytes
pH of cervical mucus	Not included in calculated score

Notes:
hpf, high-power field.
With a maximum score of 15, cervical mucus scores less than 10 represent
unfavorable mucus while those less than 5 are classified as hostile mucus (Moghissi,
1977).

critical to its interpretation. Since only preovulatory mucus will support sperm
survival and transport, testing should ideally occur during the interval between
1–2 days before ovulation through the day of ovulation. This timing is most
easily achieved through the use of urinary LH surge detection kits, scheduling
the test on the day after the surge (when fertility is optimal) 6–10 hours after
intercourse (Bronson *et al.*, 1984). At that time specimens are obtained from
the vaginal pool, the exocervix and the endocervical canal. The endocervical
specimen is evaluated to determine mucus quality (Table 18.3) and the presence
and motility characteristics of spermatozoa. If the endocervical specimen does
not contain spermatozoa, the exocervical and the vaginal pool specimens are
sequentially evaluated.

More than 10 progressively motile sperm per high-power field in good-
quality cervical mucus constitutes a normal result. Interpretation of results
where fewer sperm per high-power field or different motility is observed remains

controversial (Hull *et al.*, 1982; Jette & Glass, 1972; Collins *et al.*, 1984). When mucus quality is poor, normal survival and motility are not expected; hence the finding of poor mucus suggests that additional testing and/or therapy is indicated to improve mucus quality before sperm–mucus interaction is evaluated. Occasionally, favorable PCT results are seen in couples with abnormal semen analysis, suggesting that cervical mucus quality can compensate for some deficiencies in semen. Conversely, poor PCT results can be obtained when semen analyses are normal. Poor PCT results can be due to inappropriate timing, suboptimal ovulation, cervical or vaginal infection or inflammation, inadequate mucus production due to surgical destruction of the crypts, antisperm antibodies in either partner, or abnormalities on semen analysis.

Evaluation of uterine abnormalities

Two diagnostic tests are available to evaluate the uterine cavity for filling defects due to leiomyomata or polyps, congenital abnormalities or synechiae (Asherman's syndrome). Hysterosalpingography (HSG) is often used for initial evaluation of the uterus and tubes, since it reveals their internal contour, and can be used to document tubal patency while excluding the above uterine factors. Hysteroscopy is an invasive procedure requiring additional instrumentation and skill; it is often combined with diagnostic laparoscopy as the final stage in the diagnostic evaluation.

A properly performed and interpreted HSG is correlated with endoscopic findings, although a normal HSG does not exclude such diagnoses as endometriosis or some adnexal adhesions which do not obstruct the tube yet interfere with the normal tubo-ovarian relationship required for oocyte capture and initial transport. Indications for an HSG include the evaluation of infertility or repetitive abortion when images of the uterine cavity and fallopian tubes are required. The procedure is never done in the presence of active infection or an undiagnosed pelvic mass, and should be scheduled in the follicular phase soon after completion of a normal menstrual cycle to guard against inadvertently performing it in early pregnancy, flushing an embryo from the reproductive tract in the luteal phase or radiation exposure after ovulation. An HSG performed during the luteal phase is also more likely to show false cornual obstruction due to a thickened endometrium that obstructs the tubal ostia. Therapeutic benefits of HSG have been suggested by several controlled clinical trials, primarily when oil-based dyes are employed (Soules & Spadoni, 1982). Complications include pain during and after the procedure, allergic reactions to the contrast dye, and infection with tubo-ovarian abscess formation (Stumpf & March, 1980).

In practice, the procedure is scheduled to take place shortly after the cessation of menstrual bleeding. Many centers premedicate with an analgesic both to ensure patient comfort and to help prevent tubal spasm. In addition, some advocate prophylactic use of an antibiotic in high-risk groups such as those with a history of pelvic inflammatory disease, use of an intrauterine device (IUD), pelvic or tubal surgery, or known tubal disease. When possible, the physician caring for the patient should perform the procedure, both to allay the patient's fears and so that important information can be obtained for later use. The vagina and cervix are cleaned and one of several available cannulas is inserted into the cervical canal such that a tight seal is formed. Cervical dilatation is usually not required. Both water-soluble and oil-based contrast agents are available for HSG, the advantages of the aqueous dye being that it is quickly absorbed and less likely to cause a tissue reaction, while the oil-based dyes yield superior images.

The slow injection is monitored with fluoroscopy and a permanent record made using videotape and/or radiographs. Sufficient traction on the cervix will place the uterus perpendicular to the X-ray beam to obtain optimal images for inspection of the uterine cavity. Occasionally, it is necessary to angle the patient relative to the beam to obtain optimal images, to demonstrate that radiolucencies are injected air bubbles by their shift in position within the uterine cavity, or to facilitate the flow of dye into one of the tubes. For later evaluation, the films should include in sequence a view of the uterine cavity when it is filled but not distended with dye, when both tubes have filled but before significant spillage obscures tubal structures, and then when spillage is demonstrated confirming tubal patency. A fourth film 10–30 minutes later is used to evaluate whether dye remains in the distal tube or loculated within the peritoneal cavity, suggesting possible relative tubal obstruction or peritoneal adhesions, respectively.

Hysteroscopy is also an excellent tool for direct evaluation of the uterine cavity. A therapeutic procedure can also potentially be accomplished if adequate preparations are made for anesthesia, availability of instruments, etc. With small-diameter hysteroscopes (whether rigid or flexible), a diagnostic hysteroscopy can easily be performed in the office using oral analgesia and sedation. Clinical indications which suggest the need for hysteroscopy in addition to those mentioned above for an HSG include the evaluation of abnormal uterine bleeding and investigation of an abnormal HSG.

As with the HSG, hysteroscopy is performed after the completion of a menstrual cycle. Minimal cervical dilatation is almost always required before performing the procedure. The patient is positioned and prepared as for the HSG. Carbon dioxide gas, 0.9% saline, glycine solution and dextran are available for uterine distension. The hysteroscope is then advanced into the uterine cavity under direct vision. Complications include those of the HSG with the addition of possible uterine performation, and embolization if excessive pressures are used to instill distending media.

Evaluation of the fallopian tubes

Given their importance in gamete transport as well as the site of *in vivo* fertilization, evaluation of the fallopian tubes is a crucial step in the investigation of female infertility. There are two tests available to determine the status of the fallopian tubes, i.e., the HSG, and laparoscopy with concomitant transcervical instillation of dye.

The HSG will demonstrate opacification of the tubes if the utero-tubal junction is patent, followed by complete fill of the tube and spill of dye, indicating distal (fimbrial) patency. Furthermore, the HSG can help determine, if there is a documented tubal factor, the exact point and degree of tubal obstruction. The HSG allows examination of the endosalpinx when distal obstruction is present, preservation of which is an important determinant of possible successful tubal repair by neosalpingostomy. However, it must be emphasized that fill and spill of contrast material from the tubes does not exclude a disturbance in the tubo-ovarian relationship. Indeed, the ability of the fallopian tube to capture an oocyte or transport the embryo to the uterus can be severely disturbed by adhesions even though the tubes are patent. Thus *intrinsic* tubal disease is evident on HSG, while *extrinsic* tubal disease may be evident on the HSG examination or may only be documented with laparoscopy. The technique for performing the HSG was discussed in the previous section. Transcervical selective salpingography (TSS) using an injection catheter wedged into the cornual region can be used to confirm proximal tubal obstruction by allowing higher injection pressures while obviating the passage of dye through a contralateral patent tube (Novy *et al.*, 1988). Recannulation of the obstructed tube by passing a fine wire or an expandable balloon through the catheter can also be attempted (Thurmond & Rosch, 1990; Confino *et al.*, 1990). TSS is, however, a procedure requiring operator skill and specialized instrumentation, and is not considered a routine test for tubal patency.

Endoscopic examination of the pelvis by laparoscopy (see below) allows direct observation of the external appearance of the fallopian tubes and especially the status of the fimbriae. At the time of laparoscopy colored aqueous dye is injected transcervically, filling the uterus and then entering the tubes. Passage of the dye through the tubes and its spill from the fimbriated end can be directly observed. In addition, adhesions which interfere with tubal motility or oocyte pickup may be diagnosed *only* by this study. Hysteroscopy may occasionally be indicated to evaluate the patency and appearance of the tubal ostia. Falloposcopy, via either a transcervical or a transperitoneal approach, will some day allow direct examination of the internal structure of the fallopian tube and may allow development of novel procedures for correcting segmental tubal obstruction (Kerin *et al.*, 1992).

Evaluation of the peritoneal factor

The final step in the evaluation of the potentially infertile female is evaluation of the pelvic peritoneum, the so-called peritoneal factor. Diagnostic methods are limited at present to laparoscopy. Because of the invasive and expensive nature of this test it is usually deferred until other non-invasive studies have been completed. However, when the history suggests the possibility of adhesions (pelvic inflammatory disease, prior pelvic surgery, appendicitis, IUD use, etc.), or endometriosis (pelvic pain, dysmenorrhea or dyspareunia), laparoscopy may be warranted before other tests outlined above are completed. In the future, other imaging modalities including X-ray, radioisotopes, magnetic resonance or positron emission may be useful for evaluation of the peritoneal cavity.

Laparoscopic examination of the female pelvis was first described in 1944 using both the knee–chest position and placement of the laparoscope via the posterior cul-de-sac, and the transabdominal approach with the patient in Trendelenberg position. Not only used for diagnostic evaluation of the pelvis and abdomen, operative laparoscopy is employed for sterilization by tubal ligation, adhesiolysis, treatment of endometriosis or ectopic pregnancy, and other gynecologic and general surgical procedures. In the infertile patient, the laparoscopic examination attempts to evaluate the ovarian surfaces, patency of the utero-tubal junction and tubal fimbriae, tubo-ovarian connection for oocyte capture, external contour of the uterus (to exclude previously unrecognized uterine fibroids), and the other pelvic surfaces for evidence of endometriosis. Tubal evaluation at the time of laparoscopy is usually accomplished by transcervical instillation of a dilute colored dye solution (chromotubation) such as methylene blue, with observation of its passage into and through the tube using the laparoscope. Often the procedure is combined with hysteroscopy (especially indicated when an HSG has not been obtained) to allow examination of the uterine interior to exclude adhesions, polyps, fibroids or müllerian anomalies which could be related to infertility.

Diagnostic laparoscopy is scheduled to be performed after completion of menses but before ovulation and corpus luteum formation, since at that time the ovary is more friable and predisposed to injury with bleeding. The technique first involves administration of a general anesthetic with endotracheal intubation or administration of a regional anesthetic. Adequate relaxation of the abdominal muscles is important so that the stomach and intestines fall into the upper abdominal quadrants with the patient in dorsal lithotomy and Trendelenberg position. A uterine manipulator is first placed transvaginally to aid in manipulation of the uterus. Pneumoperitoneum is established using a needle either placed through a small abdominal incision or by transvaginal placement into the posterior cul-de-sac. The laparoscopic sleeve is then placed into the abdomen and pneuperitoneum from a subumbilical incision, allowing orientation of the laparoscope towards the pelvic organs. A second suprapubic puncture allows introduction of another instrument for retraction or elevation of structures, and the systematic examination of the pelvic reproductive organs includes evaluation of tubal patency using transcervical chromotubation. Since laparoscopy performed after completion of a basic, non-invasive infertility investigation has a significant probability of detecting a pelvic abnormality, optimally the patient and surgeon will be prepared to proceed with operative laparoscopy (e.g., adhesiolysis, laser vaporization of endometriosis) at that time. Pneumoperitoneum is then allowed to escape and the incisions closed and dressed.

Contraindications to laparoscopy include some forms of cardiac and respiratory disease where the patient may not tolerate the induction of pneumoperitoneum or the Trendelenberg position, a large pelvic mass, known significant anterior adhesions which could predispose to bowel injuries or other conditions which would potentially limit visualization of the pelvic organs (e.g., obesity). Potential complications, rare in experienced hands, include infections, vascular or visceral injuries, and burns from laser or electrosurgical instruments.

Sequence of infertility tests

A coordinated infertility investigation should not be protracted, since a delay only contributes to patient anxiety and postpones initiation of treatment. In most cases the non-invasive portions of the investigation can be completed within two to three menstrual cycles.

At the initial contact, the diagnostic sequence is discussed and individual tests scheduled as appropriate. The patient begins to evaluate the ovulatory process by determination of early follicular serum endocrine studies when indicated, and initiates BBT charting and urinary LH surge determination. After completion of the first menstrual cycle, the hysterosalpingogram can be scheduled. Since the patient should not attempt conception during the cycle when an endometrial biopsy is planned, our preference is to schedule a postcoital test in the periovulatory phase of the second menstrual cycle and the endometrial biopsy in the following cycle (using barrier contraception). Delaying the biopsy for several cycles allows confirmation of apparent ovulation, since the endometrial biopsy provides no information if it is performed in an anovulatory cycle. The physician monitors the results of tests as they are obtained, and may intervene to deviate from this sequence if results indicate that a departure is warranted. For example, the evaluation of other factors can be appropriately delayed when bilateral tubal disease is suggested by abnormalities on the hysterosalpingogram. Furthermore, it is unnecessary to evaluate sperm–mucus interaction when ovulatory function is suboptimal and will require medication to establish normal, regular ovulation. Indeed, ovulation should be established in the anovulatory patient using appropriate medication before the postcoital test and endometrial biopsy are performed, since both will be abnormal in anovulatory cycles. In the second or third cycle a second consultation is scheduled to review the results, consider treatment options available, and, if no obvious fertility factor has been identified, discuss endoscopic examination to complete the basic infertility investigation.

Conclusion

A time- and cost-effective comprehensive evaluation will uncover the etiology of infertility in nearly 90% of couples who present for evaluation. Even when the male partner is known to have a problem thought to be the cause of the couple's infertility, referral for evaluation of the female partner is indicated. Such an evaluation attempts to disclose abnormalities in the ovulatory process, cervical, uterine or tubal pathology, or abnormalities within the pelvic peritoneal cavity such as endometriosis or adhesions. Beyond the basic investigation detailed above, many specialized studies are available to evaluate further a problem determined by these screening tests. In most cases, treatment will be indicated to restore normal reproductive potential to the female partner in an attempt to maximize the benefit from treatment of the male. Many contemporary treatment modalities, such as superovulation with gonadotropin therapy, appear to enhance a woman's reproductive ability to such a degree that conception can result even when identified male factors are not completely corrected.

Some aspects of reproduction are still poorly understood, including many details of sperm–oocyte interaction, early embryo growth and development, embryo transport through the female reproductive tract, hatching from the zona pellucida, and the process of implantation. As our understanding improves, new techniques for probing these components of the reproductive process will undoubtedly emerge. What is today the basic female fertility evaluation may thus in the future be just the initial steps in a diagnostic scheme able to identify the cause of infertility with much greater precision. In turn, improved treatment results can then be expected.

References

Balasch, J., Fabreques, F., Creus, M. & Vanrell, J.A. (1992). The usefulness of endometrial biopsy for luteal phase evaluation in infertility. *Hum. Reprod.*, 7, 973–7.

Bronson, R.A., Cooper, G.W. & Rosenfeld, D.L. (1984). Autoimmunity to spermatozoa effect in sperm penetration of cervical mucus as reflected by postcoital testing. *Fertil. Steril.*, 41, 609–14.

Collins, J.A., So, Y., Wilson, E.H., Wrixon, W. & Casper, R.F. (1984). The postcoital test as a predictor of pregnancy among 355 infertile couples. *Fertil. Steril.*, 41, 703–8.

Confino, E., Tur-Kaspa, I., DeCherney, A.H., Corfman, R., Coulam, C., Robinson, E., Haas, G., Katz, E., Vermesh, M. & Gleicher, N. (1990). Transcervical balloon tuboplasty: a multicenter trial. *JAMA*, 264, 2079–82.

Corsan, G.H., Blotner, M.B., Bohrer, M.K., Sheldon, R. & Kemmann, E. (1993). The utility of a home urinary LH immunoassay in timing the postcoital test. *Obstet. Gynecol.*, 81, 736–8.

Dickey, R.P., Olar, T.T., Taylor, S.H., Curole, D.N. & Matulich, E.M. (1993). Relationship of endometrial thickness and pattern to fecundity in ovulation induction cycles: effect of clomiphene citrate alone and with human menopausal gonadotropin. *Fertil. Steril.*, 59, 756–60.

Gibor, Y., Garcia, C.J., Cohen, M.R. & Scommegna, A. (1970). The cyclical changes in the physical properties of the cervical mucus and the results of the postcoital test. *Fertil. Steril.*, 21, 20–7.

Griffith, C.S. & Grimes, D.A. (1990). The validity of the postcoital test. *Am. J. Obstet. Gynecol.*, 162, 615–20.

Hull, M.G.R., Savage, P.E. & Bromham, D.R. (1982). Prognostic value of the postcoital test: prospective study based on time-specific conception rates. *Br. J. Obstet. Gynecol.*, 89, 299–305.

Insler, V., Melmed, H., Eichenbrenner, I., Serr, D.M. & Lunenfeld, B. (1972). The cervical score. *Int. J. Gynecol. Obstet.*, 10, 223.

Jacobs, M.H., Balasch, J., Gonzalez-Merio, J.M., Vanrell, J.A., Wheeler, C., Strauss, J.F., Blasco, L., Wheeler, J.E. & Lyttle, C.R. (1987). Endometrial cytosolic and nuclear progesterone receptors in the luteal phase defect. *J. Clin. Endocrinol. Metab.*, 64, 472–5.

Jaffe, S. & Jewelewicz, R. (1991). The basic infertility investigation. *Fertil. Steril.*, 56, 599–613.

Jette, N.T. & Glass, R.H. (1972). Prognostic value of the postcoital test. *Fertil. Steril.*, 23, 29–32.

Kerin, J.F., Williams, D.B., San Roman, G.A., Pearlstone, A.C., Grundfest, W.E. & Surrey, E.S. (1992). Falloposcopic classification and treatment of fallopian tube lumen disease. *Fertil. Steril.*, 57, 731–41.

Luciano, A.A., Peluso, J., Koch, E., Maier, D., Kuslis, S. & Davison, E. (1990). Terporal relationship and reliability of the clinical, hormonal and ultrasonographic indices of ovulation in infertile women. *Obstet. Gynecol.*, 75, 412–15.

Moghissi, K.S. (1966). Cyclic changes of cervical mucus in normal and progestin treated women. *Fertil. Steril.*, 17, 663–75.

Moghissi, K.S. (1977). Significance and prognostic value of postcoital test. In *The Uterine Cervix in Reproduction*, ed. V. Insler & G. Bettendorf, pp. 231–8. Stuttgart: Thieme.

Novy, M.J., Williams, D.B., Patton, P., Uchida, B.T. & Rosch, J. (1988). Diagnosis of cornual obstruction by transcervical fallopian tube cannulation. *Fertil. Steril.*, 50, 434–40.

Noyes, R.W., Hertig, A.T. & Rock, J. (1950). Dating the endometrial biopsy. *Fertil. Steril.*, 1, 3–25.

Quagliarello, J. & Arny, M. (1986). Inaccuracy of basal body temperature charts in predicting urinary luteinizing hormone surges. *Fertil. Steril.*, 45, 334–7.

Ritchie, W.G.M. (1985). Ultrasound in the evaluation of normal and induced ovulation. *Fertil. Steril.*, 43, 167–81.

Soules, M.R. & Spadoni, L.R. (1982). Oil versus aqueous media for hysterosalpingography: a continuing debate based on many opinions and few facts. *Fertil. Steril.*, 38, 1–11.

Stumpf, P.G. & March, C.M. (1980). Febrile morbidity following hysterosalpingography: identification of risk factors and recommendations for prophylaxis. *Fertil. Steril.*, 33, 487–92.

Tal, J., Paz, B., Samberg, I., Lazarov, N. & Sharf, M. (1985). Ultrasonographic and clinical correlates of menotropin versus sequential clomiphene citrate: menotropin therapy for induction of ovulation. *Fertil. Steril.*, 44, 342–9.

Thurmond, A.S. & Rosch, J. (1990). Nonsurgical fallopian tube recanalization for treatment of infertility. *Radiology*, 174, 371–4.

Ueno, J., Oehninger, S., Brzyski, R.G., Acosta, A.A., Philput, B. & Muasher, S.J. (1991). Ultrasonographic appearance of the endometrium in natural and stimulated *in-vitro* fertilization cycles and its correlation with outcome. *Hum. Reprod.*, 6, 901–4.

Wathen, N.C., Perry, L., Lilford, R.J. & Chard, T. (1984). Interpretation of single progesterone measurement in diagnosis of anovulation and defective luteal phase: observations on analysis of the normal range. *BMJ*, 288, 7–9.

Wentz, A.C., Kossoy, L. & Parker, R.A. (1990). The impact of luteal phase inadequacy in an infertile population. *Am. J. Obstet. Gynecol.*, 162, 937–45.

World Health Organization (1991). Infertility: a tabulation of available data on prevalence of primary and secondary infertility, pp. 1–72. Geneva: WHO.

Index